TEXTBOOK OF
MAMMOGRAPHY

For Churchill Livingstone:

Publisher: Geoffrey Nuttall
Project Editor: Lowri Daniels
Copy Editor: Robin Watson
Production Controller: Neil Dickson
Sales Promotion Executive: Hilary Brown

TEXTBOOK OF
MAMMOGRAPHY

Edited by

Audrey K. Tucker MB BS FSR FRCR

Consulting Radiologist, St Bartholomew's Hospital, London;
Consultant Radiologist and Adviser, BUPA Medical Centre, London;
Consultant Radiologist, The Princess Grace Hospital, London;
Consultant Radiologist and Adviser, Marks and Spencer Health Services,
Breast Screening Programme, London, UK

CHURCHILL LIVINGSTONE
EDINBURGH LONDON MADRID MELBOURNE NEW YORK AND TOKYO 1993

CHURCHILL LIVINGSTONE
Medical Division of Longman Group UK Limited

Distributed in the United States of America by Churchill Livingstone Inc.,
650 Avenue of the Americas, New York, N.Y. 10011, and by associated
companies, branches and representatives throughout the world.

First Published 1993   Reprinted 1994 (twice)

ISBN 0-443-04208-X

British Library of Cataloguing in Publication Data
A catalogue record for this book is available from the British Library.

Library of Congress Cataloging in Publication Data
Textbook of mammography / edited by Audrey K. Tucker.
       p.   cm.
    Includes index.
    ISBN 0-443-04208-X
    1. Breast—Radiography.   2. Breast—Cancer—Diagnosis.
 I. Tucker, Audrey K.
    [DNLM: 1. Breast Neoplasms—Diagnosis.   2. Mammography.   WP 870
 T355]
 RC280.B8T457   1993
 616.99'44907572—dc20
 DNLM/DLC
 for Library of Congress   92-49320
                                                          CIP

The
publisher's
policy is to use
**paper manufactured
from sustainable forests**

Printed in Great Britain by
Butler & Tanner Ltd, Frome and London

Contents

Contributors

Jocelyn Chamberlain MB FRCP FFPHM
Director of Cancer Screening Evaluation Unit, Institute of Cancer Research, London, UK

David Cosgrove MA MSc FRCR FRCP
Consultant in Nuclear Medicine and Ultrasound, Royal Marsden Hospital, London, UK

Marigold Curling MB BS MRCS LRCP
Consultant Pathologist, St Bartholomew's Hospital, London, UK

David R. Dance MA PhD FIPSM
Consultant Physicist, The Royal Marsden Hospital, London; Honorary Senior Lecturer, Institute of Cancer Research, London, UK

Jane B. Davey MB BS
Physician, Breast Diagnostic Unit, Royal Marsden Hospital, London, UK

Peter B. Guyer DM MS FRCP FRCR DMRD
Consultant Radiologist and Honorary Senior Lecturer in Radiology, Southampton University Hospitals, Southampton, UK

Yin Y. Ng MA MBBS MRCP(UK) FRCR
Consultant and Senior Lecturer in Radiology, St Bartholomew's Hospital, London, UK

James Pemberton MB BS MRCP BSc FFR FRCR
Consultant Radiologist, St Thomas's Hospital, London, UK

Nicholas Perry MB FRCS FRCR
Consultant Radiologist, St Bartholomew's Hospital, London; Director of the Central and East London Breast Screening Service; Consultant to the European Commission—Europe Against Cancer—Breast Screening

Rosemary Toye MA MB BS FRCR
Senior Registrar in Diagnostic Radiology, King's College Hospital, London, UK

Audrey K. Tucker MB BS FSR FRCR
Consulting Radiologist, St Bartholomew's Hospital, London; Consultant Radiologist and Adviser, BUPA Medical Centre, London; Consultant Radiologist, The Princess Grace Hospital, London; Consultant Radiologist and Adviser, Marks and Spencer Health Services, Breast Screening Programme, London, UK

Elizabeth J. Wylie MBBS FRACR
Consultant Radiologist, Royal Perth Hospital, Perth, Western Australia; Consultant Radiologist, WCPU Breast Cancer Screening Service, Western Australia

Maureen Yeowell DCR(R)
Mammography Trainer, Manager—Radiography, BUPA Health Screening, London, UK

Acknowledgements

My gratitude is due to the contributors of this volume for their continued revisions as time and technical progress have advanced.

Few tasks can be completed without the support of colleagues and friends. I am indebted to the many true friends who have helped and encouraged me over the years. The late Prof. Charles Gros first stimulated my interest in mammography in Strasburg in 1968. The challenge and interest still remain. Doctor Bengt Lundgren in Gavle, Sweden, widened the perspective and I am grateful to many other Swedish friends such as Ingvar Anderson and Nils Bjurstam. In Florence, Doctors Ciatto and Rosseli del Turco especially, as well as other colleagues of the European Breast Screening Group were always enthusiastic and stimulating. In the United Kingdom my radiological colleagues, especially Drs John Price, Huw Gravelle and Eric Roebuck have always been generous with help and encouragement.

I have been extremely fortunate with the radiographers in my teams whom I cannot praise too highly. They have tried, and still continue to try, to produce the finest mammogram films that can be achieved, and to take the films that provide the right answers.

My clinical colleagues have made the challenge of breast diagnosis a pleasure, and although there are far too many to name individually, I must thank Dr Jane Davey, Mr Gilmore and Mr McKinna for superb cooperation and encouragement over the years. Finally, I must thank my long-suffering husband Dr Lewis Cannell without whom this book would never have materialized.

Introduction

A. K. Tucker

The accurate assessment of the breast as to whether it is normal or not requires the gathering of all relevant information, considerable experience and an open mind.

The efficacy of diagnostic mammography depends on

1. The optimal radiographic demonstration of the breast.
2. The perception of abnormal features.
3. The correct interpretation of these.

The diagnostic approach is relatively simple and boils down to deciding whether the appearances are normal, abnormal or equivocal. Most problems concern the equivocal appearances and what to do about them. The diagnostic algorithm is as follows: are the appearances

1. Normal.
2. Abnormal.

If abnormal, are they:
a. Benign, e.g. benign breast change, tumours, cysts, infection, haemorrhage, scars;
b. Malignant: single, multifocal, multicentric, calcification;
c. Equivocal: masses, stromal pattern, calcification.

The detection of abnormality is not always easy. Experience is needed to appreciate the wide range of both the normal and abnormal appearances. Many of the features of benign breast change (BBC) are now considered as normal variants. This concept may include benign tumours such as fibroadenomata and cysts (Hughes et al 1989).

The consistency of the basic mammographic anatomy over the years is perhaps surprising for an organ which undergoes monthly periodic cyclical change and the much more marked changes of pregnancy and lactation. Although normal glandular tissue usually involutes after the menopause the prominent duct pattern seen in benign breast change continues for life.

To achieve maximum accuracy in reporting, it is essential to have well-trained, caring radiographers, dedicated equipment, appropriate viewing facilities and good cooperation with clinical colleagues and pathologists. The radiologist relies absolutely on the radiographer, for no-one can diagnose the 'off the film' cancer. Therefore radiographers should be encouraged to take views which incorporate those areas of which the patient or clinician is suspicious. Many women present with vague signs, which should always be given due attention. Some cancers will undoubtedly be obscured in the dense breast, where microcalcification is the only sign likely to arouse suspicion. In particular, lobular in-situ carcinoma has no special radiological features and is always an incidental finding in biopsy performed for other reasons.

Approximately 50% of cancers detected at screening are impalpable and are detected by mammography alone—but regrettably, approximately 9% of palpable cancers will not show, even with optimal films and known position (Lee et al 1991). Recent advances in digital systems should not only reduce the radiation dose to the breast but also raise the possibility of computer diagnosis. While yet not technically perfect, algorithms are being developed which assist accuracy in diagnosis.

The efficiency of screening programmes in detecting breast cancer may be measured in terms of their sensitivity and specificity.

1. Sensitivity defines the accuracy of the positive mammographic diagnosis. The term therefore indicates the correct number of positive cancers diagnosed and also by inference the positive cases missed. It is a ratio of the true mammographic positive diagnoses to the total number of women with proven cancer in the screened population. The latter figure includes interval cancers and further depends on appropriate follow-up and accurate assessment of those women with negative, cancer-free diagnoses. This may present difficulties and thus limit precise accuracy.
2. Specificity indicates the rate of mammographic false-positive diagnoses in women free of cancer in the screened population. It is a reciprocal of the ratio of true negative mammographic diagnosis to the total number of healthy women screened, which includes those with false-positive X-ray diagnosis. Since the latter will be carefully assessed this is a more accurate measurement.

Sensitivity and specificity are inversely related. Higher sensitivity means that fewer cancers are missed. Higher specificity means that fewer false-positive diagnoses are made. These standard measurements can be applied to screening teams or to individual mammographers where the relative operating characteristic (ROC) curves can be calculated. These tests of screening efficiency do not apply to mammography in the symptomatic patients.

To maintain high sensitivity and specificity the viewing and reporting must be meticulous and specific. Dedicated viewing facilities with high-intensity light coned to the area of the film are desirable, and if multi-film roller viewers are used, then binoculars should be used to exclude surrounding light. Magnifying binocular viewers also help to concentrate attention, as well as magnifying the image. Routine use of a magnifying lens is often advocated for the detection of very fine, faint microcalcification. Clinical information and the knowledge of previous surgical intervention, radiotherapy and trauma will increase specificity—post-surgical fibrosis and traumatic fat necrosis are great hazards for the uninformed and unsuspecting radiologist. If the information is not supplied by the referring clinician, or the screening programme does not include physical examination, radiographers should be trained to record the necessary details.

All mammograms should be undertaken before aspiration or fine-needle aspiration (FNA) as the oedema and small haematoma caused will obscure detail and give rise to a false-positive diagnosis. Ideally, mammograms should be left for 2 weeks after FNA. When viewing mammograms it is important to inspect similar views of both right and left sides simultaneously, and they should be compared quadrant by quadrant to appreciate small differences in density or in architecture. As with most other paired organs the breasts are usually—though not invariably—symmetrical, and the commonest cause of asymmetry is previous surgery. Differences in compression between one side and the other frequently cause a difference in density, though this should be appreciated on careful viewing by the sharpness of detail. Comparison with old films is also invaluable, and is certainly the most important factor in detecting subtle changes of early malignancy in incident screening rounds. Finally, careful correlation with pathology will help to reduce both the false-positive and the false-negative rates.

REFERENCES

Hughes L E et al 1989 Radiological nomenclature in benign breast change. Clinical Radiology 40: 374–379
Wallis M G, Walsh M T, Lee J R 1991 A review of the false negative mammogram in a symptomatic population. Clinical Radiology 44: 13–15

CHAPTER 1

Clinical findings

J. B. Davey

INTRODUCTION

Disorders of the breast are common and are usually noticed by the woman herself. A lump or change in the breast tissue may only be noticed if there is patient awareness and in addition a regular practice of breast self-examination. Generations of medical students are taught the art of breast palpation early in their training but the importance of the physical breast examination as part of a general examination may easily become overlooked as more diagnostic tests are available. Antagonists of screening asymptomatic women with only mammography are also against the promotion of encouraging breast self-examination, and yet historically this is the way that breast disorders present. It is just as important to promote and teach all physicians the art of a first-class physical breast examination (Isaacs 1989) so that the clinical features of breast disease can readily be recognized and treated. The promoters of screening with mammography tend to overlook the fact that unless a clinical examination of the breast is included, then perhaps as many as 10% of cancers will be missed (Moskowitz 1983), although there is a very small percentage that is not detected by either clinical examination or mammography. Training and experience in the practice of clinical examination increases the percentage of cancers detected (Hall et al 1977). To recognize all the clinical features of breast disease a definite routine should be adhered to. It is suggested that it is important to

listen/look with palpation/listen and look again with the mammogram and then localize with palpation,

when hopefully the percentage accuracy of breast cancer diagnosis may well be over 90% (Butler 1990). Signs of change are difficult to document but important to record, especially as the change noticed by the woman herself may be the only detail available for making a diagnosis, e.g. change in nipple direction. Accurate documentation is vital and, where possible, the record used should be a photograph with marked areas rather than the usual diagram when the nipple and periareolar area is portrayed centrally in the breast rather than more inferiorly in the middle-aged woman. The detailed examination includes the skin and nipple areas, breast tissue and gland areas draining the breast (Bassett 1985). If the physical examination and history is omitted and only mammography used for the breast examination, 10–30% of cancers may not be detected (Ciatto et al 1987, Moskovic et al 1990).

THE CLINICAL EXAMINATION

Just as breast disorders are common and varied, so may breast cancer take many forms and produce many different abnormalities. The breast examination should detect the majority of the abnormalities but a clinical history to record symptoms is vital for obtaining background information. Cancer can mimic most benign disorders but symptoms usually relate more to the common benign conditions.

The clinical history

Listening to the patient's symptoms before any physical examination of the breasts is very important. This, together with the personal and family medical background, determines whether she is at a higher than average risk of breast cancer, for example, maternal family history (Lynch 1990). Where asymptomatic screening by clinical examination alone is done, details of menarche, last period, menopause, age of first pregnancy and parity, together with hormone therapy are vital because further assessment may be required following a period if the woman is premenstrual. Conversely screening programmes will detect asymptomatic cancers, making dependence on symptoms less important (Homer 1981).

Listening to the patient produces many clues to detection, and occasionally guidance to an area in question is needed if an area of suspicion is not found. It is well known that 75–80% of women with breast cancer become aware of their disease because of a lump (Haagensen 1971). Approximately 20% present with pain, nipple discharge or retraction, which are the most common symptoms apart from a lump. Skin erythema or asymmetry, axillary lymphadenopathy alone or arm oedema are rare presenting features.

The clinical examination sitting up

Inspection prior to palpation is most helpful in noting changes in contour, unequal size of breasts and nipples, skin creases, dimples or erythema. Rarely is a lump seen (Fig. 1.1) or glands visible but occasionally the woman reports findings on looking down on her breasts or looking in the mirror for change.

With the arms raised prior to palpation, skin changes are noted, especially in the inframammary fold. Moles or scars must be recorded. Placing the arms on the hips contracting the pectoralis major

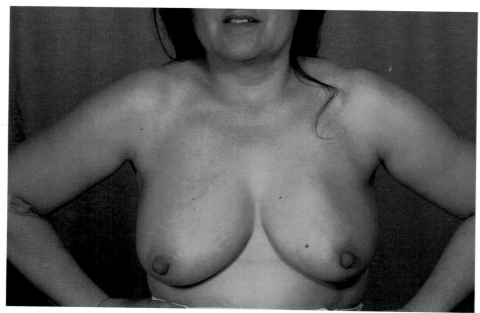

Fig. 1.1 Patient with visible lump.

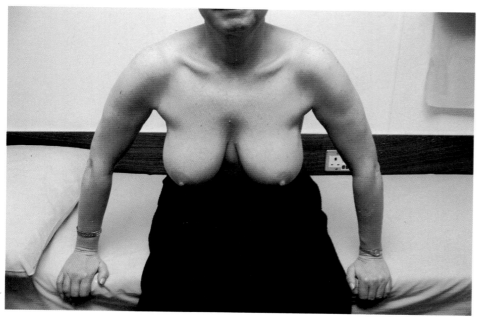

Fig. 1.2 Patient with hands on couch.

demonstrates dimples, but leaning
forward with the hands on the edge of
the couch is probably superior in this
respect (Fig. 1.2).

Palpation of breast tissue in this position is sometimes of help to confirm what is found lying down. For the larger breast it may be helpful for areas of nodularity and background breast consistency. Lifting the breast can demonstrate dimpling (Fig. 1.3*a*, *b*). The gland areas may be felt in this position or lying down according to individual preference, but feeling high up in the apex of the axilla and running the fingers down the medial wall is most productive. The supraclavicular fossa glands may be felt by standing behind the woman whereas the infraclavicular areas must be felt from the front.

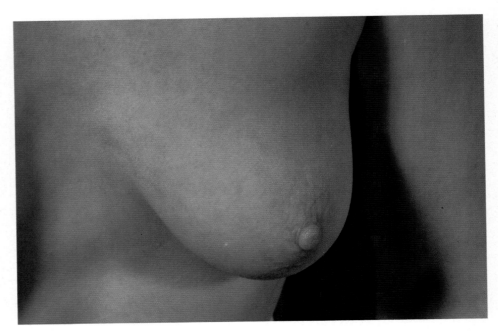

Fig. 1.3a

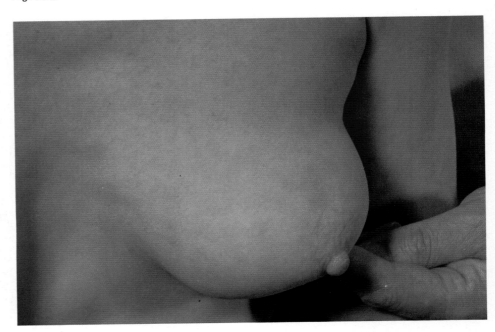

Fig. 1.3b

Fig. 1.3   *a, b* Lifting the breast to reveal dimpling.

The clinical examination lying down

Localized breast disorders are best felt lying down with the head supported by a single pillow and the arms resting comfortably above the head on the pillow. The breast tissue is spread out as thinly as possible over the chest wall. The flat of the finger tips is used and either one or both hands used simultaneously to examine one or both breasts together. Supporting the larger breast is useful but more important is turning the patient to the oblique position to concentrate on the upper outer quadrant and subareolar areas where most lumps are (Fig. 1.4). The background of breast tissue consistency is noted but it may not compare with that seen on the mammogram. The size of the mass, together with the shape, mobility and margin are recorded. Attachment to skin and fascia, tenderness and possible consistency are noted in the precise segment in which it is located.

The nipple and periareolar regions are separately checked because tiny nodules can easily be missed. Nipple retraction and its history (whether of recent origin or long-standing) must be recorded together with nipple discharge, colour and frequency. The practice of squeezing the nipple should be discouraged as it tends to produce further discharge. Scaling of the nipple is most important to record (Paget 1874).

The teaching of breast self-examination can be included at this stage. Women who already do a regular breast check should keep with their individual routine but it is important to demonstrate that there is a difference in the method of breast self-examination and the physician or nurse practitioner doing a clinical examination. The woman herself should use the examining hand flat and not the individual finger tip.

The frequency of routine clinical examination depends on a variety of factors, such as age, hormone status and frequency of mammography. It is known that annual examinations produce smaller tumours and,

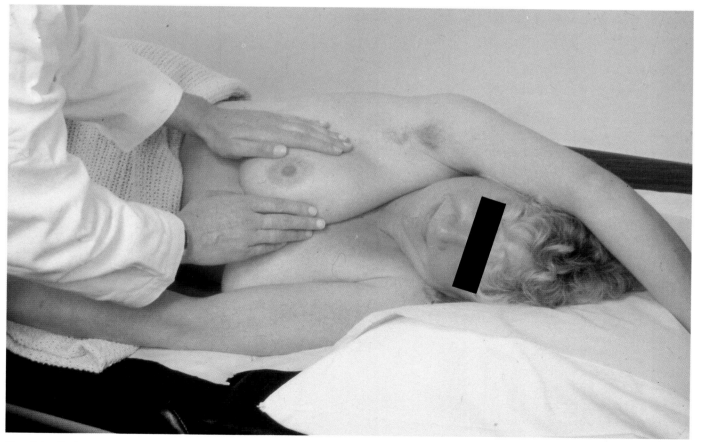

Fig. 1.4   Patient being examined in oblique position.

therefore, an improved prognosis (Senie 1981). Annual clinical examinations over the age of 40 are suggested. Looking again with the mammogram completes the examination.

CLINICAL FEATURES OF BREAST DISORDERS—BENIGN

Benign breast change

Numerous attempts have been made to classify the common benign disorders of the breast. There are also many types of benign change. Hughes et al (1987) describe a classification known as ANDI (aberrations of normal development and involution). The debate continues as to what may be accepted as a variant from the normal and what should be regarded as abnormal or pathological.

The lumpy breast is the most common problem, which previously has always been described with varying degrees as fibrocystic elements. Usually, but not always, these changes are bilateral. There is a wide variation, especially in the premenopausal woman. The site is frequently the upper outer quadrant, and in the fat depleted breast accurate clinical diagnosis is impossible without resorting to a further examination at a different time in the cycle or having further tests done, such as mammography, ultrasound or aspiration cytology (Butler 1990).

These additional tests are required with the older patients with fatty breasts where Cooper's ligaments divide the fat layer into lobules and a 'fat' lump can be felt. Following injury, fat necrosis can be a problem for the clinician and additional investigations are essential.

Without resorting to biopsy, it is difficult to know the percentage of women with benign breast change and, therefore, the likelihood of risk of developing cancer (Roberts 1984). So a consensus pathological statement was issued in 1986 (Consensus Meeting 1986) to clarify this for women undergoing biopsy. This group may be at more than average risk because of family history, for example, but the factors that produce benign breast changes may also favour the development of cancer. Further evidence of risk of breast cancer for women with benign breast change has been shown in many published articles (Brunton et al 1981).

Benign lumps

These are common, single or multiple and mobile. Attention to history is useful for the lactational galactocele or mastitis and for abscess formation. The two most common lumps beside a lipoma are fibroadenoma and cysts (Table 1.1).

The giant fibroadenoma or phylloides tumour produces a rapidly growing lump but it is nearly always benign.

Benign skin changes

Scars and skin nodules such as moles and papillomata must be documented, especially if mammography is to follow the clinical examination. Other

Table 1.1

	Fibroadenoma	Cyst
Age of Occurrence	20–40 years	30–50 years
	Single (or multiple)	Multiple (or single)
	Painless	Painless or painful
	Little change with cycle	Often size increase in premenstrual phase

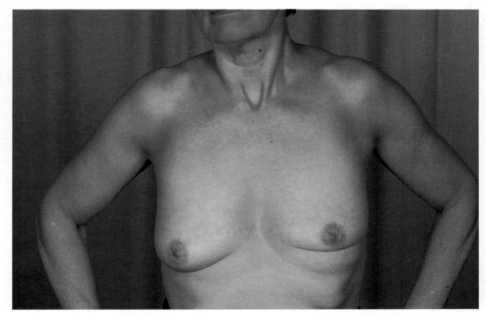

Fig. 1.5 'Congenital' crease—left breast.

skin conditions such as acne, psoriasis or eczema, particularly around the nipple, are important to record. Asymmetric vascularity and prominent vessels are noted but the main attention is focused on creases and dimples. Some creases may be congenital and dimples, although most commonly found with carcinoma, may sometimes be atrophic and, therefore, of little consequence (Fig. 1.5).

Mondor's disease
Superficial thrombophlebitis of the thoraco-epigastric vein can present with a painful crease. The thrombosed vein is usually vertical and feels like a firm piece of string with overlying skin attachment that may look suspicious of underlying malignancy (Tabar & Dean 1981) (Fig. 1.6).

The nipple
Nipple change is more often a sign of malignant disorder than benign. Benign causes of retraction are associated with duct ectasia and fat necrosis. Inversion is usually long-standing and must not be mistaken for retraction. Palpation of the subareolar area is frequently soft and there appears to be an absence of breast tissue causing the edge to resemble a localized nodule. This is similar to oval fatty lumps in the inframammary ridge. Gentle squeezing of the nipple completes the examination. Commence low down and test any nipple discharge with haemostix to see if it is blood-stained (Fig. 1.7). If discharge is not spontaneous, squeezing should be discouraged. Creamy discharge suggests fibrocystic change.

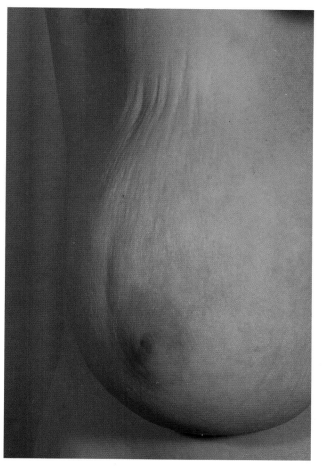

Fig. 1.6 Mondor's disease—right breast.

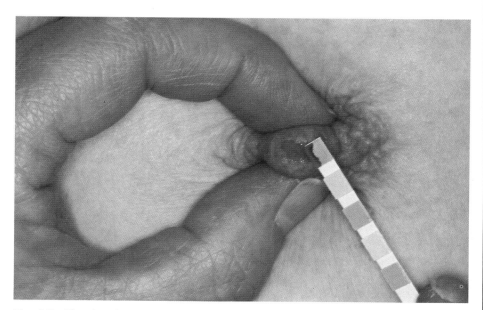

Fig. 1.7 Blood-stained nipple discharge.

CLINICAL FEATURES OF BREAST DISORDERS—MALIGNANT

Breast cancer classification is as complex as benign breast change. A simple pathological system would include three varieties: non-invasive, invasive and Paget's disease of the nipple. The presenting feature or symptom in the majority of cancers is a lump, which would not be covered by this classification; yet a lump in a woman of middle years may be considered as cancer until proved otherwise. Asymptomatic screening, however, would follow the more pathological classification if the clinical examination is omitted and screening is carried out by mammography only.

The malignant lump

Usually painless, a lump is the most common presenting symptom and sign of cancer. It is rarely visible (Fig. 1.1) but may be seen by the patient looking down or by the physician looking at the patient. Women may report a thickening or change in breast tissue consistency and yet an obvious lump is palpable to the physician. Conversely some lumps are varied in outline and quite large at presentation. Mobility is variable but some tethering either to skin or deep tissues may be present. An irregular margin is common but smooth surfaces are found in some malignant lumps. Clinical examinations detect more lumps as size increases but detection increases if more care and attention is paid to the detail of clinical examination. Experience and skilled tuition is imperative for detection of malignant

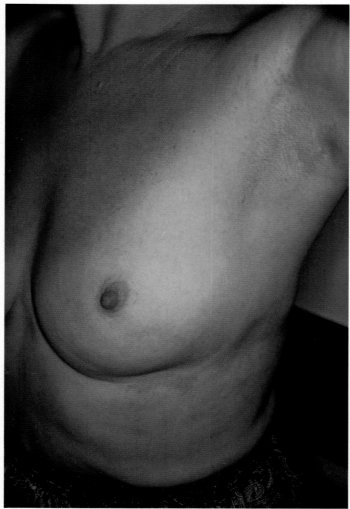

Fig. 1.8a

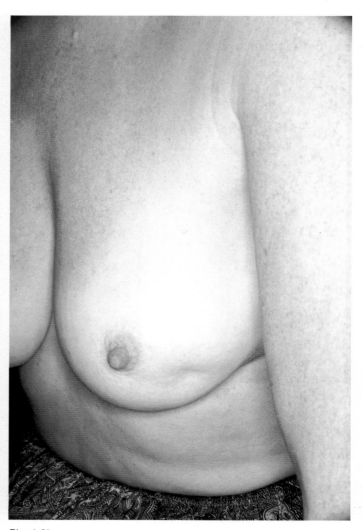

Fig. 1.8b

Fig. 1.8   *a, b* 'Malignant' dimpling of left breast.

lumps because the variation of signs and symptoms of breast cancer is great (Hall 1977).

Malignant skin change

Skin dimpling, a classical finding of cancer for the physician, is rarely reported by the patient. She may notice skin thickening or thickening deep in the breast and sometimes erythema or an increased vascular pattern. Peau d'orange or 'orange peel skin', often quite extensive, is found in the lower half of the breast since it results from dependent oedema of the skin. This is due to either a deep-sited tumour, axillary gland obstruction or accompanying erythema with an inflammatory diffuse carcinoma. Ulceration is less common still but can be an initial presenting factor with or without haemorrhage.

Flattening of the breast or a change of skin contour is not common but the carcinoma may be of insidious and painless onset, so signs may be quite gross at presentation (Fig. 1.8—this patient having a negative mammogram; the patient had also noticed her left breast to be smaller than the right by looking down onto the breast rather than looking at herself in the mirror as shown in the photograph).

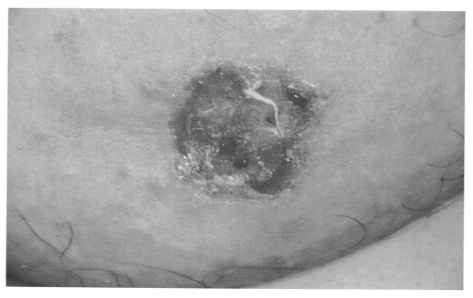

Fig. 1.9 Paget's disease of nipple showing total destruction.

The malignant nipple

Paget's disease of the nipple is more commonly recognized as eczema; first being described by Sir James Paget in 1874. The nipple may become flattened or retracted prior to ulceration or simple eczematous scaly changes only may be found. A mammogram must always be carried out to detect the commonly associated intraductal carcinoma which may not be palpable or invasive duct carcinoma, either of which may be palpable some distance from the nipple. Much variation in nipple appearance is found including total destruction (Fig. 1.9).

Retraction of the nipple is often associated with a malignant mass on palpation. Benign causes are senile duct ectasia and fat necrosis. It is important not to confuse recent retraction with long-standing or even congenital inversion of the nipple.

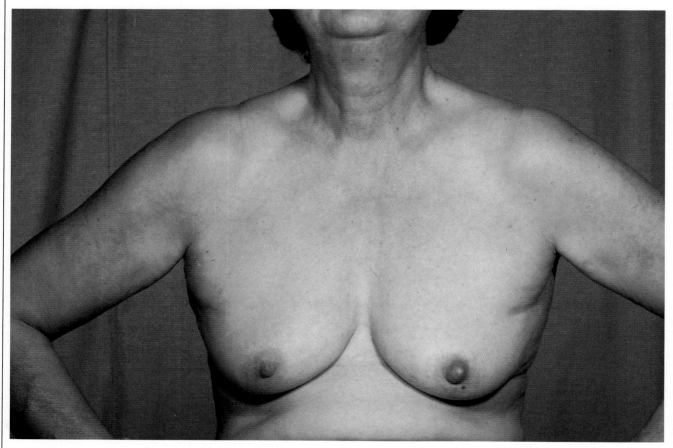

Fig. 1.10   Difference in size of nipples.

Enlargement of the nipple without ulceration is an uncommon presentation of breast cancer, difference in size of nipples being the only abnormality on the mammogram (Fig. 1.10). Nipple discharge occurs in about 10% of women with breast cancer. It may be watery, serous or blood-stained (Leis 1985). The watery or serous discharge should be checked by haemostix for blood, and cytology of nipple discharge may be helpful. Nipple discharge is more commonly associated with benign conditions.

BREAST DISORDERS IN PREGNANCY

Normal breast enlargement and engorgement makes detection of breast disorders more complicated. Benign lumps are more common than cancer but it is essential to establish a diagnosis. Aspiration and cytology may be more useful than mammography. Simple fibroadenomata may increase in size quite rapidly and cause pain. The galactocele may also be painful.

Breast cancer often has nodal involvement at the time of diagnosis but the prognosis is similar to that of the woman who is not pregnant at

diagnosis (Van der Vange & Van Dorgen 1991) so detection when the cancer is small and localized is important. Treatment rather than observation of a breast lump in pregnancy is imperative.

DISORDERS IN THE MALE BREAST

Gynaecomastia, either unilateral or bilateral, is the most common disorder of the male breast. In a teenage youth it is often associated with excessive milk drinking. A clinical history is especially important with regard to hormonal changes and also family history.

Breast cancer comprises 1% of all cancer cases in the USA in men and at an older age than women. It is more common in the left breast than the right and is said to carry a poorer prognosis (Hodson et al 1985) because it is more advanced at diagnosis than in the female. Clinical features are similar to the female, i.e. a painless lump at presentation or nipple discharge. The differential diagnosis is with unilateral gynaecomastia.

THE FINAL CLINICAL ASSESSMENT

It is the responsibility of the clinician to make the final assessment for diagnosis prior to treatment. Three results from the clinical examination emerge: suspicious of carcinoma; equivocal; or benign and non-suspicious. This must be a quality assessment involving teamwork, the understanding of results from other diagnostic tests and guidance for follow-up appointments.

Traditionally, the clinical findings have been all-important and still have a major role in assessment for extent of disease, on which staging depends. Nowadays, few clinicians fail to accept that mammography can detect impalpable tumours. Prognosis for cure correlates inversely with tumour size. This is a great incentive for careful clinical examination which, like other tests, must never be done in isolation.

REFERENCES

Bassett A A 1985 Physical examination of the breast and breast self-examination. In: Miller A B (ed) *Screening for cancer*. Academic Press, New York, pp 271–291

Brunton L A, Vessey M P, Flavel R et al 1981 Risk factors for benign breast disease. American Journal Epidemiology 113: 203–214

Butler J A, Vargas H I, Worthen N et al 1990 Accuracy of combined clinico-mammographic-cytologic diagnosis of dominant breast masses: a prospective study. Archives of Surgery 125(7): 893–895

Ciatto S, Cataliotti L, Distante V 1987 Nonpalpable lesions detected with mammography: review of 512 consecutive cases. Radiology 165: 99–102

Consensus Meeting 1986 Is fibrocystic disease of the breast precancerous? Archives of Pathology and Laboratory Medicine 110: 171–173

Haagensen C D 1971 Disease of the breast. W B Saunders, Philadelphia

Hall D C, Goldstein M K, Steingh G H 1977 Progress in manual breast examination. Cancer 40: 364

Hodson G R, Undaneta L F, Al-Jurf A S et al 1985 Male breast carcinoma. American Surgery 51: 5147–5149

Homer M J 1981 Nonpalpable mammographic abnormalities: timing the follow-up studies. American Journal of Radiology 136: 923

Hughes L E, Mansel R E, Webster D J T 1987 ANDI—a new perspective on benign breast disorders. Lancet ii: 1316–1318

Isaacs J H 1989 Clinical Obstetrics and Gynaecology 32(4): 761–767

Koss L 1979 Diagnostic cytology and its histopathic bases, 3rd ed. J B Lippincott, Philadelphia

Leis H P, Cammarata A, La Raja R D 1985 Nipple discharge significance and treatment. Breast 11: 6

Lynch H T, Watson P, Conway T A et al 1990 Clinical/genetic features in hereditary breast cancer. Breast Cancer Research and Treatment 15(2): 63–71

Moskovic E, Sinnett H D, Parsons C A 1990 The accuracy of mammographic diagnosis in surgically occult breast lesions. Clinical Radiology 41: 344–346

Moskowitz M 1983 Screening for breast cancer. How effective are our tests? A critical review CA/A. Cancer Journal for Clinicians 33: 26–29

Moskowitz M, Russell P et al 1975 Breast cancer screening. Preliminary report of 207 biopsies performed in 4128 volunteer screenees. Cancer 36: 2245

Paget J 1874 On disease of the mammary areola preceding cancer of the mammary glands. St Bartholomew's Hospital Report 10: 87–89

Roberts M M, Jones V, Elton R A et al 1984 Risk of breast cancer in women with a history of benign breast disease of the breast. British Medical Journal 288: 275–278

Senie R T, Rosen P R, Lesser M L, Kinne D 1981 Breast self-examination and medical examination related to breast cancer state. American Journal of Public Health 71: 583–590

Tabar L & Dean P B 1981 Mondor's disease. Clinical mammographic and pathological features. Breast 7: 18

Van der Vange N & Van Dorgen J A 1991 Breast cancer and pregnancy. European Journal of Surgical Oncology 17: 1–8

CHAPTER 2

Physical factors in mammography

D. R. Dance

INTRODUCTION

X-ray mammography is a difficult technique and the quality of the mammographic image is critically dependent upon the imaging equipment employed and the way which it is utilized. Inadequate breast compression, poor positioning or the use of the wrong image receptor or X-ray tube will all result in a suboptimal image. However, equipment is available which is specifically designed for mammography and images of excellent quality can be obtained at a moderately low dose to the breast. This chapter describes such equipment and the physical principles which govern its design, performance and utilization. Within the United Kingdom, guidelines have been published by the Department of Health which indicate the performance necessary for some of the components of the mammographic system (Department of Health and Social Security 1987, Department of Health (DH) 1990) and reference will be made to these guidelines where appropriate.

In mammography there are four physical parameters which must be considered when assessing the performance of the imaging system. Contrast is important because of the need to see small differences in soft tissue density. Resolution is important because of the need to visualize microcalcifications as small as 100 μm that are often associated with abnormality (Mills et al 1976). Dose is important because of the small risk of carcinogenesis associated with the examination (National Commission on Radiation Protection and Measurements (NCRP) 1986, Feig & Ehrlich 1990) and noise is important because the dose is ultimately limited by the need to achieve an adequate

signal-to-noise ratio in the image. The relation between these parameters is sometimes complex and dependent upon the performance of several components of the imaging system, and we shall find that it is necessary to compromise between them.

THE COMPONENTS OF THE MAMMOGRAPHIC IMAGING SYSTEM

The modern mammographic X-ray set (Fig. 2.1) is a dedicated unit with a low-energy X-ray spectrum and a small focal spot. The use of a non-dedicated unit is *not* recommended as this will almost certainly lead to images of inferior quality. The radiation field from the dedicated unit is collimated to avoid unnecessary irradiation of other body tissues, and the focal spot is often positioned above the edge of the radiation field closest to the patient with the cathode–anode axis running in the direction chest wall to nipple. This choice of geometry ensures the visualization of the maximum amount of tissue and, because of the 'heel effect', provides a greater incident photon flux at the chest wall than at the nipple, thus making partial compensation for the increased absorption of photons by the thicker regions of the compressed breast.

The X-ray set may be angled to achieve any desired radiographic projection and the patient is usually examined standing. The breast rests on or against a support plate and is compressed onto this plate using a plastic paddle. The compression pressure can be applied manually but power-assisted compression is generally preferred because this allows the radiographer to use two hands to position the breast. The shape and rigidity of the compression plate are

important contributory factors to the quality of the compression. The support plate should have a high X-ray transmission and is often constructed from a carbon-fibre composite. In many cases this support will form the front of a tunnel which receives the image receptor, but in some cases it will form the front face of the cassette which contains the image receptor.

The contrast of the mammographic image is significantly degraded by scatter and the use of a mammographic anti-scatter grid is recommended (DH 1990). Both stationary and moving grids are available and these are normally incorporated within the cassette and cassette tunnel, respectively. The standard image receptor used in mammography is the high-resolution mammographic screen-film combination. The Xerox receptor has decreased in popularity although it is still in use in some centres.

The transmission of X-ray photons through the breast varies considerably with breast thickness, and composition and the final part of the mammographic system is the automatic exposure control device. The detector for this device is placed after the image receptor, and two or more positions within the radiation field should be available to cope with different imaging situations.

An important accessory of the more expensive systems that have a second (very fine) focus, is the magnification bridge, which is used to elevate the breast away from the image receptor and hence to provide a magnified image. This plate should also have a high photon transmission.

PHYSICAL PROPERTIES OF THE BREAST

The composition and size of the female breast vary widely. It may be composed predominantly of adipose or glandular tissues and its compressed thickness can range between 2 and 8 cm or even more with a median value of about 5 cm. When compressed, it has a projection which is approximately D-shaped with an area of between 35 and 250 cm² (Dance & Davis 1983). For the largest breasts it may be necessary to use a larger film format or more than one exposure.

In the mammographic energy range, the principal interactions of X-ray photons with tissue are Compton scattering and the photoelectric effect, with Compton scattering preponderating at the higher energies and the photoelectric effect at the lower energies. At 20 keV, for example, 60% of the interactions are photoelectric and the mean distance between photon interactions is 1.6 cm. Adipose tissues have a lower density and higher X-ray transmission than fibroglandular tissues but the difference in transmission between carcinoma and glandular tissue can be small (Johns & Yaffe 1987), and it is important to image at a low photon energy to obtain adequate soft tissue contrast. Figure 2.2 gives two examples of the variation of contrast with (monoenergetic) photon energy: 1 mm of fibroglandular tissue viewed against a background of 'average' breast tissue and a 100 µm calcification viewed against the same background. Both curves show a rapid fall-off with increasing photon energy: there is a decrease of a factor of six in contrast between 15 and 30 keV. Furthermore, the glandular tissue contrast falls below 0.01 for energies above 27 keV. This result is for a model calculation,

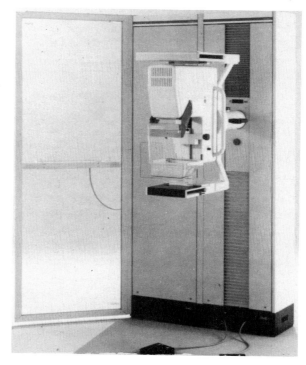

Fig. 2.1 A typical mammographic X-ray set (Siemens Mammomat 2). Photograph courtesy of Siemens Medical Engineering.

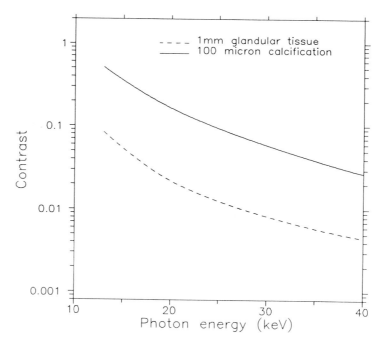

Fig. 2.2 Variation of contrast with photon energy. The upper curve is for a 0.1 mm calcification (assumed to be calcium hydroxyapatite) and the lower curve is for 1 mm glandular tissue. Contrast degradation due to scatter and the resolution of the imaging system have been ignored.

but it clearly indicates the need to use a low photon energy for mammography and the fact that if the energy is too high, the contrast of some structures will fall below the threshold for recognition.

Because mammographic X-ray spectra are low energy, the dose within the breast decreases rapidly with increasing depth. For a 6 cm-thick compressed breast the exit depth dose can vary between 1% and 13%, depending upon beam quality (Hammerstein et al 1979). It is important therefore to specify breast dose using a quantity which is representative of the dose to the whole organ. It is believed that the glandular tissues within the breast (including acinar and ductal epithelium and associated stroma) are the most sensitive to radiation-induced

carcinogenesis, and Hammerstein et al (1979) suggested that the mean dose to the glandular tissues within the breast is an appropriate dosimetric quantity. This suggestion has been widely adopted and its use is recommended by the NCRP (1986), the International Commission on Radiological Protection (1987) and the Institute of Physical Sciences in Medicine (1989).

The main factors which affect the dose to the breast are the composition and thickness of the organ, and the X-ray photon energy. The influence of breast area is small (Dance 1980). Figures 2.3 and 2.4 show the variation of the mean glandular dose with (monoenergetic) photon energy for breast thicknesses of 2 and 8 cm, and the dependence on composition for a 5 cm-thick breast (Dance 1990), respectively. There is a rapid increase of dose with decreasing

photon energy and with increasing breast thickness, and a marked dependence on the glandularity of the breast. It is clear that there is a severe dose penalty associated with the use of very low photon energies and that a compromise must be reached between the requirements of high image contrast and low dose.

X-RAY TUBE

The optimal photon energy for X-ray mammography is dependent upon the choice of image receptor. For screen-film imaging Jennings & Fewell (1979), Dance & Day (1981) and other authors have predicted optimal energies based on estimates of the signal-to-noise ratio in the image. These estimates vary with breast thickness, but demonstrate that the conventional mammographic X-ray

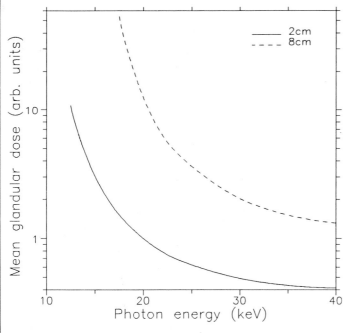

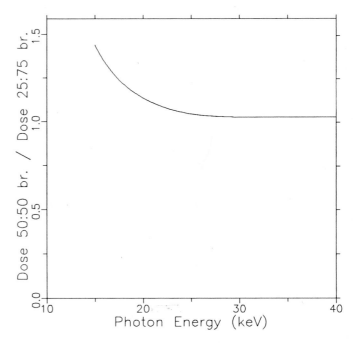

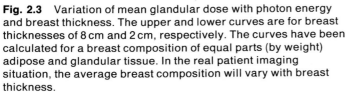

Fig. 2.3   Variation of mean glandular dose with photon energy and breast thickness. The upper and lower curves are for breast thicknesses of 8 cm and 2 cm, respectively. The curves have been calculated for a breast composition of equal parts (by weight) adipose and glandular tissue. In the real patient imaging situation, the average breast composition will vary with breast thickness.

Fig. 2.4   The dependence of mean glandular dose on breast composition. The curve plotted is the ratio of the mean glandular dose values for breasts 5 cm thick with compositions 50 : 50 by weight and 25 : 75 by weight adipose and glandular tissues, respectively.

spectrum obtained from a molybdenum target with a 30 μm molybdenum filter is well matched to the task of imaging all but the largest breasts. The molybdenum spectrum is shown in Fig. 2.5 and its main features are the characteristic K X-ray lines at 17.4 and 19.6 keV and the bremsstrahlung background, which is heavily attenuated by the molybdenum filter above its K-edge at 20.0 keV. At this energy, there is a large increase in the molybdenum photoelectric cross-section due to the threshold for the ejection of K-shell electrons being reached. Peak potentials in the range 25–30 kV are normally used depending upon local preference and breast size and density. In general, a lower kV will be used for an examination without a grid. Molybdenum target X-ray tubes generally have a beryllium exit window to avoid undue hardening of the beam, and the 30 μm molybdenum filter corresponds to the minimum allowed filtration (National Radiological Protection Board 1988). The half-value layer measured with the compression cone in place will generally be in the range 0.32–0.40 mm of aluminium.

Not all mammographic X-ray sets used for screen-film mammography have a molybdenum anode. In some cases a molybdenum/tungsten or a tungsten target is used instead. The resulting spectrum is also filtered by a K-edge filter (Beaman et al 1983, Bakir et al 1984, Sabel et al 1986) and can offer a dose reduction but at some sacrifice in contrast. Different K-edge filters can be used at different breast thicknesses so that a softer spectrum is used for the smaller breasts. Three filter materials are suitable: molybdenum (K-edge at 20.0 keV), rhodium (K-edge at 23.2 keV) and palladium (K-edge at 24.4 keV). Beaman et al (1983) have reported a dose reduction of about 50% using a tungsten target/palladium filter, which is a combination well suited to imaging large breasts.

A tungsten target is also used for imaging with the Xerox receptor. In this case, because of the low sensitivity of this receptor, it is necessary to use a much harder spectrum, at the expense of some loss in image quality, and a higher potential (40–50 kV). Additional filtration is used (a total of 2 or 3 mm of aluminium) at a half-value layer of 1.6 mm aluminium or more.

To achieve a short exposure time, and to reduce the effects of movement unsharpness and reciprocity law failure, it is desirable that a tube current of at least 100 mA is available for contact mammography (DH 1990). A typical exposure for a 5 cm-thick breast imaged using a mammographic screen-film receptor, a grid and an X-ray set with a molybdenum target is about 50 mAs and the exposure time is then about 0.5 s.

The exposure time will increase with increasing breast thickness and density and an exposure-time exposure-current product of at least 600 mAs should be available (DH 1990). The use of a high-voltage waveform with low ripple is recommended.

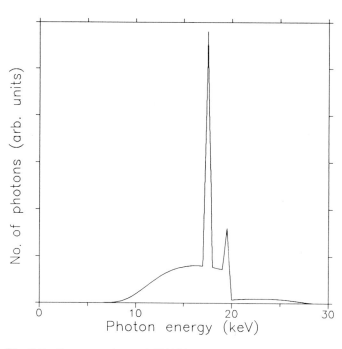

Fig. 2.5 X-ray spectrum at 28 kV for an X-ray tube with a molybdenum target and a 30 μm molybdenum filter. The spectrum is based on the work of Birch et al (1979).

IMAGING GEOMETRY AND FOCAL SPOT SIZE

There are three contributions to the overall unsharpness in the mammographic image: intrinsic blurring in the image receptor; blurring due to the finite size of the focal spot, and blurring from movement. If the breast is well compressed and there are no mechanical vibrations from the movement of the grid, the latter contribution should be small and is usually neglected in the analysis of system performance. The overall unsharpness then depends upon the image magnification, the focal spot size and the receptor unsharpness. A typical value for the receptor unsharpness is about 100 μm, and Fig. 2.6 shows how the overall unsharpness depends upon magnification for this particular value. Curves are given for four focal spot sizes. (It should be noted that these curves are for true focal spot sizes rather than nominal focal spot sizes. A tolerance of a factor of 1.5 is generally allowed between the nominal and measured values.) For each curve in the figure, magnifications that result in an overall unsharpness of less than 100 μm represent an improvement in resolution. It will be seen therefore that magnification can only minimize the unsharpness significantly if the focal spot is small enough. If the focal spot is too large, magnification will increase the unsharpness, and the magnification should then be kept as close as possible to 1 by increasing the focus film distance and minimizing the object–film distance. For contact mammography, which is usually done at a focus film distance of 60 cm, a true focal spot size of 0.6 mm (0.4 mm nominal) or less is desirable. The upper surface of an 8 cm-thick breast is then imaged at a magnification of × 1.15 and gives an acceptable overall unsharpness of 120 μm. It is noted that a limiting focal spot size of 0.5 mm (measured) is specified in DH (1990).

As pointed out above, magnification mammography will only produce a significant improvement in sharpness if a small focal spot size is used. A 0.2 mm (measured) focal spot size will produce only small improvements in sharpness and 0.1 mm (measured) focal spot size is preferred. The use of larger focal spot sizes for magnification is not recommended. For the 0.1 mm (measured) focal spot size, a magnification of × 1.5–2 is suggested.

As well as the above benefit of improved sharpness for magnification mammography, there is a decrease in the image noise and an improvement in contrast. The latter improvement occurs because the air-gap used for the magnification technique also provides some scatter rejection, but this must be offset in practice against the fact that the grid is usually removed for the exposure. There are, however, two important disadvantages of the magnification technique: it is necessary to take more than one exposure to fit the image of the entire breast on a single film, and there is a dose increase of a factor of two or three. Magnification is therefore not used for the initial films, but it finds an important role in providing further information when appropriate at a higher resolution and at a reduced noise level.

COMPRESSION

We have seen already that firm compression is important in mammography because it reduces breast dose and prevents or reduces movement unsharpness, but it also produces several other benefits.

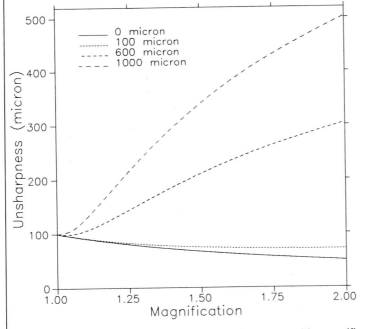

Fig. 2.6 Variation of the overall image unsharpness with magnification and focal spot size. The unsharpness has been estimated for a receptor unsharpness of 100 μm and (actual) focal spot sizes of 0, 100, 600 and 1000 μm.

Geometric unsharpness is reduced because all structures within the breast are closer to the image receptor. Image contrast is also improved and for two reasons: the quantity of scattered radiation leaving the bottom of the breast is reduced and the X-ray spectrum reaching the image receptor is softer. In addition, the visualization of overlapping structures within the breast is better because the amount of overlap is reduced. Finally, because the tissue path length will be quite similar for much of the image, it is easier to fit the photon pattern leaving the breast within the latitude of the image receptor.

ANTI-SCATTER GRIDS

Photon scatter is important in mammography because it causes a significant loss of image contrast. The magnitude of the scatter is not strongly influenced by photon energy but it does vary with breast thickness, producing contrast losses of 20% and 50% for breast thicknesses of 2 and 8 cm, respectively (Dance & Day 1984). Because of this loss of contrast, the use of anti-scatter grids has become well established and two different types of mammographic grid are presently available: a stationary grid with a line density of about 80 lines/cm and an aluminium interspace material (Chan et al 1985), and a moving grid with a line density of about 30 lines/cm and an interspace material of paper or cotton fibre (Barnes 1979, Dance & Day 1984). A comparison of the performance of these two grids has been made by Alm Carlsson et al (1989). Because the stationary grid has an aluminium interspace, it attenuates the primary photons more than the stationary grid and requires a dose some 30% higher. Furthermore, since the thickness of

the stationary grid is restricted because of its high primary attenuation, it only has a grid ratio (ratio of grid height to width of interspace) of 3.5, whereas this ratio for the moving grid is 5.0. As a consequence, the moving grid is better at stopping scattered photons and it offers better contrast. It is strongly recommended for imaging medium to large breasts where it produces a very noticeable improvement in contrast (53% for an 8 cm compressed breast thickness, with a dose increase of a factor of 2.1). For the smaller breast, the improvement is less significant, amounting to some 17% for a 2 cm breast with a dose increase of a factor of 1.7, and the use of a slightly lower X-ray tube potential and no grid can be considered.

IMAGE RECEPTORS

Screen-film receptors

The screen-film combination is the standard image receptor used in X-ray mammography. If an appropriate combination is used with well-controlled processing, then films can be obtained that offer good contrast and resolution at a reasonably low dose.

Resolution and contrast. The majority of the blackening of the mammographic film is caused by light-fluorescent photons emitted by the phosphor following the absorption of an incident X-ray photon. Direct absorption of the incident X-ray photon by the film emulsion causes only a few per cent of the total film blackening. The light-fluorescent photons produced by the phosphor are emitted isotropically and spread laterally as they pass from phosphor to emulsion. The magnitude of this lateral spread is proportional to the

distance between the point of emission of the fluorescent photons and the emulsion, and this distance should be reduced as much as possible. This can be achieved by using a single emulsion film and a single screen placed behind the film and in contact with the emulsion. This configuration avoids the crossover effect associated with the use of double-screen double-emulsion systems, and brings the production point of the fluorescent photons as close as possible to the screen. It is essential to maintain good film-screen contact and this is readily achieved using modern mammographic cassettes. The lateral spread can also be reduced by decreasing the phosphor thickness and introducing light-absorbing dyes or pigments into the screen. This will also reduce the sensitivity of the receptor, and a compromise has to be found between the resolution and speed of the system. With a typical mammographic screen-film combination, it should be possible to see calcifications as small as 100–200 μm.

In recent years mammographic receptors have been introduced which use a double-screen double-emulsion combination. The emulsions used contain grains of tabular form (to reduce the effects of crossover) and the screens form an asymmetric pair. Kimme-Smith et al (1987) have reported on one such combination which offers a reduction in dose of about 50% but at the cost of inferior visibility of (simulated) calcifications, increased image noise (quantum mottle) and reduced contrast in regions of dense parenchyma.

Mammographic screen-films have a high contrast, a narrow latitude and are exposed to a high density so that in the region of the image close to the edge of the breast, the optical density can be 3.0 or even higher. To view such films it is essential to use a special mammographic light box in a darkened room and to mask all glare from regions of the light box not covered by film. Figure 2.7 shows the film characteristic for two mammographic screen films. With such steep characteristics, it is very important to use the correct exposure so that all regions of the breast lie on the steep part of the curve rather than in the toe or shoulder regions. Automatic exposure control and careful control and monitoring of film processing are mandatory, and a dedicated mammographic processor is recommended.

The shape of the film characteristic and the film speed are strongly influenced by the processing temperature and time, and the use of extended processing, which can reduce dose by about 35% whilst maintaining or improving contrast, is popular.

Screen sensitivity. Mammographic screens have a fluorescent layer of either calcium tungstate or a rare earth phosphor such as terbium-activated gadolinium oxysulphide. The sensitivity of the screen is governed by its X-ray absorption characteristics and light production efficiency. The X-ray absorption efficiency is quite high: for the Kodak Min-R screen with 34 mg/cm² gadolinium oxysulphide, the energy absorption efficiency at 20 keV is about 70% and similar values.obtain for tungstate phosphors. However, the light production efficiency of rare earth phosphors is 15–18%, whereas for tungstate phosphors this efficiency is only 3.5% (Stevels 1975). The rare earth phosphor can in principle have a higher sensitivity, but in practice, mammographic systems are noise-limited and sensitivity has to be sacrificed to reduce quantum mottle, and the differences in speed between different mammographic screen-film systems can be small.

Film sensitivity. The spectrum of the light-fluorescent photons emitted by the screen depends upon the phosphor used. The light emitted by the gadolinium oxysulphide phosphor is predominantly green whereas that from calcium tungstate is blue (Stevels 1975). For maximum sensitivity the spectral response of the film should be matched to the light emitted by the screen and an orthochromatic film should be used with the rare earth phosphor. It is necessary to use a special safelight for green sensitive emulsions.

Dose. Table 2.1 gives typical values for the mean glandular breast dose and entrance air kerma for breasts imaged using a mammographic screen-film receptor for a range of conditions. The variation of incident air kerma with breast thickness is greater than that of the mean glandular dose. This is because the change in exposure with change in thickness is partially compensated by the change in the mass of the breast itself.

Choice of screen-film combination. There are many mammographic screen-film combinations available commercially, and new combinations are continually introduced as manufacturing techniques are refined. The choice of the optimum system is both subjective and difficult, and may be different for different requirements (e.g. high- and low-contrast resolution). Comparisons based on tests using phantoms (e.g. Law & Kirkpatrick 1990, Kimme-Smith et al

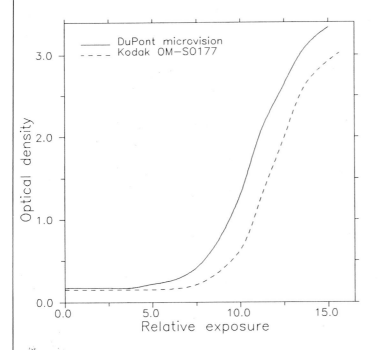

Fig. 2.7   Film characteristics for Dupont microvision and Kodak OM-SO-177 film when developed at 35°C for 3 min. The characteristics are based on Kimme-Smith et al (1990) and were measured using a sensitometer emitting green light.

1990) provide useful guidance, but these must always be supplemented with tests based on clinical images.

Xerox receptors

Xeroradiography is a dry non-silver photographic process which can enhance fine detail but shows poor large area contrast. It has the special advantage of producing an edge-enhanced image with good visualization of small differences in local contrast (Dance & Davis 1983) and a decade ago was regarded by some as the mammographic image receptor of choice. However, the Xerox receptor has a lower sensitivity than the mammographic screen-film combination and a higher associated breast dose (by a factor of three or more) even when a higher-energy spectrum is used. Furthermore, the quality of the film image has improved considerably following the introduction of the mammographic anti-scatter grid and improvement in mammographic screens and films, and Xeroradiography is now little used in the United Kingdom.

AUTOMATIC EXPOSURE CONTROL

In mammography the radiation exposure is normally controlled by a radiation detector located after the image receptor. The detector monitors the X-rays transmitted by the receptor, and the exposure is terminated when the signal recorded by the monitor reaches a predefined level. Unfortunately, the X-ray spectrum reaching the detector varies considerably with the size and composition of the breast, and the signal recorded provides only an approximate indication of the energy absorbed in the screen. Moreover, the overall sensitivity of the screen-film combination (and hence the density on the film) also depends upon exposure time because of reciprocity law failure. Accurate automatic exposure control is therefore difficult, and in early mammographic X-ray sets it was not possible to compensate automatically for these effects. Overall film density varied with breast size and composition and it was necessary to compensate by adjusting the density control when imaging larger or denser breasts. For some of the latest automatic exposure control systems, however, more than one detector is used (LaFrance et al 1986) and the density is accurately controlled.

DOSE AND RISK

It is essential that in any breast screening programme, the number of breast cancers induced is considerably exceeded by the number of cancers detected, particularly since estimates of breast cancer induction rate are model-dependent and uncertain. Fortunately, risk estimates have come down in recent years following the adoption of a relative risk model, and allowance for the variation of risk with age at exposure (National Institute of Health 1985). Using these new risk estimates, Feig & Ehrlich (1990) have

Table 2.1 Mean glandular dose values and incident air kerma (without backscatter) for breasts imaged using an X-ray spectrum from a molybdenum target filtered with 30 μm molybdenum at 28 kV

Breast thickness (cm)	Condition	Incident air kerma (mGy)	Mean glandular dose (mGy)
3.0	Grid	2.7	0.9
4.5	Grid	5.2	1.2
7.0	Grid	15.7	2.2
4.5	No grid	2.6	0.6
4.5	×2 magnification	16.9	3.9

HVL (half value layer) with compression cone in place 0.37 mm aluminium.

Table 2.2 Losses and gains in life expectancy for multiple annual screenings of 100 000 women

Age at entry (years)	Years' screening	Risk 20%	Risk 60%	Benefit 20%	Benefit 60%	Benefit/risk 20%	Benefit/risk 60%
50	25	12.9	6.5	12 623	37 869	978	5826
55	20	6.6	3.3	10 097	30 291	1530	9179
60	15	2.8	1.4	7442	22 325	2658	15 946
65	10	2.8	0.5	4792	14 377	5324	28 754

Data taken from Feig and Ehrlich (1990).
Dose per exam 1.0 mGy.

calculated the gains and losses in life expectancy associated with breast cancer detection and radiogenic breast cancer induction for multiple annual screenings. Table 2.2 gives an extract from their results. The two percentage columns under the heading 'Risk' assume that subsequent screenings will reduce loss due to radiogenic cancers by the percentages indicated, and give the years of life lost through radiogenic cancers. The columns under the heading 'Benefit' give the reduction in years lost due to spontaneously occurring cancers assuming these same percentages. The table demonstrates very clearly that the benefit risk ratio is substantial.

REFERENCES

Alm Carlsson G, Dance D R, Persliden J 1989 Grids in mammography: optimisation of the information content relative to radiation risk. Report ULi-RAD-R-059, University of Linkoping, Sweden, pp 1–59

Bakir Y Y, Roebuck E J, Whelpton D, Worthington B S 1984 Film-screen combinations for mammography. British Journal of Radiology 57: 653

Barnes G T 1979 Characteristics of scatter. In: Logan W W, Muntz E P (eds) Reduced dose mammography. Masson, New York, pp 223–242

Beaman S A, Lillicrap S C, Price J L 1983 Tungsten anode tubes with K-edge filters for mammography. British Journal of Radiology 56: 721–727

Birch R, Marshall M, Ardan G M 1979 Catalogue of spectral data for diagnostic X-rays. HPA, London

Chan H-P, Frank P H, Doi K, Iida N, Higashida Y 1985 Ultra high strip density grids: a new antiscatter technique for mammography. Radiology 154: 807–815

Dance D R 1980 The Monte Carlo calculation of integral radiation dose in xeromammography. Physics in Medicine and Biology 25: 25–37

Dance D R 1990 An introduction to the physics of mammography. In: Physics in Diagnostic Radiology, IPSM report 61. Institute of Physical Sciences in Medicine, York, pp 1–11

Dance D R, Davis R 1983 The physics of mammography. In: Parsons C A (ed), Diagnosis of breast disease. Chapman & Hall, London, pp 76–100

Dance D R, Day G 1981 Simulation of mammography by Monte Carlo calculation—the dependence of radiation dose, scatter and noise on photon energy. In: Drexler G, Eriskat H, Schibilla H (eds) Patient exposure to radiation in medical X-ray diagnosis. EUR7438, CEC, Brussels, pp 227–243

Dance D R, Day G J 1984 The computation of scatter in mammography by Monte Carlo methods. Physics in Medicine and Biology 29: 237–247

Department of Health 1990 Revised guidance notes for health authorities on mammographic X-ray equipment requirements for breast screening, Report STD/90/46. Department of Health, 14 Russell Square, London

Department of Health and Social Security 1987 Guidance notes for health authorities on mammographic equipment requirements for breast screening, Report STD/87/34. DHSS, 14 Russell Square, London

Feig S A, Ehrlich S M 1990 Estimation of radiation risk from screening mammography: recent trends and comparison with expected benefits. Radiology 174: 638–647

Hammerstein G R, Miller D W, White D R, Masterson M E, Woodard H Q, Laughlin J S 1979 Absorbed radiation dose in mammography. Radiology 130: 485–491

Institute of Physical Sciences in Medicine 1989 The commissioning and routine testing of mammographic X-ray systems, IPSM Report 59. Institute of Physical Sciences in Medicine, York

International Commission on Radiological Protection 1987 Statement from the 1987 Como meeting of the ICRP. Annals of the ICRP 17: No. 4, ICRP Publication 52. Pergamon Press, Oxford

Jennings R J, Fewell T R 1979 Filters-photon energy control and patient exposure. In: Logan W W, Munz E P (eds) Reduced dose mammography. Masson, New York, pp 212–222

Johns P C, Yaffe M 1987 X-ray characterisation of normal and neoplastic breast tissues. Physics in Medicine and Biology 32: 675–695

Kimme-Smith C, Bassett L W, Gold R H, Roe D, Orr J 1987 Mammographic dual-screen–dual-emulsion film combination: visibility of simulated microcalcifications and effect on image contrast. Radiology 165: 313–318

Kimme-Smith C, Bassett L W, Gold R H, Zheutlin J, Gornbein J A 1990 New mammography screen-film combinations: imaging characteristics and radiation dose. American Journal of Roentgenology 154: 713–79

LaFrance R, Gelskey D E, Barnes G T 1986 A circuit modification which improves mammographic phototimer performance. Paper presented at the 72nd Scientific Assembly of the Radiological Society of North America

Law J, Kirkpatrick A E 1990 Further comparisons of films, screens and cassettes for mammography. British Journal of Radiology 63: 128–131

Millis R R, Davis R, Stacey A J 1976 The detection and significance of calcifications in the breast. A radiological and pathological study. British Journal of Radiology 49: 12–26

National Commission on Radiation Protection and Measurements 1986 Mammography—a user's guide, Report 85. NCRP Publications, Bethesda, Maryland

National Institute of Health Ad Hoc Working Group to develop radio-epidemiological tables. NIH Publication 85-2748. NIH, Bethesda, Maryland

National Radiological Protection Board, Health and Safety Executive and Health Departments 1988 Guidance notes for the protection of persons against ionising radiation arising from medical and dental use. HMSO, London, p 17

Sabel M, Willegroth F, Aichinger H, Dierken J 1986 X-ray spectra and image quality in mammography. Electromedica 54: 158–165

Stevels A L N 1975 New phosphors for X-ray screens. Medicamundi 20: 12–22

CHAPTER 3

Mammography positioning technique

Maureen Yeowell

INTRODUCTION

Mammography has been proved to be the single most important breast imaging technique, both for symptomatic and asymptomatic women. In screening asymptomatic women, the purpose is to detect abnormalities that require further evaluation, while symptomatic women with a known palpable lump or a suspicious area of the breast require diagnostic problem solving mammography.

The radiographer's attitude towards the patient should be carefully considered. It should be professional, pleasant, sympathetic and the manner projected should be friendly and reassuring throughout the mammography examination. The patient might be embarrassed, or display various other emotional reactions, such as fear, anger awkwardness or an inability to follow any instructions given. These patients present the radiographer with the greatest challenge to a professional attitude. Thoughtful handling is important to enable the patient to relax and cooperate during the examination.

It must be emphasized that mammography has to be adapted to the individual needs of the patient, though in the context of primary breast screening one should perhaps be thinking of women rather than patients. There is no absolute standard technique and adaptation is necessary for different equipment. The height of the radiographer and the length of her arms will need to be considered in the way the technique is performed. With practice, a perfect technique can be obtained despite difficulties. As many as possible of the variations have been covered in this chapter, but given sufficient enthusiasm others may well be invented.

Quality assurance is essential for all aspects of mammography:— equipment; image recording systems; processing; radiographic and radiological skills must be considered. Mammography is very dependent on correct technique and radiographers should be trained to the highest standards to enable excellent images with maximum diagnostic information, optimal detail and contrast, to be consistently produced. Even with good technique 5–10% of breast cancers are not detected by mammography. The density of the cancer may be less than glandular tissue and very small tumours may be difficult to detect in a nodular breast.

Inferior quality and poor positioning technique will limit the interpretation skills of the radiologist. Technical errors should not be accepted or ignored by either radiographer or radiologist. Identification letters should be placed in the axillary region, well away from the breast. They should be correctly orientated to avoid confusion between the oblique and extended craniocaudal views.

COMPRESSION

Compression of the breast is necessary to avoid the thick part of the breast near the chest wall being under-exposed and the thin part near the nipple being over-exposed. Overlapping structures are separated and lesions are brought nearer to the film, improving detail. Reduction of movement, radiation dose and shorter exposure times result from firm compression.

The necessity for compression must be explained to the patient. Symptomatic women generally accept compression without complaint in order to obtain an accurate diagnosis, but asymptomatic women fear that compression may be harmful to the breast. The women may not return for screening if the procedure is found to be unacceptably painful.

The patient should be informed of the procedure, the coldness of the film support, and it should be stressed that the examination may be uncomfortable, but should not be painful. The patient must be asked to say if the compression is unacceptable. The breasts are more likely to be painful and swollen prior to a menstrual period, and toleration of firm compression at this time will be less. Compression is checked by squeezing the sides of the breast between the fingers and thumb. If the breast is firm, then it is sufficient.

POSITIONING TECHNIQUE

When the compression plate is applied, some of the posterior portion of the breast is omitted from each view (Fig. 3.1). The hemispherical-shaped breast curves around the chest wall extending from the lateral margin of the sternum to the axilla, and overlies the pectoral muscle. Although the oblique view should demonstrate the whole of the glandular tissue, the geometry between the breast, the shape of the thoracic wall and the straight edge of the film support may make it difficult to project all the breast tissue in one view. It may therefore be necessary to take two or more views. Any lesion seen must be demonstrated in at least two views. Magnification of the usual mammographic views may be required to evaluate specific areas within the breast.

The breast tissue should always cover the automatic exposure chamber, and with some mammographic equipment, it may be necessary to alter the position of the chamber according to the size of the breast. The views described are:

a. Mediolateral oblique
b. Craniocaudal (medial and lateral rotation)
c. Extended craniocaudal (lateral extension)
d. Extended craniocaudal (medial extension)
e. Axillary view
f. Lateral (mediolateral, lateromedial)
g. Specialized views
h. Spot compression
i. Magnification.

Evaluation criteria are listed, and pitfalls and their prevention are discussed for each view described.

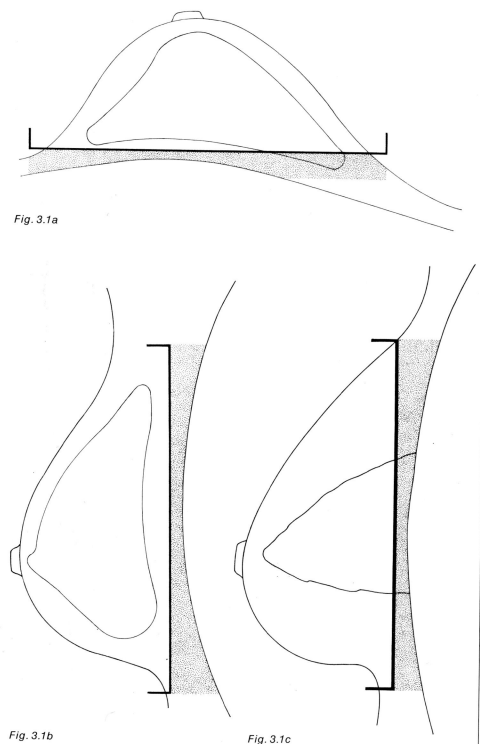

Fig. 3.1a

Fig. 3.1b

Fig. 3.1c

Fig. 3.1   Shaded areas represent the posterior area omitted in each view when compression is applied. *a* Craniocaudal view; *b* oblique view; *c* lateral view.

Fig. 3.2 Lateral-oblique view. 1 Identification and date, 2 anatomical letter in axillary region, 3 whole breast imaged, 4 skin pores demonstrating adequate compression, 5 nipple in profile, 6 pectoral muscle level with nipple and at correct angle, 7 inframammary fold.

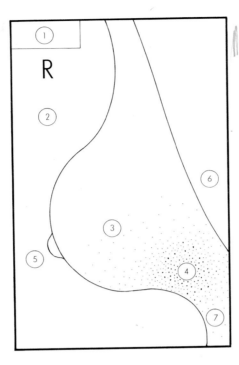

EVALUATION CRITERIA

Oblique view (Fig. 3.2)

1. Identification and date

2. Anatomical letter in axillary region

3. Whole breast imaged

4. Skin pores demonstrating adequate compression

5. Nipple in profile

6. Pectoral muscle level with nipple and at correct angle

7. Inframammary fold

8. Correct exposure

9. Correct processing

10. Absence of axillary and other skin folds

11. Absence of movement

12. Absence of processing and handling artefacts.

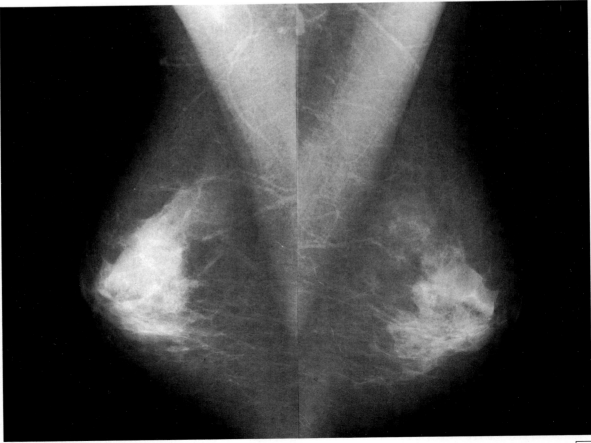

L   R

Fig. 3.4 Oblique views.

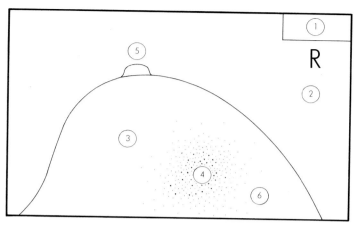

Fig. 3.3 Craniocaudal view. 1 Identification and date, 2 anatomical letter in axillary region, 3 whole breast imaged, demonstrating retromammary space, 4 skin pores demonstrating adequate compression, 5 nipple in profile.

Craniocaudal view (Fig. 3.3)
1. Identification and date
2. Anatomical letter in axillary region
3. Whole breast imaged demonstrating retromammary space
4. Skin pores demonstrating adequate compression
5. Nipple in profile
6. Correct exposure
7. Correct processing
8. Absence of skin folds
9. Absence of movement
10. Absence of processing and handling artefacts.

When the films are viewed together they should be a mirror image of each other (Figs 3.4 and 3.5).

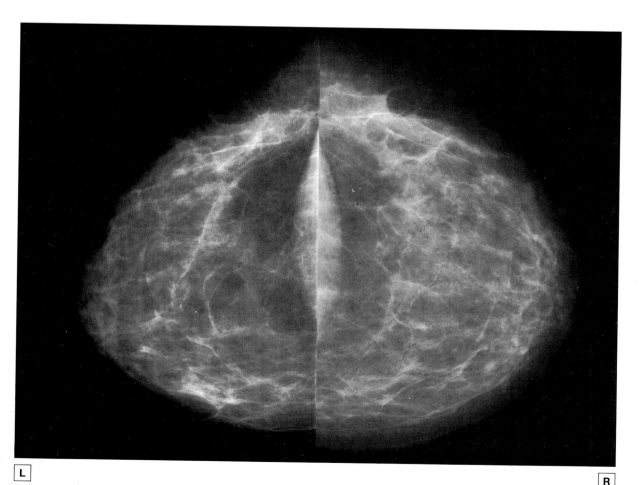

Fig. 3.5 Craniocaudal views.

MEDIOLATERAL OBLIQUE VIEW

The Forrest Report (Department of Health and Social Security 1986) recommends the mediolateral oblique view for screening, as this single view demonstrates the maximum amount of breast tissue. The axillary tail, pectoral muscle and inferior portion of the breast are visualized. The breast should be parallel to the pectoral muscle, so that compression will displace the breast forward onto the film. Most abnormalities are found in the upper outer quadrant and this view clearly demonstrates the area.

The machine is usually angled at 45°, but to demonstrate the maximum amount of breast tissue and pectoral muscle the angle may need to be varied with the individual from 35° to 60°. The smaller the breast the steeper the angle required. The patient stands facing the machine angled at 45° with the breast to be examined in front of the film support. The arm is placed along the top of the film support with the flexed elbow resting behind it. The height of the machine is then adjusted so that the maximum amount of breast tissue is included. The radiographer should stand at the patient's opposite shoulder, and one hand is then placed against the ribs to slide the breast forward. The breast is held with the palm of the hand on the lateral aspect and the thumb on the medial aspect (Fig. 3.6). The patient is leaned forward and the breast extended upwards and outwards. At the same time, using the other hand, the patient's arm is raised to lift and extend the shoulder so that the corner of the film support is in the posterior part of the axilla (Fig. 3.7). The hand supporting the breast is rotated to cup it in the palm, holding the upward and outward position (Fig. 3.8). The posterior axillary skin fold and other skin folds are removed at this stage with the other hand. The opposite side of the body is rotated away very slightly to avoid hurting the ribs and sternum as the compression is applied.

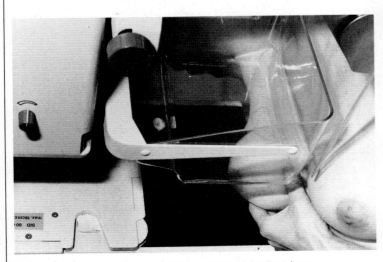

Fig. 3.6   The breast is held with the palm of the hand on the lateral aspect and the thumb on the medial aspect.

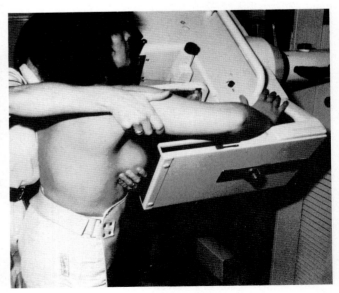

Fig. 3.7   The patient's arm is raised to lift and extend the shoulder, while the breast is held in the other hand.

When the compression plate touches the breast, the body is rotated inwards again to demonstrate the maximum amount of posterior breast tissue. The hand is removed when compression is almost complete, and to avoid the breast dropping, the breast can be gently nudged up using the finger and knuckle area (Fig. 3.9).

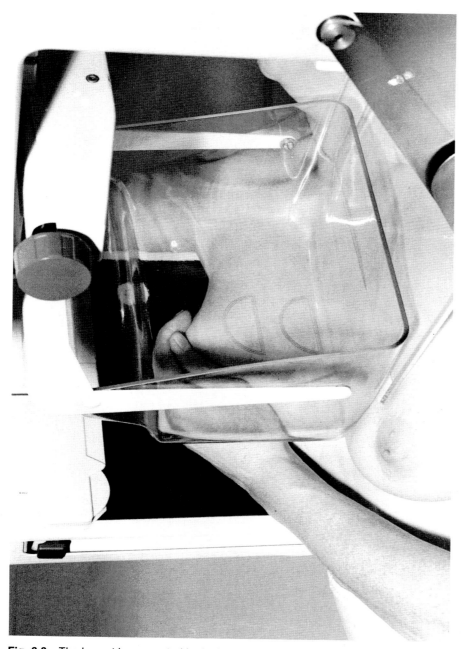

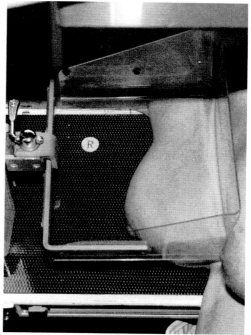

Fig. 3.8 The breast is supported in the hand and the upward and outward position maintained.

Fig. 3.9 The axilla, axillary tail, maximum breast tissue and inframammary angle are imaged. Reproduced with permission from POSTRAD (Lancaster).

A good-quality image is obtained when the axilla, axillary tail, breast tissue and pectoral muscle at the correct angle, level with the nipple are demonstrated. The nipple should be approximately one-third of the way up the film. When films are viewed as a mirror image, the pectoral muscle should meet forming a deep 'V' with the breasts matching at the inferior border (Fig. 3.10).

Pitfalls and prevention

Inaccurate exposure. This is prevented by ensuring the glandular tissue is centralized over the automatic exposure chamber.

Insufficient breast demonstrated. The height of the film support must be correct and the breast must not be released before adequate compression is applied to hold the position, preventing loss of the axillary area or the inferior border. The patient must stand well in front of the film support with the feet and hips in line with the rest of the body facing the machine, and the radiographer's hand must slide forward from the rib cage to bring the maximum amount of breast onto the film. The shoulder and arm must be extended over and the patient encouraged to relax and lean in towards the machine to fully demonstrate the pectoral muscle.

Nipple not in profile. To prevent this happening with 'normal'-type breasts, the patient must not stand too far in front of the film support otherwise the nipple will rotate under the bulk of the breast. The nipple will lie above the bulk of the breast if the patient stands too close or behind the film support.

Inadequate compression. This is often due to the compression being applied to the whole of the axillary

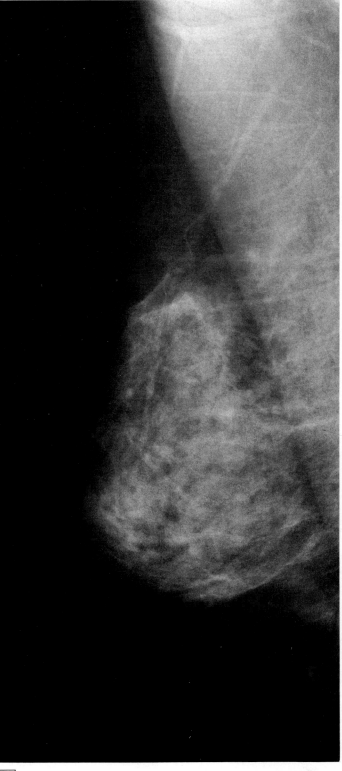

R

Fig. 3.10   Lateral-oblique view.

area, immediately below the head of the humerus, and including the posterior skin folds. It can be prevented when the top edge of the cassette is placed so that it lies no less than 1 cm below the head of the humerus and the posterior skin fold removed before compression is applied. The breast must be checked for firmness, or it will drop, poor detail will be obtained and the skin pores will not be well demonstrated.

Skin folds. Skin folds are prevented from being trapped between the film support and lateral aspect of the breast by removing them gently while the breast is supported and maintained in position before full compression. The inframammary fold should not be visualized through overlapping breast tissue. This is prevented by ensuring the patient is not standing too close to the film support and by lifting the breast up.

CRANIOCAUDAL VIEW

In the craniocaudal view abnormalities demonstrated are seen medial or lateral to the nipple. The medial aspect of the breast is sometimes not completely demonstrated in the oblique view and it may be preferred to emphasize this area in the craniocaudal view by rotating the breast towards the lateral aspect. The lateral aspect of the glandular tissue, where much of the pathology occurs, is more clearly demonstrated by rotating the breast medially. The technique described allows the maximum amount of glandular tissue to be included with very little loss of the medial aspect of the breast.

The patient faces the mammography machine with the tube parallel to the floor, and the body is rotated 15–20° so that the side to be examined is brought close to the film support with the arm resting on the abdomen or side of the machine to relax the pectoral muscle (Fig. 3.11). The patient's head is turned parallel to the tube and away from the side under examination. The breast is lifted up to form a right angle with the body and the machine is then raised to make contact with the breast at the junction of the inframammary angle and chest wall (Fig. 3.12). The hand is gently removed, leaving the nipple in profile in the midline of the breast tissue. The shoulder is gently pressed down so that the outer quadrant of the breast is brought into contact with the film support. The breast is held at the sides between the fingers and thumb, with

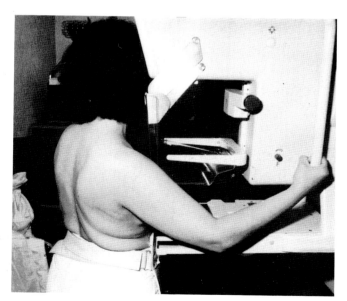

Fig. 3.11 The patient is rotated 15–20° so that the side to be examined is brought close to the film support.

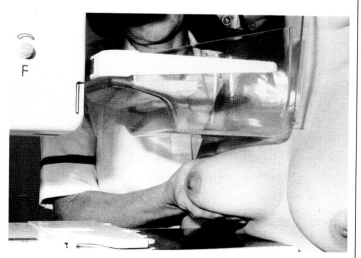

Fig. 3.12 The breast is lifted to form a right angle with the body.

the index and middle finger on top, and is then gently stretched across the film support (Fig. 3.13). The patient is gently pushed in towards the machine using the other hand on her back.

Compression is applied slowly, and when the plate makes contact with the breast at the chest wall margin the fingers are gradually brought forward towards the nipple and removed when

compression is almost complete. The patient is then gently rotated in, so that the medial aspect is fully included. Any skin folds at the lateral aspect can be removed after compression by being gently eased out. The patient presses the other breast in against her body, away from the direction of the beam, with her hand to avoid inclusion on the film (Fig. 3.14).

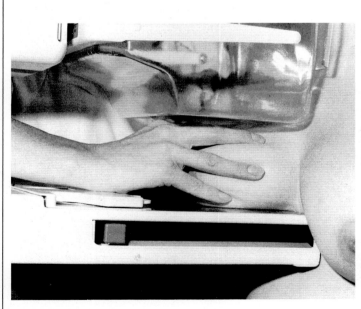

Fig. 3.13 The breast is held at the sides between the fingers and thumb, with the index and middle finger on top.

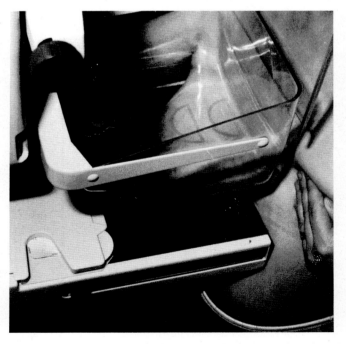

Fig. 3.14 The patient presses the other breast in against her body to avoid inclusion on the film.

A good-quality image is obtained when the nipple is shown towards the 11 o'clock position for the right breast or the 1 o'clock position for the left breast, allowing the maximum amount of glandular tissue to be demonstrated (Fig. 3.15).

Pitfalls and their prevention

Inaccurate exposure. Usually prevented by ensuring the breast is centralized over the chamber of the automatic exposure control.

Insufficient breast demonstrated. Overextending the breast laterally prevents the medial posterior portion of the breast being demonstrated, and insufficient lateral extension results in cut-off of the glandular tissue. If the breast is not stretched forward enough, and the patient not leaned inwards, the posterior breast tissue will be prevented from being demonstrated.

Nipple not in profile. This can generally be prevented by ensuring the film support is at the correct height. If it is too high, the nipple lies above the midline of the breast and the posterior inferior portion will not be demonstrated. If the film support is too low, the nipple will lie below the midline and the superior posterior portion of the breast will not be demonstrated.

Inadequate compression. Underpenetration and lack of detail is produced with inadequate compression. The firmness of the breast should be checked by hand.

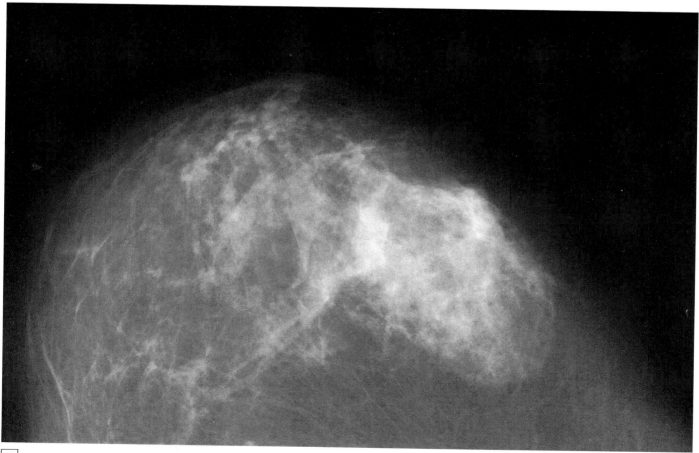

R

Fig. 3.15 Craniocaudal view.

EXTENDED CRANIOCAUDAL (LATERAL EXTENSION)

Lesions in the upper outer quadrant of the breast on the lateral oblique view are not always demonstrated on the routine craniocaudal, but the extended craniocaudal view will show the outer quadrant and axillary tail. The procedure requires the patient to lean backwards about 35–45°. Another technique with the film support angled approximately 5° down medially will often provide sufficient information. The patient faces the machine and is then rotated 45° so that the breast to be examined is positioned at the correct height with the nipple in profile and level with the medial edge of the film support (Fig. 3.16). The patient's arm is placed along the side of the support and holds the machine. Standing behind the patient, the breast is lifted up and extended over the film to demonstrate as much tissue as possible (Fig. 3.17). The patient leans back approximately 35–45° with the shoulder depressed to enable the outer quadrant and axilla to make contact with the film support. The patient's other hand holds the machine to maintain balance. (Fig. 3.18). The arm is further extended and with the radiographer gently pushing her back, the patient leans in, allowing the breast to rotate in to demonstrate the posterior margin of the breast. The breast is held, with the nipple in profile, until compression is almost

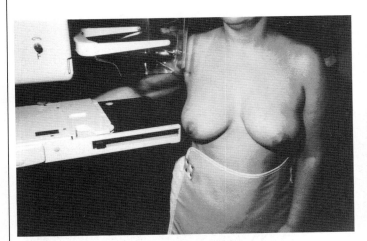

Fig. 3.16 The patient is rotated 45° to the machine.

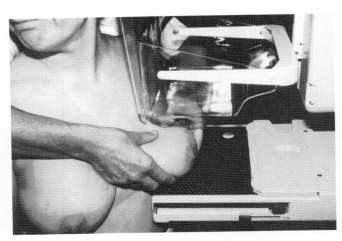

Fig. 3.17 Standing behind the patient, the breast is lifted up and extended across the film.

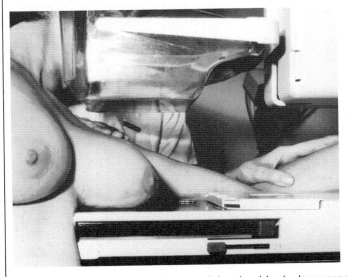

Fig. 3.18 The patient leans back and the shoulder is depressed.

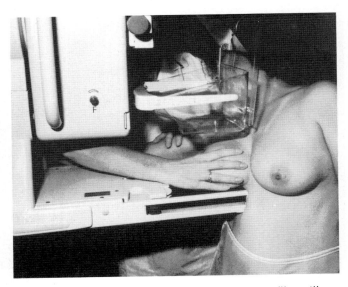

Fig. 3.19 The breast is held with the nipple in profile until compression is almost complete.

complete, fitting into the angle created by the head of the humerus and rib cage (Fig. 3.19). The axilla and outer quadrant are demonstrated, although not all the medial aspect is seen (Fig. 3.20).

A good-quality image is obtained when the axilla, axillary tail, pectoral muscle and maximum amount of breast tissue are demonstrated (Fig. 3.21).

Pitfalls and prevention

Inaccurate exposure. The main area of glandular tissue should be positioned over the automatic exposure chamber to prevent underpenetration.

Insufficient breast demonstrated. Prevention of loss of breast tissue, axillary tail and axilla is achieved by ensuring that the nipple is at the medial edge of the film support before the patient leans backwards. Care must be taken not to overextend the view, thus rotating the lesion off the film.

Nipple not in profile. The height of the film support must be at the level of the inframammary crease. The patient must lean inwards, allowing the breast to rotate onto the film support; this will ensure that the nipple will be in profile.

Inadequate compression. This is prevented by checking the firmness of the breast and by ensuring that the compression plate is not obstructed by the head of the humerus.

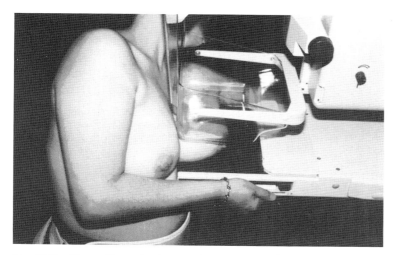

Fig. 3.20 The axilla and outer quadrant are demonstrated.

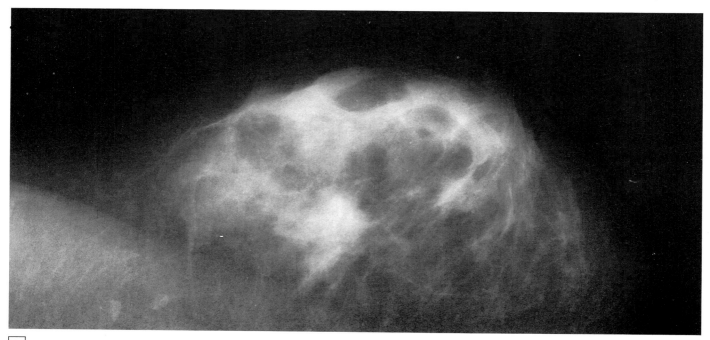

L

Fig. 3.21 Extended craniocaudal view (lateral extension).

EXTENDED CRANIOCAUDAL VIEW (MEDIAL EXTENSION)

Lesions in the medial portion of the breast can be viewed with the breast rotated so that more of the medioposterior portion is projected on to the film. It will sometimes be necessary, and particularly for small breasts, to use manual exposure to avoid a flash exposure.

The patient faces the machine with the sternum approximately 8–9 cm from the medial edge of the unaffected breast. Both breasts are lifted up to allow the film support to fit in the inframammary angle (Fig. 3.22). The patient is lightly pushed in towards the machine and the affected breast is gently stretched in and rotated laterally while compression is applied, enabling the medial aspect of the breast to be visualized (Fig. 3.23). The medial aspects of both breasts are seen. (Fig. 3.24).

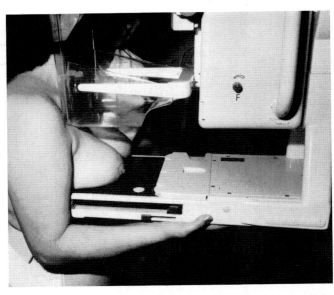

Fig. 3.22   Both breasts are placed on the film support with the sternum approximately 8–9 cm from the medial edge of the unaffected breast.

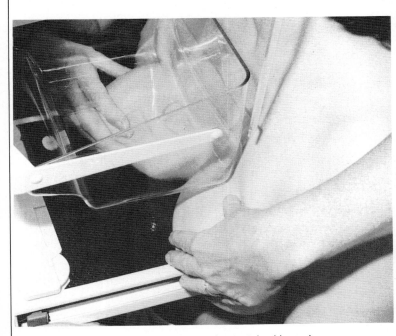

Fig. 3.23   The affected breast is gently stretched in and rotated laterally.

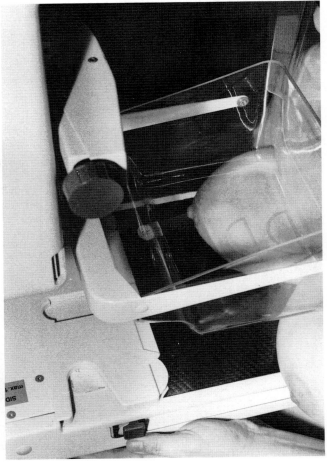

Fig. 3.24   The medial aspects of both breasts are seen.

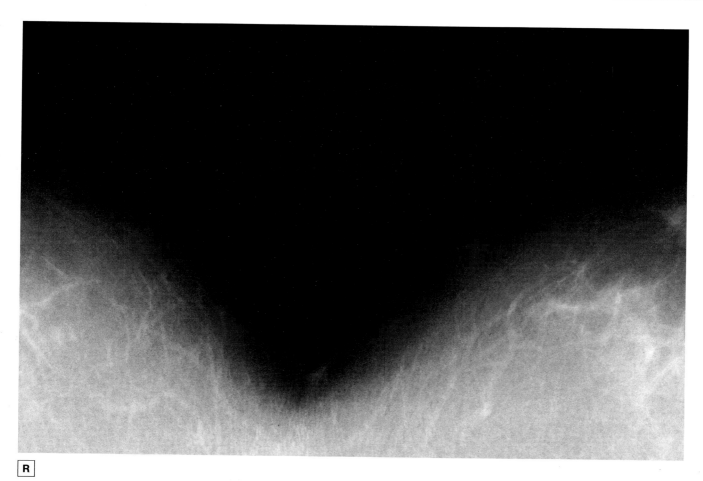

R

Fig. 3.25   Extended craniocaudal view (medial extension).

A good-quality image is obtained when the maximum amount of the medioposterior part of the breast is visualized and also some of the medial aspect of the other breast (Fig. 3.25).

Pitfalls and prevention

Inaccurate exposure. Underpenetration is prevented by accurately positioning the breast over the automatic exposure chamber. When manual exposure is selected, note the mAs obtained from the craniocaudal view and use the same factors.

Insufficient breast demonstrated. To prevent loss of the inner quadrant of the breast, the patient must be leaned inwards and the medial portion extended towards the lateral aspect.

Nipple not in profile. The film support must be level with the inframammary angle and the breast lifted up and extended to prevent the nipple not being in profile.

Inadequate compression. This is prevented by checking the firmness of the breast.

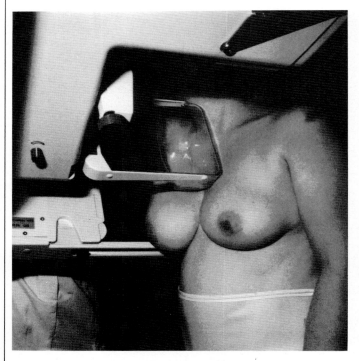

Fig. 3.26 The shoulder is positioned in front of the cassette to demonstrate the axillary area.

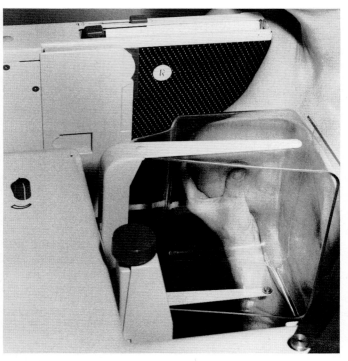

Fig. 3.27 The breast is held with the palm of the hand on the lateral aspect and the thumb on the medial aspect.

AXILLARY VIEW

The axillary tail of the breast and some of the axilla are seen on the mediolateral oblique view. However, in some cases an additional view of the upper axilla may be required, e.g. postmastectomy patient.

A localized axilla compression plate is used for preference. The machine is rotated into the lateral oblique position. The shoulder is positioned in front of the cassette with the soft tissue covering the automatic exposure chamber. Firm compression cannot be applied, but the soft tissue of the entire axillary area is visualized (Fig. 3.26).

LATERAL VIEW

The breast is examined from either the lateromedial or mediolateral direction at 90° to the craniocaudal view. The lateral view often clarifies areas of suspicion, asymmetrical densities, and is essential for localization of an impalpable lesion which is shown superior or inferior to the nipple on the oblique view.

It is generally accepted that more breast tissue is shown in the mediolateral view, and most of the pathology occurs in the outer half of the breast which makes this the preferred view for routine procedures.

Accurate assessment of lesions is obtained with reduced geometric unsharpness and improved detail, when the lesion is brought close to the film. The position of the lesion seen in

the craniocaudal view should be carefully studied to decide which of the two lateral views should be taken.

Mediolateral

The machine is rotated so that the tube and film support are vertical. The patient stands facing the tube column, with the film support against the lateral aspect of the breast and the corner placed in the posterior part of the axilla. The arm is placed behind the film support, holding the machine to maintain position. The height is adjusted to include the inferior portion of the breast. The radiographer's hand is placed against the side of the rib cage and slides forward to hold the breast with the palm of the hand on the lateral aspect and the thumb on the medial aspect (Fig. 3.27). The hand is rotated to cup the breast in the palm of the hand and the breast is lifted upwards and

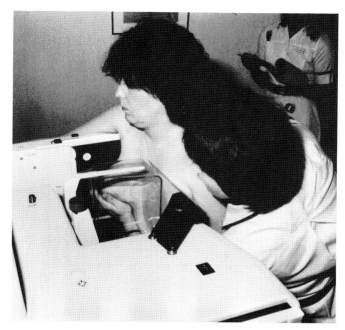

Fig. 3.28 The breast is lifted upwards and extended outwards.

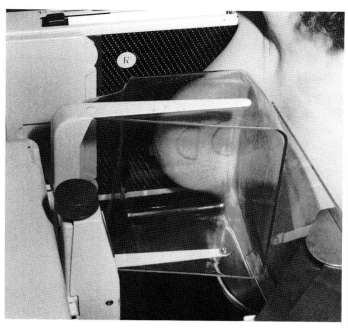

Fig. 3.29 Compression is made with the nipple in profile and the inframammary angle visualized.

extended outwards, ensuring that the nipple is in profile (Fig. 3.28). The patient is gently pushed inwards at the same time with the other hand. The opposite shoulder is carefully rotated back to allow the compression plate to be brought in contact with the breast, then pushed forward. The hand still holds the breast, and any trapped skin folds are removed with the other hand. The breast is supported with the knuckle area of the hand and removed to complete compression (Fig. 3.29).

A good-quality image is obtained when the nipple is in profile, and when the maximum amount of breast tissue including some pectoral muscle, the inferior border of the breast and inframammary skin fold are visualized (Fig. 3.30).

Pitfalls and prevention

Inaccurate exposure. This is prevented by ensuring the breast tissue is positioned over the automatic exposure chamber.

Insufficient breast demonstrated. The hand slides the breast forward from the rib cage to gain full demonstration of the breast tissue.

Nipple not in profile. This is prevented by ensuring that the patient is not standing too far in front of the film support, when the nipple will be under the midline of the breast, or too far behind, which will result in the nipple lying above the midline of the breast.

Skin folds. Trapped skin between the lateral aspect of the breast and film support must be gently removed to prevent folds overlying and obscuring breast tissue, prior to full compression.

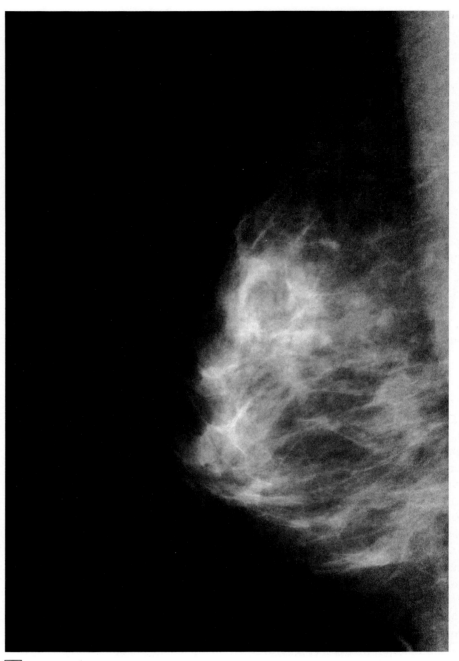

R

Fig. 3.30 Mediolateral view.

LATEROMEDIAL VIEW

The patient faces the machine with the edge of the film support in contact with the sternum. The arm of the affected side is raised to rest over the machine, and the body rotated in to allow the breast to make contact with the film support. The breast, with the nipple in profile, is supported in the palm of the hand with the thumb on the lateral aspect, and then extended upwards and outwards as compression is applied (Fig. 3.31). The fingers are removed to nudge the breast up for final compression (Fig. 3.32).

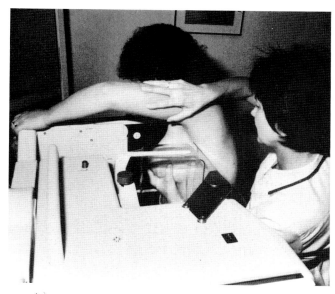

Fig. 3.31 The breast is held up and the arm raised.

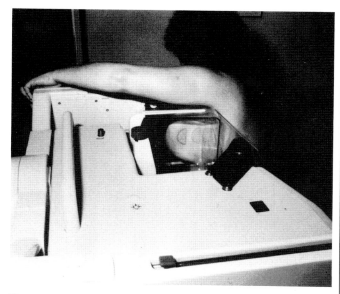

Fig. 3.32 Compression completed.

A good-quality image is obtained when the maximum amount of breast, the inferior border, some pectoral muscle and the inframammary skin fold are included (Fig. 3.33). To demonstrate a lesion in the upper quadrants of the breast, the arm must be placed in front of the film support for the mediolateral or lateromedial view.

Pitfalls and prevention

Insufficient breast demonstrated. To prevent this, the patient must be gently pushed in towards the film as much as possible.

Nipple not in profile. The body is rotated into an oblique position if the arm is pulled over too much, causing the nipple to lie under the midline of the breast.

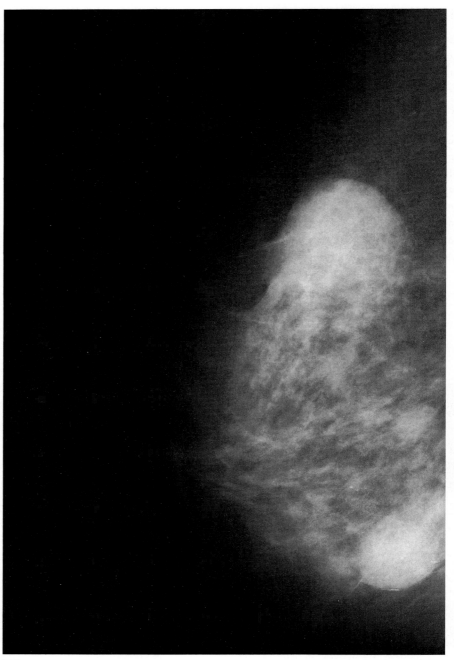

L

Fig. 3.33 Lateromedial view.

PROBLEMS AND SOLUTIONS

LARGE BREASTS

Large breasts should be examined using 24 × 30 cm film whenever possible to limit the radiation dose, the number of exposures, and to reduce the time in performing the procedure. If this is not available, it is necessary to take several films to cover the entire breast.

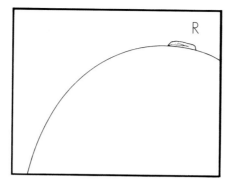
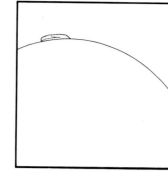

Fig. 3.34 Craniocaudal view.

Craniocaudal view

The breast is rotated medially to demonstrate the lateral portion, and then rotated laterally to demonstrate the medial portion. In both these views the nipple area may be demonstrated at the extreme edge of the film. Failure to demonstrate the nipple area adequately will necessitate a view specifically for the nipple area only (Fig. 3.34).

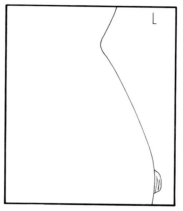
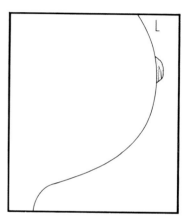

Fig. 3.35 Oblique view.

Mediolateral oblique view

The axillary area and upper quadrant of the breast is demonstrated by allowing the breast to rest naturally or with a little upward lift. The nipple should be included at the lower border of the film if possible. The breast is then lifted upwards and outwards to demonstrate the inferior portion of the breast, with the nipple at the upper border of the film. These two views will generally allow sufficient overlap of the breast tissue to demonstrate the entire breast. A specific view of the nipple area should be taken if not fully visualized (Fig. 3.35).

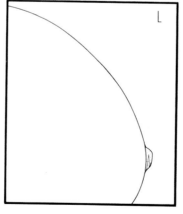
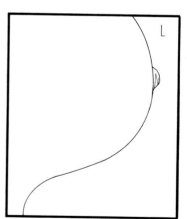

Fig. 3.36 Lateral view.

Lateral view

The breast is examined in a similar way to the mediolateral oblique view (Fig. 3.36).

SMALL BREASTS

Small breasts can be difficult to position. It is important that the patient relaxes as much as possible to demonstrate the maximum amount of tissue. It may be necessary to take the arm completely in front of the film support to include the posterior skin folds in order to fully visualize the breast tissue. In the oblique view, poor compression is avoided by ensuring that the compression plate is not too near the head of the humerus.

Underpenetration is avoided in all views by ensuring the automatic exposure chamber is covered with breast tissue. A manual exposure must be used if this is not possible.

MALE BREASTS

These are often no more difficult to demonstrate than the small female breast. In all views the breast must be carefully positioned over the automatic exposure chamber. The pectoral muscle is usually well demonstrated in the mediolateral oblique view (Fig. 3.37).

DIFFICULT-TO-IMAGE PATIENTS

In some circumstances the ideal position is not achieved, and it may be necessary to modify the usual views. A nipple might not be projected in profile when there is an associated mass, surgery, or unusually sited nipples. A view of the nipple area only should be taken if this happens. Patients with a depressed sternum or pronounced ribs should have a lateromedial view, a lateromedial oblique and a craniocaudal view.

IMPLANTS

Two or more views may be necessary to demonstrate the breast tissue surrounding implants. Manual exposures must be selected to avoid overpenetration. It may be advisable to do a trial exposure. It should also be remembered that films with implants must be viewed obscuring the light transmitted through the implant. The usual oblique and craniocaudal views are taken. A lateral view demonstrates the posterior portion of a firmly encapsulated breast. For these views firm contact is made, but firm compression is *not* applied. It is possible to obtain more breast tissue

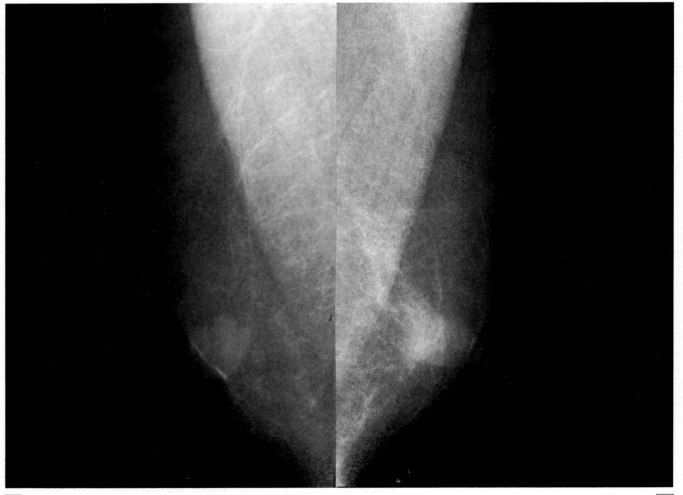

L   R

Fig. 3.37   Male breasts—oblique views.

and improved image detail by modifying the usual views (Eklund 1989). The breast tissue is pulled over and in front of the implant and compression is carefully applied. This causes the implant to be flattened and pushed back against the chest wall, allowing the breast tissue to be visualized (Fig. 3.38).

ADDITIONAL VIEWS

Additional views should be taken to provide increased diagnostic information on routine two-view examinations when the results are inconclusive, or when a lesion is seen only in one view.

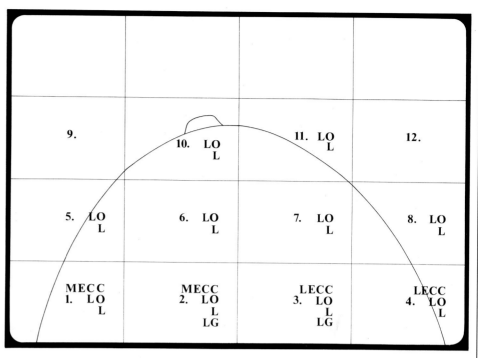

Fig. 3.39 A guide to the views which will be most likely to show pathology in different areas of the breast, as related to the oblique view. L, lateral; LO lateral-oblique; LG, lumpogram; CC, craniocaudal; LECC, lateral extension craniocaudal; MECC, medial extension craniocaudal.

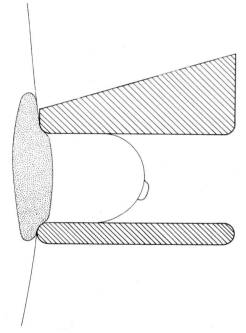

Fig. 3.38 The breast tissue is compressed in front of the implant, which is pushed back and flattened against the chest wall.

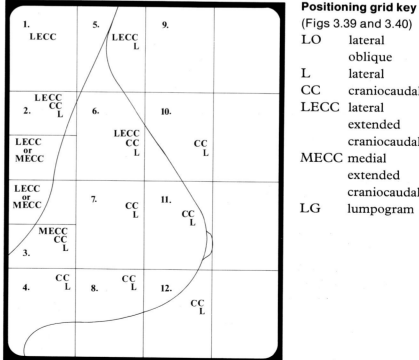

Positioning grid key
(Figs 3.39 and 3.40)

LO	lateral oblique
L	lateral
CC	craniocaudal
LECC	lateral extended craniocaudal
MECC	medial extended craniocaudal
LG	lumpogram

Fig. 3.40 A guide to the views which will be most likely to show pathology in different areas of the breast, as related to the craniocaudal view. For abbreviations see Fig. 3.39.

SPECIALIZED VIEWS

Specialized views should be taken
when necessary to provide increased
diagnostic information.

Angling

Doubtful lesions seen in the oblique or
craniocaudal view should be repeated
first, as the difference in projection
might disperse the superimposed
breast tissue to confirm or negate an
abnormality. Further evaluation may
be obtained by changing the degree of
obliquity in the mediolateral oblique
position, or by angling the machine
(Anderson 1986). The machine is
rotated 10° in one or both directions in
the craniocaudal position and the
breast compressed in the usual way
(Fig. 3.41).

Rolling

Another method of evaluating the area
is by 'rolling' the breast in the
craniocaudal position (Kopans 1989).
This separates the overlapping
structures or a suspected abnormality
into a different position on the film.
The breast is placed in the
craniocaudal position on the film
support and then rolled about the axis
of the nipple. The superior part of the
breast is rotated medially while the
inferior part is rotated laterally, and
then compression is applied. If the
lesion is seen to move medially then it
lies in the superior part of the breast,
and if laterally, then the lesion is in the
inferior part of the breast (Fig. 3.42).

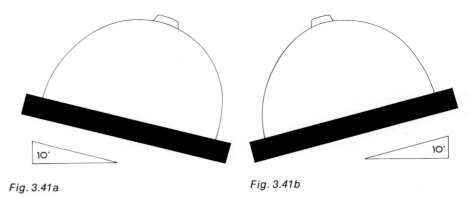

Fig. 3.41a   Fig. 3.41b

Fig. 3.41   The tube and film support are angled 10° in either direction.

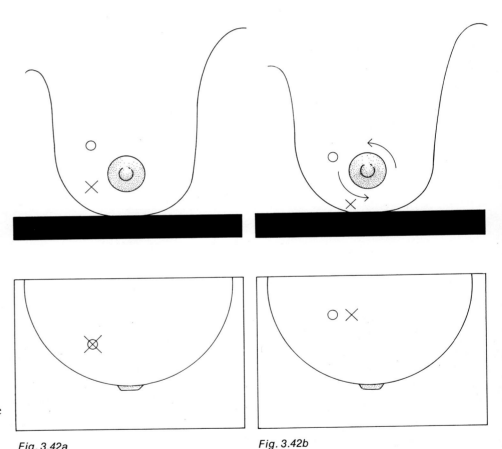

Fig. 3.42a   Fig. 3.42b

Fig. 3.42   The superior part of the breast is rotated medially while the inferior part is rotated laterally.

Tangential view

Tangential views can be used to demonstrate skin lesions, an area of dimpling, or where there is a palpable lump seen in one view only. A spot compression plate and a 'D'-shaped mask are used. The film is angled so that it is parallel to an imaginary line from the 'lump' to the nipple (Fig. 3.43).

Lumpogram

A 'lumpogram' can be performed when a lesion high against the chest wall is demonstrated on the oblique and lateral views, but not clearly on the craniocaudal view (Sickles 1988). The breast is pressed up against the film support, creating a bulge or lump of breast tissue which is then firmly compressed to demonstrate the lesion (Fig. 3.44).

Skin lesions

Skin lesions can sometimes be confused with a true lesion in the breast. A small wire marker, secured with tape around the lesion, is clearly outlined on the mammography film in any view (Fig. 3.45).

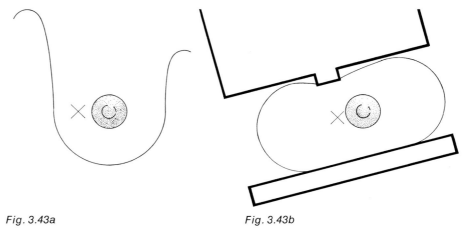

Fig. 3.43a　　　　　　　　*Fig. 3.43b*

Fig. 3.43　The film is angled so that it is parallel to an imaginary line from the 'lump' to the nipple.

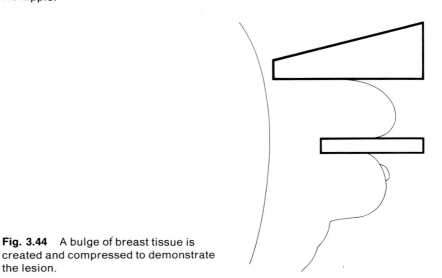

Fig. 3.44　A bulge of breast tissue is created and compressed to demonstrate the lesion.

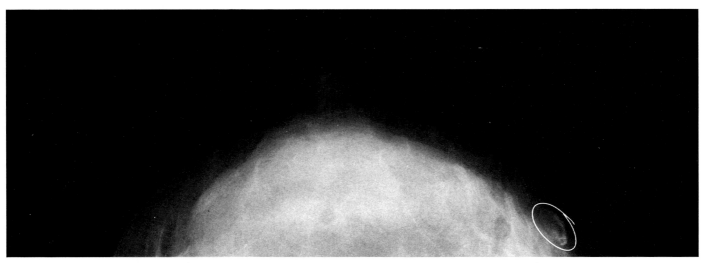

R

Fig. 3.45　Skin lesion.

Spot compression

A small compression cone and a 'D'-shaped mask is used. Scattered radiation is reduced and contrast is increased as pressure is applied to a small volume of the breast. Overlapping structures are spread out and excellent detail of abnormal areas is obtained (Fig. 3.46). This technique will produce superior quality images and should be used if magnification is unobtainable (Fig. 3.47). Less radiation is required than with magnification, which is particularly relevant for younger women.

Magnification

Magnification requires a very small focal spot size of 0.1–0.15 mm for a magnification factor of 1:1.5–1:2.

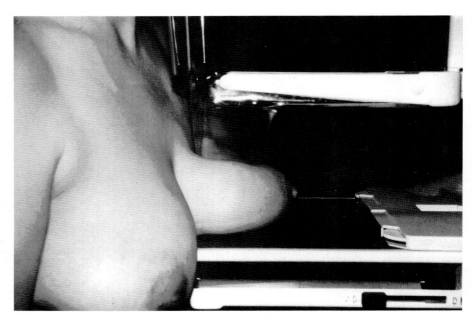

Fig. 3.46   A small compression cone is used.

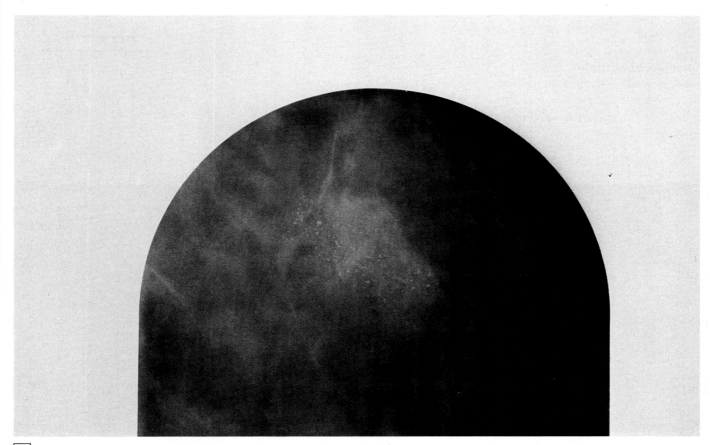

R

Fig. 3.47   Spot compression.

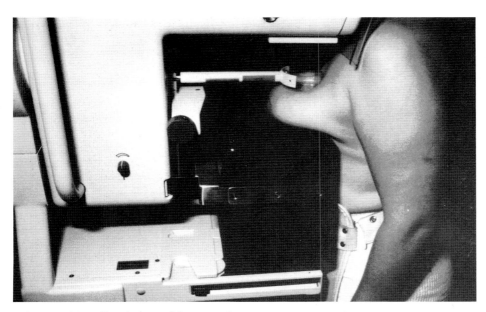

Fig. 3.48 Magnification—paddle cone view.

Increasing the distance between the breast and film produces an enlarged image with improved demonstration of the breast architecture. Reduction of scatter and improved contrast is obtained with the air-gap technique, so the grid is normally removed.

Magnification is of value to routine mammography when the original diagnosis is equivocal. It facilitates a definitive diagnosis, as more accurate diagnostic information regarding distribution, shape, structure of calcifications and masses is revealed. However, there is an increased radiation dose of 1.5–4 times that of conventional mammography, and so collimation is preferred to limit the film of radiation to a specific area (Fig.

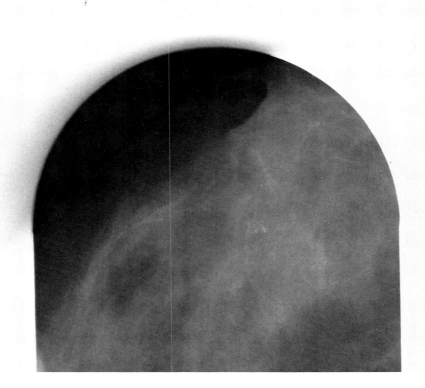

L

Fig. 3.49 Magnification is of value when original diagnosis is equivocal.

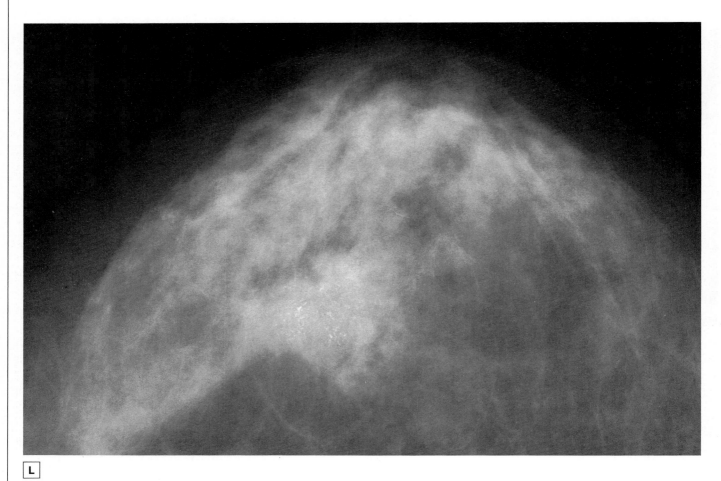

L

Fig. 3.50   Magnification—whole breast.

3.48). Magnification can be performed in any of the standard positions which demonstrate the lesion. Full (Fig. 3.49) or paddle magnification can be obtained (Fig. 3.50).

REFERENCES

Andersson I 1986 Mammography in clinical practice. Vol. 62, No. 2, Kodak
DHSS 1986 Breast cancer screening. DHSS Report of Working Group chaired by P Forrest. HMSO, London
Eklund G W 1989 Technique for improved imaging of the augmented breast. In: Problems and solutions for the breast imaging technologist.
Harvard Medical School, Massachusetts General Hospital
Kopans D B 1989 Breast imaging. Lipincott, Philadelphia
Sickles E A 1988 Practical solutions to common mammographic problems. In: Problems and solutions for the breast imaging technologist. Harvard Medical School, Massachusetts General Hospital

CHAPTER 4

Quality assurance

D. R. Dance

INTRODUCTION

The importance of quality assurance in diagnostic radiology has long been recognized, both for screening and diagnosis. In mammography, the imaging constraints of high contrast, excellent resolution, low noise and low dose are all important. The use of the wrong equipment, badly set up or calibrated equipment or inadequately trained staff can be expected to result in the loss of diagnostic information or an unnecessarily high breast dose. Quality assurance must therefore be regarded as an essential part of the mammographic system. This is reflected in the appearance of a 'Eurostandard' for mammography (Commission of the European Communities (CEC) 1989) and the establishment of national quality assurance programmes or recommendations. In the United Kingdom, guidelines have been produced for the establishment of quality systems for mammography (Department of Health (DH) 1989a) and detailed descriptions of test procedures have been given by the Institute of Physical Sciences in Medicine (IPSM 1989). Test procedures have also been described by the American Association of Physicists in Medicine (AAPM 1990), Moores et al (1987) and the British Institute of Radiology (BIR 1988).

In this chapter we discuss the components of the mammographic quality system and some of the tests which should be made on mammographic X-ray equipment. It is not possible to give an exhaustive treatment of these tests here and the reader should consult the above references for a more detailed discussion of methodology.

THE QUALITY SYSTEM

Quality assurance, management and control

Quality assurance can be defined as all those planned and systematic actions necessary to provide adequate confidence that a product or component will satisfy given requirements for quality (British Standards Institution (BSI) 1987). It has two important aspects: quality management, which is that part of the management function which determines and controls quality policy; and quality control which is the set of operations necessary to maintain or improve quality.

The mammographic quality system will therefore include the assignment of responsibility, the establishment of standards, staff training, proper documentation of procedures, and the quality control of the equipment and its use at installation and throughout its working life. Quality control should include the monitoring of the performance of both the radiographer and the radiologist.

Objectives

The objectives of a radiological quality system are (International Electrotechnical Commision 1988) as follows.

1. To achieve and maintain radiological information of adequate quality for medical diagnostic purposes.
2. To minimize the radiation dose to the patient consistent with achieving adequate quality.
3. To maximize cost containment by minimizing wastage of time and resources.

These rather general statements need to be made much more specific before they can be implemented in the practical situation. In the United Kingdom Breast Screening Programme they have been re-expressed in terms of 'outcome' objectives (DH 1989a), which are limits or standards for quantities which can be measured. Examples of such standards would include upper and lower limits for breast dose, minimum scores for imaging a test phantom, an upper limit on the number of reject films and figures which relate to the number of cancers detected per million women screened and the benign to malignant biopsy ratio. The difficulty here is knowing where to set the standard and it is important that the quality system is dynamic and changes as experience develops.

Organizational features

For an effective and well-organized quality system it is essential to appoint a senior member of staff as quality manager. This person should be responsible for the implementation of quality policy, the production of a quality assurance manual and the monitoring and review of the quality control programme in relation to the results obtained locally, nationally and internationally. The quality manager should be assisted in this task by a quality assurance committee, with representatives of all appropriate staff groups.

The quality manual plays a key role in the quality system. It should include the names of those responsible for the various aspects of the quality system, details of acceptance, commissioning and routine test procedures (see the following section) and of equipment maintenance and repair. It should list the limiting values for each test, the test frequency and the corrective action which should be taken if the test results are outside the limiting values.

Some of the routine tests described in the quality manual will be performed frequently and are designed to be quick and easy to do. It is usually most convenient if these are done by the radiographer, whereas other tests, which are done less frequently and may require more complex equipment or special expertise, are often done by a medical physicist or medical physics technician. Electrical and mechanical checks at the acceptance of the equipment are often done by an X-ray engineer. In all cases it is important that the results of the tests are conveyed to staff and appropriate action taken.

Technical aspects of the quality system

The technical quality programme comprises the steps specification, acceptance testing, commissioning and routine testing of the X-ray equipment (IPSM 1989 and Fig. 4.1). The choice of mammographic equipment is the extremely important first step in this process, and in the United Kingdom the Department of Health has given a specification for mammographic screening equipment (Department of Health and Social Security (DHSS) 1987, DH 1990) and for illuminators for viewing breast screening mammograms (DH 1989b) as well as general technical requirements for X-ray equipment (DH 1989c). Both the specification and technical requirements should form part of the purchase contract.

Once the equipment has been installed, it must be tested to ensure that it performs according to its specification (acceptance testing). This can be done by the manufacturer, who

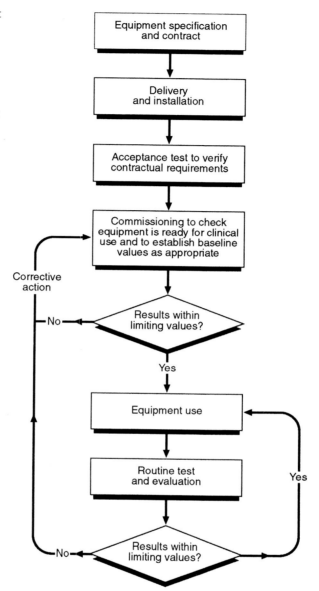

Fig. 4.1 Tests of the X-ray equipment. Reproduced with permission of the Institute of Physical Sciences in Medicine (1989).

demonstrates the performance of the equipment to the customer or by the customer himself. Commissioning comprises the tests which are carried out to ensure that the equipment is ready for clinical use. It includes measurements to provided baseline values against which subsequent routine checks can be compared and

the process of optimizing the performance of the system.

Once the system is in clinical use, its performance must be monitored by a series of routine tests. Some of the tests are done daily, some weekly and others six-monthly or annually. After repair work or service of the equipment, some of the tests may need to be repeated to establish new baseline values. It is very important that limits of acceptability are established for each test and that appropriate action is taken if the results of the test are outside these limits. Equally, the values of the tests themselves must be assessed: as noted previously, the quality system must be dynamic and responsive to feedback from monitoring, review and evaluation (DH 1989a).

TESTS OF MAMMOGRAPHIC X-RAY EQUIPMENT AND ITS USE

The selection of the tests which are included in the mammographic quality system is very important, and the tests themselves will only be useful if the appropriate limiting values are set and a suitable programme of action laid down for when these values are exceeded. Table 4.1 provides an outline list of tests and test frequencies, and some of the more important of these tests are discussed below. In most cases the detailed methodology is not given and the reader should refer to IPSM (1989) and AAPM (1990) for further information. Tests of the Xerox receptor are not included in this chapter.

Many of the tests described necessitate the use of calibrated equipment. It is important to ensure that the equipment used is suitable for mammographic X-ray qualities and has an appropriate calibration. For example, the use of an ionization chamber suitable for general radiography, and which does not have a calibration for mammographic qualities, can easily lead to an underestimate of dose by 40% (Clark et al 1991).

Table 4.1 Mammographic quality control tests and test frequencies

Test	Frequency
Safety	
Electrical safety	12
Mechanical safety and function	3–12
Radiation safety inspection	12
Radiation safety measurements	6–12
X-ray set performance	
kV	6
Focal spot size	12
Output	6
Timer	12
AEC	6
Grid film	12
Screen-film system, processing and viewing	
Screen-film contact	12
Cassette speed	6
Cassette light tightness	12
Safelights	12
Sensitometry	D
Processing parameters	W 3–12
Viewing boxes	3–12
Test phantom	D–W
Breast dose	
Full measurement	6
Check with test phantom	D–W
Reject analysis	M–3

D = daily, W = weekly, M = monthly, 3 = 3 monthly, 6 = 6 monthly, 12 = 12 monthly.

The frequencies are intended as guidance only. Where a range is given this may be because there are several tests under a given heading or simply that the user should consider the range indicated.

Tests of the X-ray set

Safety. It is essential that the electrical, mechanical and radiation safety of the equipment be checked at installation and at regular intervals thereafter. The requirements for electrical safety are laid down in TRS89 (DH 1989c) and in British Standard 5724, Part 1 (BSI 1979). Mechanical checks will include a careful check of the power-assisted system for breast compression, for which

a. there must be no slackness that could lead to uneven compression
b. automatic and emergency release mechanisms must function correctly
c. the maximum compression force should not exceed 200 N.

The requirements for radiation safety are laid down in the Ionising Radiation Regulations (Her Majesty's Stationary Office (HMSO) 1985, 1988), and the Approved Code of

Practice (Health and Safety Commission (HSC) 1985) and Guidance Notes (National Radiological Protection Board (NRPB) 1988) which accompany the 1985 Regulations. Radiation safety checks must include an inspection of the function and layout of the exposure controls and warning lights, an asessment of the X-ray filtration by a measurement of half-value layer, and estimations of tube leakage and the transmission through the lead protective screen and the table. A minimum tube filtration equivalent to 0.5 mm aluminium or 0.03 mm molybdenum is required (NRPB 1988). It is also important to check that the X-ray field is appropriately collimated and aligned with the film cassette so that the radiation is restricted to only the tissues which are being examined.

Tube performance. The contrast obtainable in mammography is critically dependent on tube voltage and it is essential that this quantity be correctly calibrated and regularly monitored. A 2 kV change in tube voltage will produce approximately a 10% change in image contrast and it is desirable that the tube kV be controlled to within ± 1 kV of its nominal value. The preferred method of measurement is to use a digital kV meter specially designed for mammography. Such instruments are quick and easy to use but an overall measurement frequency of 6 months is sufficient because changes in image contrast will also be identified from test phantom measurements.

The focal spot size should be measured at commissioning and annually thereafter. It should be measured at 28 kV and at the most-used value of the tube current. It must

agree with its specification within the tolerances given in IPSM (1989). Although the resolution of the system is critically dependent on this parameter, frequent checks are not needed because the resolution will be monitored as part of the test phantom measurements. The preferred method for measuring focal spot size is to use a slit camera, but it is also possible to use a pin hole. In both cases it is important to make the measurement using the reference axis specified by the tube manufacturer, because the effective focal spot size will change with the target viewing position in the image plane.

The output of the X-ray tube should be checked every 6 months, including tests on reproducibility for repeat exposures, constancy since the last measurement and variations with mA, mAs and tube voltage. Results outside tolerance can indicate the loss of a filter or problems with the high-voltage waveform or generator. Tests should be made for the tube currents and tube potentials used for both contact and magnification procedures.

Mammography is performed under automatic exposure control but there may be occasions when manual exposure is required. Manual exposure is also used when checking the performance of the equipment. It is important therefore to check the exposure time over the range of settings available. A digital timer is suitable for this purpose but the user must be aware that this will measure the radiation waveform and small systematic errors may occur.

Grid. The performance of an anti-scatter grid can be specified in terms of the Dose Increase (or Bucky) Factor and the Contrast Improvement

Factor. These factors are simply the ratios of the relevant quantity with and without the grid and they should be measured at acceptance to ensure that they conform with the grid specification. It is also useful to check the uniformity of the grid using a plain radiograph of a uniform Perspex phantom which is taken with grid movement disabled. Examination of the image with a magnifying glass provides a check on line density whereas poor uniformity can indicate a fault in construction or incorrect focusing of the lead lamellae within the grid. In this connection it is important to check that a grid of the correct focal length is used.

Automatic exposure control. A good automatic exposure control (AEC) system will prove to be reliable, give reproducible results and will produce similar density on the film for a wide range of breast thicknesses, compositions and exposure conditions. As noted in Chap. 2, some of the earlier AEC systems did not cope well with variation in breast composition and thickness, and it is important to provide a careful specification for this component of the system.

The AEC system must be tested at acceptance for variation with exposure conditions including with and without grid, standard and magnification geometries, changes in tube current and voltage, and the position of the detector that controls the AEC exposure. The test exposures should be made with a Perspex slab phantom 4 cm thick and the same cassette should be used for each exposure. The optical density should be measured at the same position on each of the resulting radiographs, a variation of $\pm 10\%$ of the mean value being acceptable. The reproducibility of the AEC should also be tested by making repeat exposures (range of $\pm 5\%$ desirable) and the variation of optical density with breast thickness tested using exposures of Perspex slabs 2, 4, 6 and 8 cm thick (limiting value $\pm 10\%$ of the value for 4 cm Perspex). An appropriate subset of these measurements should be repeated at six-monthly intervals.

Overexposure of the breast is prevented in the event of failure of an AEC system by an override timer. This timer will terminate the exposure after a preset time interval and should be regularly tested by making an exposure with a lead sheet protecting the AEC detector. The function of the AEC system is also checked by the regular exposure of the test phantom.

Tests of the screen-film system, processing and viewing

Cassettes. Screen-film contact should be tested before a cassette is used clinically, and annually thereafter. A contact test tool is placed on the top surface of the cassette and radiographed. Uneven density patches on the resulting film indicate poor contact. Cassette speed should be checked every 6 months. A 4 cm Perspex phantom is exposed using each cassette and the post-exposure mAs is recorded in each case. Providing the AEC is functioning well, the densities at a fixed position on the resulting films should all be within ± 0.1 OD and the recorded values of the post-exposure mAs should be within $\pm 10\%$ of their mean value. Any cassettes producing results outside these limiting values should be rejected. The light tightness of each cassette should also be checked.

Processing. The control of film processing is critical to the mammographic quality. It is strongly recommended that a dedicated processor is used, because the requirements for processing a single emulsion mammographic film are different from those for conventional double emulsion films, particularly if extended processing is used. It has been pointed out by Hendrick (1990) that if the processing activity is too low (less than 50 films per day), incorrect developer replenishment may occur.

The most important test of the processor is sensitometry. When a new film is introduced it can be useful to measure the film characteristic using a sensitometer based on (preferably) X-ray or light exposure. A light sensitometer must be used daily to monitor the performance of the processor. The resulting film is measured on a densitometer (or a sensi-densitometer which combines the function of both instruments) to assess the speed and contrast of the system as well as measure the background fog level. It is usual to choose a step (S1) on the sensitometric strip which corresponds to an optical density of about 1.0 above background base + fog (B) as a measure of the speed of the system. Contrast is assessed as the difference in optical density S2 − S1 between the step S1 and a second step S2 of density about 2.0 above background. The quantities S1 − B, S2 − S1 and background are plotted (Fig. 4.2) and appropriate action taken if they are outside of the limiting values. It can also be helpful to monitor the processor temperature and replenishment rate, and baseline values of quantities such as specific gravity, pH, and residual hypo should also be measured.

Viewing. The light output of the film viewing boxes should be measured at least annually, and a simple visual check carried out every 3 months. The luminance can be measured with a photometer or a light output meter and should be at least 5500 lux. The variation in intensity across the light field should be no more than 10%. The ambient light level in the viewing room should not exceed 86 lux (IPSM 1989).

Tests of the system

Test phantoms. The acceptability of the mammographic image is often assessed by a skilled radiologist based on his experience of other mammograms and possibly by comparison with reference 'standards of excellence'. Images of test phantoms provide complimentary information about the performance of the system in terms of measurable physical parameters such as high- and low-contrast resolution, and enable both the comparison of different imaging systems and the long-term monitoring of the performance of a particular system, although any given phantom may not be well suited to both of these objectives because of their differing requirements for complexity and ease of interpretation.

A good test phantom should approximately simulate the size and X-ray attenuation of the breast so that it can be exposed under automatic exposure control to reproduce a clinical exposure. It should contain a sufficiently wide range of high- (e.g. simulated microcalcification) and low-contrast features of clinical relevance to provide discrimination between different mammographic imaging systems. The features which test the resolving power of the system should be placed at the top of the phantom where they maximize geometric unsharpness and present the greatest challenge to the system.

Most test phantoms contain a series of objects of varying contrast and size to facilitate a subjective assessment of system performance, but it is also valuable to make objective measurements using a densitometer. Simple examples of this are checking the constancy of the film density at a fixed point on the image and the constancy of the system contrast by measurements on the image of a radiographic step wedge. For more sophisticated comparisons, it is also possible to measure modulation transfer functions and noise power spectra.

Test phantoms have been produced by many workers (e.g. Tonge & Davis 1978, White & Tucker 1980, Yaffe et al 1986). Commercial phantoms have been produced by, for example, Agfa, CGR, DuPont, FAXIL at Leeds, Kodak, Nuclear Associates, RMI and Victoreen. Unfortunately few of these phantoms test the system at the full range of optical densities present in a clinical mammogram, and many offer insufficient discrimination even at a single density. The ideal phantom has yet to be developed.

In order to build on common experience, it is desirable that the same phantom be used in many different centres for assessing system performance. In the United States the ACR phantom has been used for accreditation purposes (Hendrick 1990), in Sweden the CGR phantom is used for performance comparison, and in the United Kingdom imaging standards have been based on the Leeds TOR mammographic phantom developed at FAXIL (DH 1989a, Cowen & Coleman 1990).

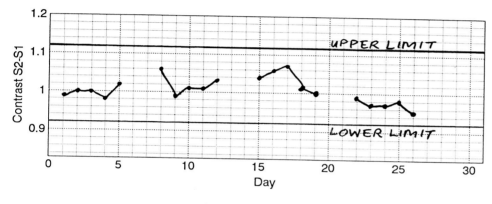

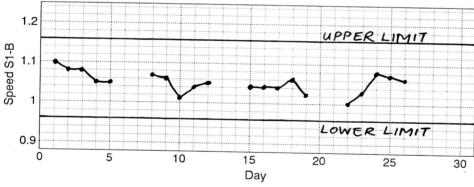

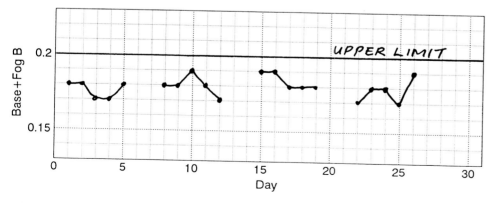

Fig. 4.2 Chart showing results of daily sensitometry. The upper curve gives a measure of contrast, the middle curve a measure of speed and the lower curve is the base + fog level. Limiting values are set at ±0.1 OD from the mean value for contrast and speed and at 0.20 OD for base + fog.

The main details of the Leeds phantom are shown in Fig. 4.3. It comprises (Cowen & Coleman 1990) a semicircular test plate which is positioned on top of 4 cm Perspex. The test plate contains two line-pair test objects positioned at right angles and capable of measuring up to 20 cycles/mm, simulated calcifications of varying sizes and contrasts, and 6 mm objects of varying contrast to test low-contrast resolution. There is also a low-contrast bar pattern and a step wedge to facilitate a densitometric assessment of contrast. The phantom has met with some criticism because of its discrimination range, but is widely used for frequent checks on image quality, and is of value in comparing the performance of different systems.

Radiation dose. Breast dose should be kept as low as reasonably practicable consistent with achieving appropriate image quality, and its value should be regularly monitored. Any significant change in dose will reflect a change in the operating point of the mammographic equipment. For example, a shift from a tube potential of 28 kV to a tube potential of 30 kV will reduce the dose for a 45 mm-thick breast by about 14%.

It is noted in Chap. 2 that breast dose should be quoted as the mean dose to the glandular tissues within the breast, and that this dose will vary with both breast composition and thickness. To compare doses in different centres, it is necessary therefore to make measurements for a standard breast, and the IPSM (1989) has suggested the use of a standard breast phantom for this purpose. This phantom simulates a breast 4.5 cm thick of adipose and glandular tissue composition (equal parts by weight). Because of the expense of constructing

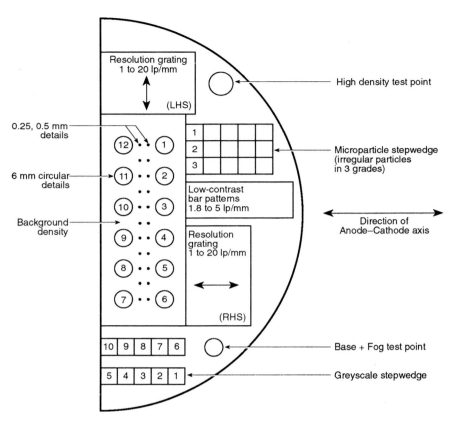

Fig. 4.3 Main details of the Leeds TOR (MAX) phantom. Reproduced with permission of the Institute of Physical Sciences in Medicine (from Cowen & Coleman 1990).

such a phantom, measurements are made of the incident air kerma required to correctly expose a 4 cm-thick Perspex phantom, and conversion factors (Dance 1990) are used to relate this reading to the mean glandular dose for the standard breast. This procedure is time-consuming and should be done at the commissioning of the equipment and at intervals of 6 months, as indicated in Table 4.1. For an imaging system employing a screen-film receptor and a grid, IPSM (1989) gives an upper dose limit of 3.0 mGy, although it is likely that this should be reduced, and AAPM (1990) gives an upper dose limit of 1.8 mGy for a slightly different breast model. For systems without a grid these dose limits should

be halved. Notwithstanding these limits, it is important to establish the dose obtained by others using similar equipment, and to explore the reasons for any differences.

For more frequent checks of breast dose it is sufficient to monitor the constancy of the mAs per exposure of a simple phantom. The phantom used to check image quality will be suitable for this purpose and the mAs given can be recorded whenever the phantom is used. Recording the mAs is easy for more modern units that provide a post-exposure indication of this quantity, but for older units, a more complicated procedure is necessary (IPSM 1989); an alternative approach would be to use TLD (thermo-luminescent dosimetry). Limiting values of $\pm 10\%$ of the average value are appropriate for both the frequent and less frequent tests of breast dose.

It is also of interest to study breast dose for the population of patients being examined. A simple approach is to note the post-exposure mAs and compressed breast thickness for a series of patients. A similar methodology to that described above for the standard breast phantom can be used to estimate breast dose for the mean or mode of the patient series or indeed for the complete series. This procedure can only be approximate because of the lack of knowledge of the breast composition for any patient, but the results will provide a basis for monitoring changes in the patient population or breast compression.

Reject analysis. The analysis of rejected films is an essential component of the quality system. It provides a monitor of both the performance of the equipment and its correct use by the radiographer. All reject films should be kept and classified according to the reason for rejection (for example overexposure, underexposure, patient movement, poor positioning). The results should be analysed and discussed with a view to improving performance. In our institution we have also found it helpful to determine the reject rate for particular mammography units and for individual radiographers. A reject rate of not more than 3% is both desirable (DH 1989a) and achievable.

REFERENCES

American Association of Physicists in Medicine 1990 Equipment requirements and quality control for mammography. AAPM Report 29. American Institute of Physics, New York

British Institute of Radiology 1988 Assurance of quality in the diagnostic X-ray department. British Institute of Radiology, London

British Standards Institution 1979 British standard medical electrical equipment Part 1: Specification for general safety requirements. BS5724, Part 1. British Standards Institution, London

British Standards Institution 1987 British standard quality vocabulary, Part 1: International terms. BS4778, Part 1. British Standards Institution, London

Commission of the European Communities 1989 Quality criteria for diagnostic radiographic images—breast. In: Moores B M, Wall B F, Eriskat H, Schibilla H (eds) Optimisation of image quality and patient exposure in diagnostic radiology. BIR Report 20. British Institute of Radiology, London, p 278

Clark M J, Delgardo A, Hjardemaal O, Kramer H M, Zoetelief J 1991 The CEC extended intercomparison programme of dose meters used in diagnostic radiology—presentation of the results of the intercomparison programme. Paper presented at CEC Seminar on dosimetry in diagnostic radiology, Luxembourg, March 1991

Cowen A R, Coleman N J 1990 Design of test objects and phantoms for quality control in mammographic screening. In: Physics in Diagnostic Radiology. IPSM Report 61. Institute of Physical Sciences in Medicine, York, pp 30–36

Dance D R 1990 Monte Carlo calculation of conversion factors for the estimation of mean glandular dose. Physics in Medicine and Biology 35: 1211–1219

Department of Health 1989a Guidelines on the establishment of a quality assurance system for the radiological aspects of mammography used for breast screening. Report of a sub-committee of the Radiological Advisory Committee of the Chief Medical Officer. Department of Health, London

Department of Health 1989b Guidance notes for health authorities on

illuminators for breast cancer screening mammograms. Report STD/88/30. Department of Health, London

Department of Health 1989c Technical requirements for the supply and installation of equipment for diagnostic imaging and radiotherapy. Report TRS89. Department of Health, London

Department of Health 1990 Revised guidance notes for health authorities on mammographic X-ray equipment requirements for breast screening. Report STD/90/46. Department of Health, London

Department of Health and Social Security 1987 Guidance notes for health authorities on mammographic equipment requirements for breast screening. Report STD/87/34. DHSS, London

Health and Safety Commission 1985 Approved Code of Practice. The protection of persons against ionising radiation arising from any work activity. HMSO, London

Hendrick R E 1990 Standardisation of image quality and radiation dose in mammography. Radiology 174: 648–654

Her Majesty's Stationery Office 1985 The Ionising Radiations Regulations 1985. Statutory Instrument 1985, No. 1333. HMSO, London

Her Majesty's Stationery Office 1988 The Ionising Radiations (Protection of Persons undergoing Medical Examination or Treatment) Regulations 1988. HMSO, London

Institute of Physical Sciences in Medicine 1989 The commissioning and routine testing of mammographic X-ray systems. IPSM Report 59 Institute of Physical Sciences in Medicine, York

International Electrotechnical Commission 1988 Quality assurance in diagnostic X-ray departments, Part 1: General aspects (draft report)

Moores B M, Henshaw E T, Watkinson S A, Pearcey B J 1987 Practical guide to quality assurance in medical imaging. Wiley, Chichester

National Radiological Protection Board, Health and Safety Executive and Health Departments 1988 Guidance notes for the protection of persons against ionising radiation arising from medical and dental use. HMSO, London, p 17

Tonge K A, Davis R 1978 A phantom designed to compare the quality of

various mammographic images. British
Journal of Radiology 51: 731–733

White D R, Tucker A K 1980 A test object
for assessing image quality in
mammography. British Journal of
Radiology 53: 331–335

Yaffe M J, Johns P C, Nishikawa R M,
Mawdsley G E, Caldwell C B 1986
Anthropomorphic radiologic phantoms.
Radiology 158: 550–552

CHAPTER 5

The normal breast

J. Pemberton, Yin Y. Ng

INTRODUCTION

The mammary glands are essentially modified sweat glands which appear in a rudimentary form during the second month of human fetal development. The glandular components are derived from the mammary line which extends from the axilla to the groin in the embryo. In the pectoral region of the future upper chest wall the mammary line thickens to become the mammary ridge. This invaginates and from this ingrowth 15 or 20 solid buds arise which extend from the deep surface into the mesodermal tissues beneath them. Each bud represents a future lobe of the breast and further division produces the lobules. The original solid stalk becomes cannalized during the eighth month of intrauterine life to form the lactiferous ducts. These are surrounded by a sheath formed by the underlying mesoderm. Interlobar and connective tissue septa are formed and separate the adjacent lobes. A certain amount of fatty tissue is laid down within the breast during the fifth month. About the time of birth the pit from which the ectodermal buds originated becomes raised above the surface to form the nipple, and the lactiferous ducts now open at the apex of the nipple instead of into the floor of the original pit or depression.

Summary:
Ectodermal milk ridge appears on embryonic trunk;
5 weeks: thoracic portion becomes mammary ridge;
8 weeks: ectodermal cells become invaginated;
16 weeks: epithelial buds develop and branch;
20 weeks: branched epithelial tissues cannalize under hormonal influence;
32–40 weeks: parenchymal differentiation occurs;
40 weeks: nipple areolar complex develops.

DEVELOPMENTAL ABNORMALITIES

Congenital

Supernumerary nipples may occur anywhere along the line of the primitive milk ridge, which in the fetus extended obliquely from the axilla to the groin. Rarely accessory breast tissue also develops, usually as an isolated island of tissue in the axillary region but occasionally in the inferior part of the breast. Such accessory axillary breast tissue is present in 2–6% of women (Vorherr 1974). It may present as a palpable mass or axillary thickening (Adler et al 1987). When there are no signs of a nipple or lactation, the diagnosis is rarely made, and the findings often attributed to a lipoma (Greer 1974). The diagnosis is usually obvious mammographically, best shown on the oblique or extended craniocaudal view. An accessory axillary breast is separate from the bulk of the parenchyma as distinct from the

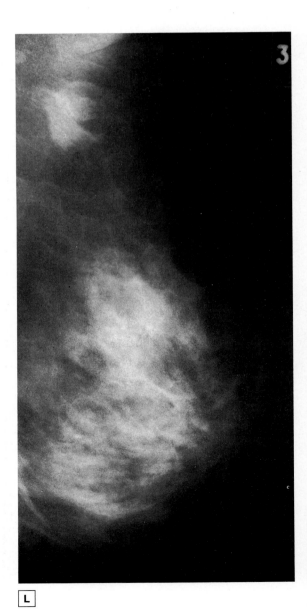

Fig. 5.1 Axillary breast presenting as a palpable mass. *a* With dense parenchyma. *b* With fatty parenchyma. *c* Same case with axillary view to show accessory nipple (arrowed).

L

Fig. 5.1a

relatively frequent 'axillary tail of Spence', which represents a direct extension from the outer margin of the main mass of glandular tissue. The parenchyma may be dense or fatty and an accessory nipple may be apparent (Fig. 5.1). Carcinoma and benign breast lesions have been reported in axillary breast tissue (Andrews 1929, Raudin 1934, Rawls 1942, DeCholnoky 1951).

Hypoplasia of one or both breasts may occur. If unilateral the opposite breast is either hyperplastic or normal. There is, in addition, the very rare Poland's syndrome in which there is hypoplasia of one breast, the thorax and pectoral muscles on that side. Other congenital abnormalities include amastia or congenital absence of the breast or amazia, when the breast tissue is absent but a rudimentary nipple is present.

Acquired

Underdevelopment of the breast tissue may occur from a variety of causes. These include trauma, radiotherapy or breast biopsy. The latter has on occasion inadvertently caused removal of the breast bud and hence the breast has been unable to develop during puberty.

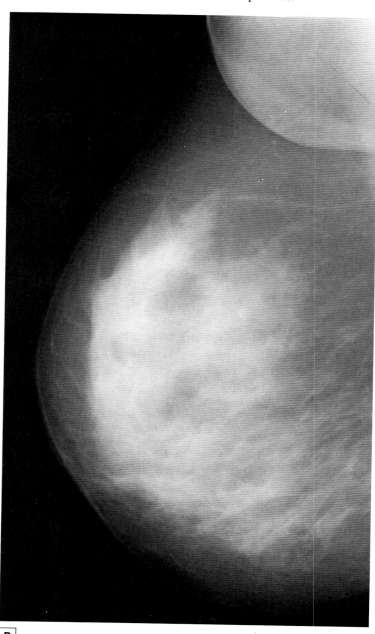

R

Fig. 5.1b

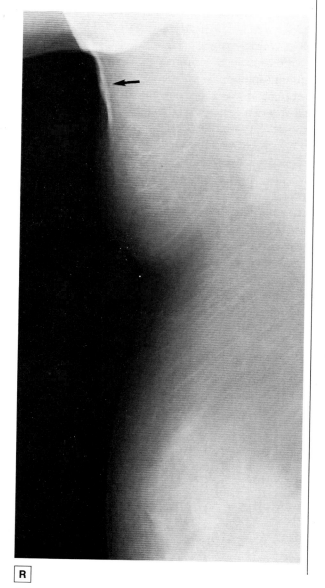

R

Fig. 5.1c

SURFACE ANATOMY

The adult female breast lies vertically from the 2nd to the 6th rib and in the transverse plane from the lateral border of the sternum to the mid-axillary line. The gland lies on the superficial fascia which covers the muscles pectoralis major, serratus anterior and the external oblique. Almost a third of the breast extends laterally beyond the anterior margin of the axilla, and the so-called axillary tail reaches as far laterally as the posterior axillary line.

The nipple lies in the centre of the breast and is a conical protrusion of skin, on the surface of which the lactiferous ducts terminate. The often-quoted anatomical position of the 4th intercostal space is of no value, for clearly this varies with the degree of the development of the breast tissue. The nipple is surrounded by a circular pigmented area, the areola, the surface of which has a pimply appearance due to the presence of sebaceous glands (Montgomery's tubercles). The areolar muscle consists of smooth muscle fibres disposed in a circular and radiating manner. During suckling the nipple is stimulated, causing the fibres to contract and the nipple to become erect.

GROSS ANATOMY

The breast is made up of essentially three distinct components. The most important is the glandular tissue arranged in lobes, and between these lobes fibrous tissue runs and fatty tissue is deposited. There is no distinct capsule but the subcutaneous tissues which envelop the gland send septa into it to act as a supporting framework for the various lobules. Fibrous processes arising in the fascia that covers the gland pass forwards to both the skin and nipple. These fibrous bands are at their most developed in the upper part of the breast where they are known as the suspensory ligaments of Cooper. The glandular tissue consists of some 15–20 lobes. The lobes are in turn composed of lobules which are connected by areolar, vascular and ductal tissues. The lobules themselves consist of rounded alveoli which open into the branches of the lactiferous ducts. The latter coalesce to form larger ducts which then end in excretory or lactiferous ducts. The latter vary in number from 15 to 20 and converge towards the areola, beneath which they form saccular dilatations named the lactiferous sinuses. The lactiferous ducts then turn forwards to the base of the nipple and exit at separate orifices on the surface of the nipple.

MALE BREAST

The male breast has a rudimentary duct system similar to that of the female breast until puberty. After puberty the female breast under hormonal influence undergoes a further development whereas normally in the male the rudimentary and undeveloped ductal system of the gland persists. Exceptionally there may be development of the male gland during adolescence, producing the so-called pubertal gynaecomastia. This is usually a temporary condition and the swelling regresses after a few months. Occasional cases of persistence into adult life have been recorded. Adult gynaecomastia may result from a variety of causes which in broad terms may be classified as:

1. Iatrogenic, e.g. oestrogen or antihypertensive therapy
2. Gonadal
3. Intersex states
4. General metabolic causes such as cirrhosis, malnutrition and haemodialysis.

VASCULAR SUPPLY AND DRAINAGE

The arterial supply to the breast is the lateral mammary branch of the lateral thoracic artery, the anterior cutaneous or perforating branches of the internal mammary artery and branches are also derived from the 2nd to the 6th intercostal arteries. The veins describe an anastomotic circle around the base of the nipple, the so-called circulus venosus. From the circulus small veins take the blood to the circumference of the gland before terminating in the axillary and internal mammary veins.

LYMPHATIC DRAINAGE

This is particularly important because it is by this route that the spread of malignant disease may occur. There is both a superficial and a deep plexus of lymphatic vessels (Fig. 5.2). The superficial plexus lies beneath the skin superficial to the gland. It receives afferent vessels from the gland and sends its efferent lymph to lymph nodes in the pectoral and infraclavicular chains, and other vessels pass to the deep plexus that lies in the deep fascia on which the mammary gland rests. It is this plexus which receives directly most of the lymphatic drainage of the breast. The efferent vessels from the deep plexus drain as follows.

1. To the pectoral group of nodes.

2. To the sub-scapular group of nodes.

3. From both the above groups channels pass directly and via the central group to the lateral axillary and apical nodes.

4. To the infraclavicular lymph nodes, which in turn communicate with the apical lymph nodes and the postero-inferior group of deep cervical nodes.

5. To the internal mammary chain and onwards to the mediastinal group.

6. Others cross the costal margin and drain into the subdiaphragmatic plexus.

7. There is a significant communication with the deep lymphatic plexus of the contralateral breast.

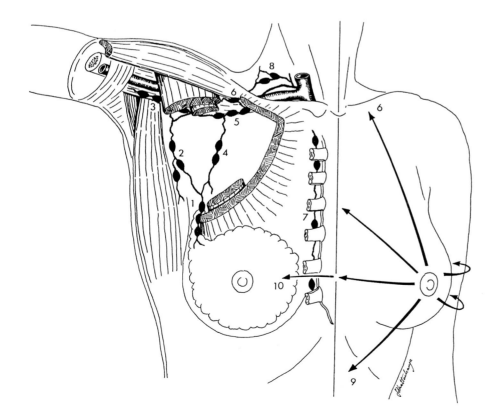

Fig. 5.2 The lymphatic drainage of the breast. Lymph node groups and drainage areas are numbered as follows:
1, pectoral nodes; 2, subscapular nodes; 3, lateral axillary nodes; 4, central nodes; 5, apical nodes; 6, infraclavicular nodes; 7, internal mammary nodes; 8, posterior-inferior group of deep cervical nodes; 9, subdiaphragmatic plexus; 10, communication to contralateral breast plexus.

NERVOUS SUPPLY

The breast is supplied by the anterior and lateral cutaneous branches from the 4th, 5th and 6th intercostal nerves. These nerves supply afferent and sympathetic fibres to the breast tissues. The secretory function is essentially under hormonal control but afferent impulses associated with suckling are involved in the reflex secretion of prolactin and oxytocin.

HORMONES AND THE BREAST

Both the initial growth and the subsequent development of the breast at puberty takes place under the influence of oestrogen and progesterone produced by the ovaries. During pregnancy the corpus luteum and placenta produce oestrogen and progesterone, and under the stimulation of these hormones there is both proliferation and development of the mammary tissues. Other hormones that are believed to stimulate the growth of the mammary glands are prolactin somatomammotrophin (lactogenic hormone) and adrenal corticosteroids.

At parturition the corpus luteum degenerates, the placenta is lost and the level of the circulating oestrogen and progesterone falls dramatically. Milk secretion is generated by the increased production of prolactin and the secretion of adrenal cortical steroids. The act of suckling sets up a reflex mechanism which inhibits the release of prolactin inhibiting factor (PIF) and thus causes the release of prolactin from the anterior pituitary gland. The same impulses also cause the release of oxytocin, and this stimulates the myoepithelial cells of the mammary gland causing them to contract and eject milk from the glands. In the absence of suckling milk secretion stops and the mammary glands begin to regress. The glandular tissue returns to an inactive form.

After the menopause the mammary gland tissue atrophies or involutes. Ovarian hormones are no longer stimulated and the secretory cells of the alveoli degenerate. Some ductal tissue, however, remains. The connective tissue components also degenerate; there is a decrease in the number of stromal cells and collagen fibres. Hence the mammographic parenchymal patterns essentially reflect the relative densities of the various component tissues of the breast. These patterns will alter as the hormonal environment of the breast is altered.

WOLFE CLASSIFICATION OF BREAST PARENCHYMAL PATTERNS

Wolfe has described four parenchymal patterns of the breast (Wolfe 1976, 1983a) based on the relative amounts of fat, epithelial and connective tissue densities as seen mammographically. These have been classified as follows:

1. N1: normal. The breast parenchyma is of low density and has a large proportion of fat. No ducts are visible (Fig. 5.3)

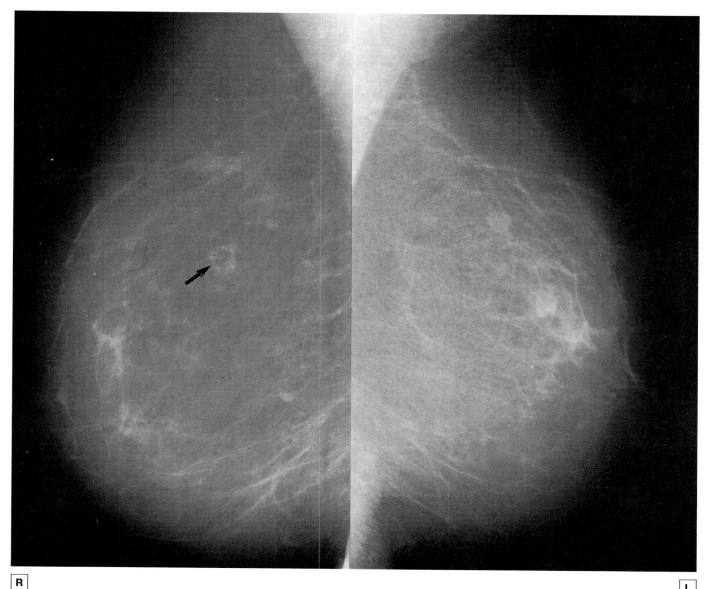

R

L

Fig. 5.3   Normal fatty breast with intramammary lymph node (arrow). Lateral oblique view.

2.   P1: the parenchyma is composed chiefly of fat, with a prominent duct pattern in the anterior portion of the breast but involving less than one-quarter of the breast volume (Fig. 5.4)

3.   P2: prominent duct pattern which involves more than one quarter of the breast volume and with which there is often an associated nodular component (Fig. 5.5)

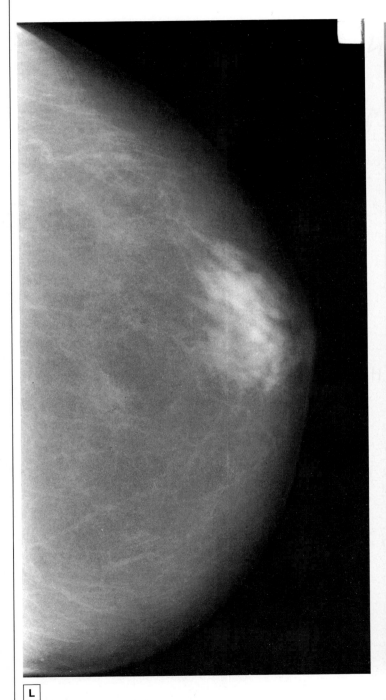

Fig. 5.4   Craniocaudal view showing a P1 pattern.

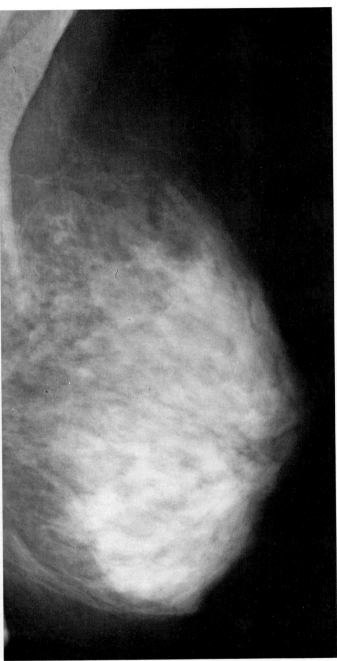

Fig. 5.5   Lateral-oblique view showing a P2 pattern, i.e. prominent ducts occupying more than 25% of the volume of the breast.

4. DY: increased density of the
breast parenchyma with or without
areas of nodularity. The density often
obscures the underlying duct pattern
(Fig. 5.6)

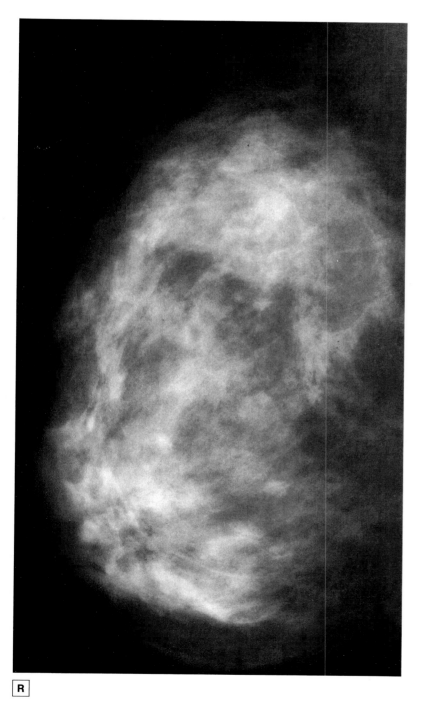

R

Fig. 5.6 Lateral-oblique view showing a DY pattern.

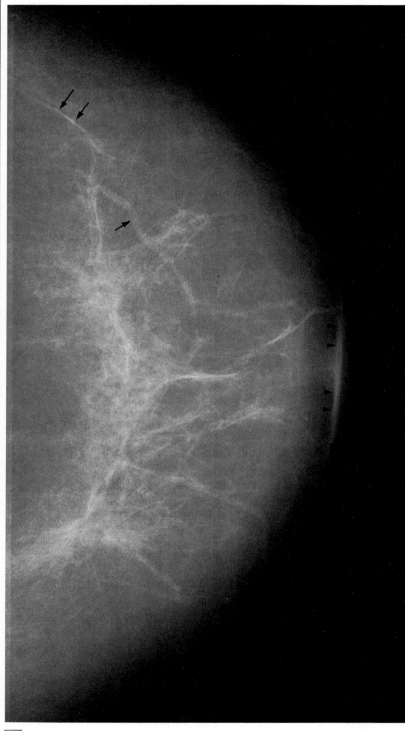

R

Fig. 5.7   Features seen in the normal breast. Arrowheads outline the areola with centrally converging ducts leading to the nipple. Single arrow points to a blood vessel. Double arrow indicates supporting ligament of Astley Cooper.

Figures 5.7 and 5.8 illustrate the radiological anatomy of the normal breast. Trabeculae are to be distinguished from ducts (Fig. 5.9); the former being curvilinear, whereas ducts have a definite cross-sectional diameter with a nodular component. This latter feature, together with the fact that ducts converge on the nipple, helps to distinguish ducts from blood vessels (Fig. 5.10). Ducts may 'coalesce' due to a large amount of periductal collagenosis with obliteration of the surrounding fat, resulting in a homogeneous breast density. Wolfe states that this radiographic homogeneity of prominent ducts is not to be mistaken for a DY pattern.

The demonstration of an association between background breast parenchymal pattern and risk of developing breast cancer, although most probably not of the magnitude originally demonstrated by Wolfe, is widely accepted by radiologists and surgeons. Wolfe (1976) first suggested that a P2 or DY pattern was associated with a significantly increased risk of developing breast cancer. This association was attributed to an increased frequency of high-risk

Fig. 5.8a

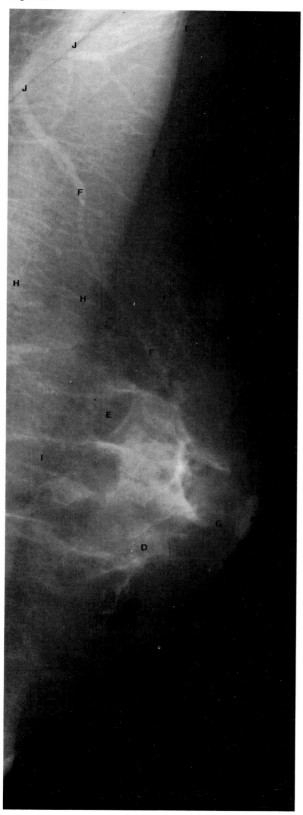

R

epithelial proliferative lesions (Page et al 1985) found in P2 and DY patterns. More recent studies of the relation between Wolfe pattern and histological appearances have failed to confirm this association (Urbanski et al 1988). The radiological appearances of background patterns clearly cannot be attributed to microfocal epithelial changes. The epithelial structures present in the breast are usually situated in fibrous tissue, but the proportions cannot be assessed separately. At present it is not possible to identify the precise mechanism of the relationship between mammographic background pattern and breast cancer risk.

Fig. 5.8a & b. Right breast lateral-oblique film. A, nipple; B, areola; C, skin; D, glandular tissue; E, fat; F, vessel; G, duct; H, Astley Cooper ligament; I, pectoralis muscle; J, skin fold.

Fig. 5.8b

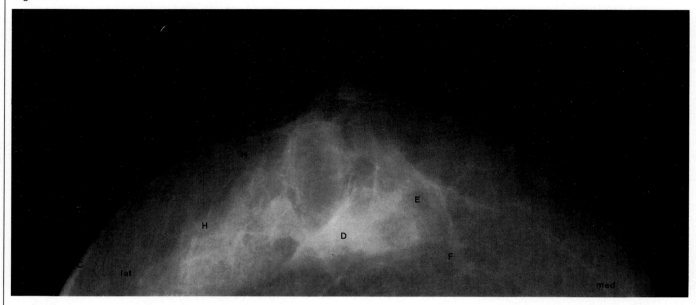

Fig. 5.8a & b.   Right breast lateral-oblique film. A, nipple; B, areola; C, skin; D, glandular tissue; E, fat; F, vessel; G, duct; H, Astley Cooper ligament; I, pectoralis muscle; J, skin fold.

The major contributory factors to alterations in breast stroma are described under the following three headings.

Age

The developing breast has a dense mammographic parenchymal patern due to stromal and ductal proliferation (Fig. 5.11). With maturity the parenchyma assumes a relatively transparent appearance due to fat replacement with involution (Fig. 5.12). There is a tendency for DY patterns to be replaced by P2, P1 or possibly N1.

Parity

Nulliparous women have a different hormone status to parous women. They have higher morning prolactin levels, higher oestrogen levels and lower levels of progesterone (Bernstein et al 1985, Brinton et al 1983). Breasts of nulliparous women involute more slowly than those of multiparous woman. There is therefore longer maintenance of DY and P2 patterns. Multiparity has a long term effect on mammographic appearances. The breasts of women who have borne three or more children involute earlier in life (Kaufman et al 1991).

Hormone replacement therapy (HRT)

HRT is thought to inhibit the involution of the normal breast that should occur naturally with the ageing process. Women on HRT may therefore have persistence of the DY, P2 parenchymal patterns on their mammograms for a longer period than women who do not undergo replacement therapy (Kaufman et al 1991). The importance of this finding in assessing any predisposition to breast malignancy will be considered in Chapter 13, as indeed will the increased incidence of breast malignancy in the upper outer quadrant. The glandular parenchyma in this quadrant is usually the last to involute (Parsons 1983). Asymmetrical involution of the fibroglandular parenchyma is seen in 3–5% of otherwise normal breasts (Kinne & Kopans 1987, Kopans et al 1989), and may lead to confusion with mass lesions (Fig. 5.13). It is worthwhile noting here that if the

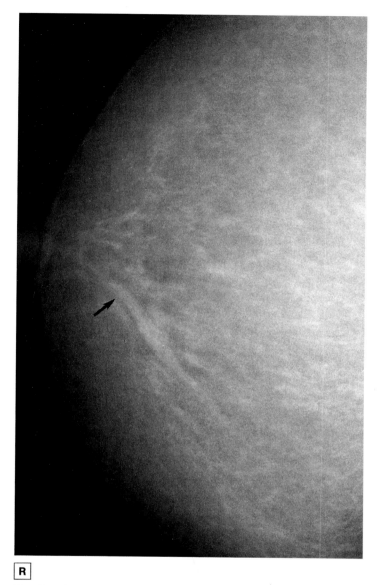

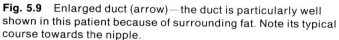

Fig. 5.9 Enlarged duct (arrow)—the duct is particularly well shown in this patient because of surrounding fat. Note its typical course towards the nipple.

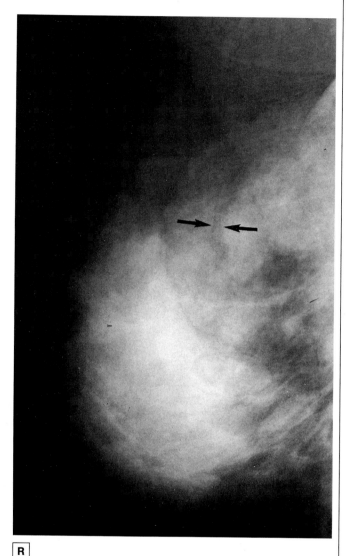

Fig. 5.10 Blood vessel (arrows) surrounded by fat, as distinct from duct (see Fig. 5.7).

asymmetrical area is relatively small, say under 2 cm, is of increased or variable density and produces architectural distortion, it should be regarded with suspicion (Kopans et al 1989). A previous biopsy may also lead to parenchymal asymmetry.

HISTOLOGY OF BREAST TISSUE OF ADULTS AND NON-PREGNANT FEMALES

If the breast tissue is examined under low magnification the lobules of the breast may be seen to form islands of glandular tissue within a mass of dense fibrous and adipose connective tissue. If higher magnification is employed the lobules are seen to consist of

alveolar ducts lined by cuboidal epithelium and supported by a prominent basement membrane. Myoepithelial cells form a discontinuous layer and lie between the duct lining cells and the basement membrane. During adulthood the duct epithelium is subject to the influence of the ovarian hormones and undergoes cyclical changes. In the early part of the cycle the lumina of the ducts are not clearly evident but later they become more prominent and may be seen to contain an eosinophilic secretion. The intralobular connective tissue is dense and fibrous whereas the connective tissue within the lobule is loose, highly cellular, relatively free from fat and contains a rich network of capillaries.

Acknowledgement
We wish to thank Dr Ian Ellis for his contribution on the association between breast parenchymal pattern and risk of developing breast cancer, and Dr J Bhattacharya for his drawing of the lymphatic drainage.

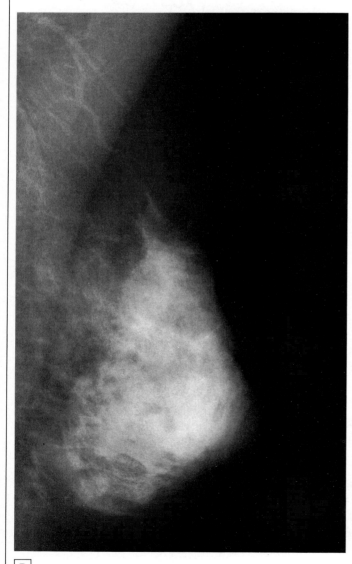

R

Fig. 5.11 Premenopausal breast.

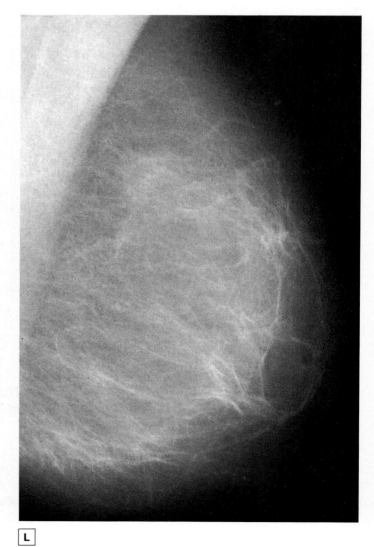

L

Fig. 5.12 Postmenopausal breast.

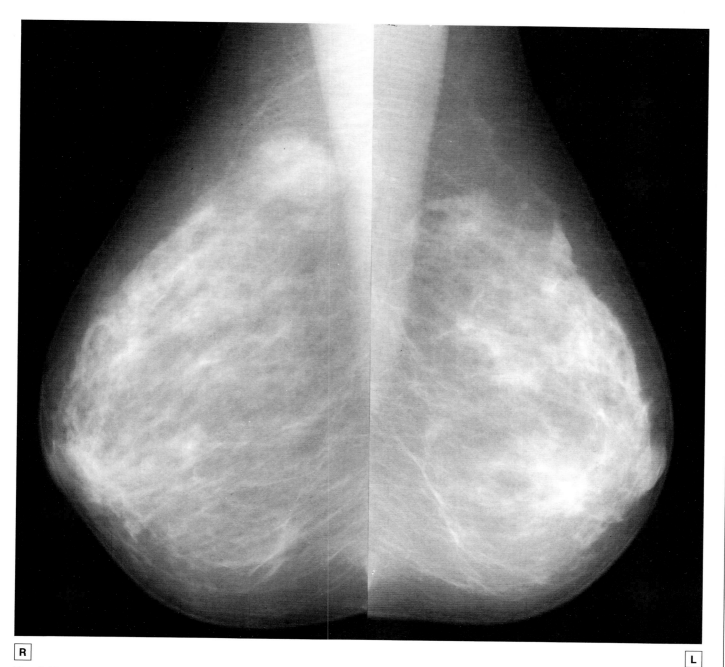

R

L

Fig. 5.13 Asymmetrical involution of the breast parenchyma, with more breast tissue in the right axillary tail. Biopsy showed normal breast tissue only.

REFERENCES

Adler D D, Rebner M, Pennes D R 1987 Accessory breast tissue in the axilla: mammographic appearance. Radiology 163: 709–711

Andrews E 1929 Multiple carcinomata in aberrant breast tissue. Surgical Clinics of North America 9: 333–335

Brinton L A, Hoover R, Fraumeni J F Jr 1983 Reproductive factors in the etiology of breast cancer. British Journal of Cancer 47: 757–762

DeCholnoky T 1951 Accessory breast tissue in the axilla. New York State Journal of Medicine 51: 2245–2248

Greer K E 1974 Accessory axillary breast tissue. Archives of Dermatology 109: 88–89

Kaufman Z, Garstin, W I H, Hayes R, Michell M J, Baum M 1991 The mammographic parenchymal patterns of women on hormonal replacement therapy. Clinical Radiology 43: 389–391

Kinne D W, Kopans D B 1987 Physical examination and mammography in the diagnosis of breast disease. In: Breast diseases. J B Lippincott, Pennsylvania, ch 3

Kopans D B, Swann C A, White G et al 1989 Asymmetric breast tissue. Radiology 171: 639–643

Page D L, Dupont W D, Rogers L W, Rados M S 1985 Atypical hyperplastic lesions of the female breast. A long term follow-up study. Cancer 55: 2698–2708

Parsons C A 1983 Diagnosis of breast disease. Chapman and Hall, London

Raudin J S 1934 Carcinoma arising in accessory breast tissue. Surgical Clinics of North America 14: 139–141

Rawls J L 1942 Extramammary breast carcinoma. Virginia Medical Monthly 69: 448–449

Urbanski S, Jensen W M, Cooke G, McFarlane D, Shannon P, Kmikov V, Boyd N F 1988 The association of histological and radiological indicators of breast cancer risk. British Journal of Cancer 58: 474–479

Vorherr H 1974 The breast. Academic Press, New York

Wolfe J N 1976a Breast patterns as an index of risk for developing breast cancer. American Journal of Radiology 126: 1130–1139

Wolfe J N 1976b Risk for breast cancer development determined by mammographic parenchymal pattern. Cancer 37: 2486–2492

Wolfe J N 1976c Breast parenchymal patterns and their changes with age. Radiology 121: 545–552

Wolfe J N, Saftlas A F, Salne M 1987 Mammographic parenchymal patterns and quantitative evaluation of mammographic densities. A case–control study. American Journal of Radiology 148: 1087–1982

CHAPTER 6

Malignant disease

Elizabeth Wylie

INTRODUCTION

Primary carcinoma is by far the most common malignancy seen in the female breast. Secondary carcinoma, sarcoma and lymphoma are also seen occasionally. With improved mammographic techniques, in-situ ductal carcinoma is being detected with increasing frequency, especially in screening programmes. Invasive carcinoma can also now be detected at very early stages, when the mass is only a few millimetres in size. Multifocal disease can often be detected, with satellite tumours occurring up to 3 cm from the primary lesion. Mammography should always be performed before segmental and local resections, to exclude occult multicentric disease.

PATHOLOGY

Breast carcinoma may be non-invasive (in-situ) with an intact basement membrane, or invasive with tumour cells extending into the adjacent parenchyma and stroma. Most are now thought to be derived from the terminal duct lobular unit. In any institution, the proportion of in-situ to invasive carcinomas detected by mammography depends on whether the patients are symptomatic or referred from a screening programme. Rosen (1987) noted that 3% of symptomatic carcinomas, and 8–22% of carcinomas detected in the first screening round, were in-situ tumours. Invasive ductal carcinoma 'not otherwise specified' is responsible for at least 75% of breast cancers (Teng 1986). The ratio of epithelial cells to stroma is very variable, although the stromal element is usually extensive.

Some cellular tumours, such as mucinous and medullary carcinomas, have little stroma and grow in a nodular fashion, pushing into the surrounding breast and forming a mass with smooth outlines on mammography. However, cellular infiltrating ductal carcinomas need not be well-circumscribed. Each individual breast carcinoma is composed of a heterogeneous population of cell types including fibroblasts, leucocytes, and blood vessels, which may affect their mammographic appearance and prognosis. These are discussed in the section on types of breast malignancy (p. 108).

AN APPROACH TO MAMMOGRAPHIC INTERPRETATION

Mammographic signs of malignancy may be divided into 'major' and 'minor' signs. 'Major' signs include a stellate mass, clustered microcalcification which has characteristics suspicious for malignancy, and localized stromal distortion or asymmetry of parenchyma in the absence of previous surgery. 'Minor' signs include associated skin or nipple changes, change in vascularity, asymmetry of the duct pattern particularly affecting one segment, and enlarged round and dense axillary lymph nodes.

Stellate mass

The most typical sign of a carcinoma is a stellate mass. 50% of invasive carcinomas less than 10 mm diameter, and 88% of those greater than 10 mm, present as an abnormal mass on mammography (Andersson 1981). 84% of malignant tumour masses are stellate (Barth 1979). Ductal and tubular carcinomas show this pattern of growth, spreading into the surrounding parenchyma and inducing a desmoplastic stromal fibrous and elastic reaction (Freundlich et al 1989) (Fig. 6.1). Lobular carcinoma may also produce a stellate tumour, but this occurs less frequently (Mendelson et al 1989). Egan (1988) states that these desmoplastic tumour types are associated with the worst prognosis.

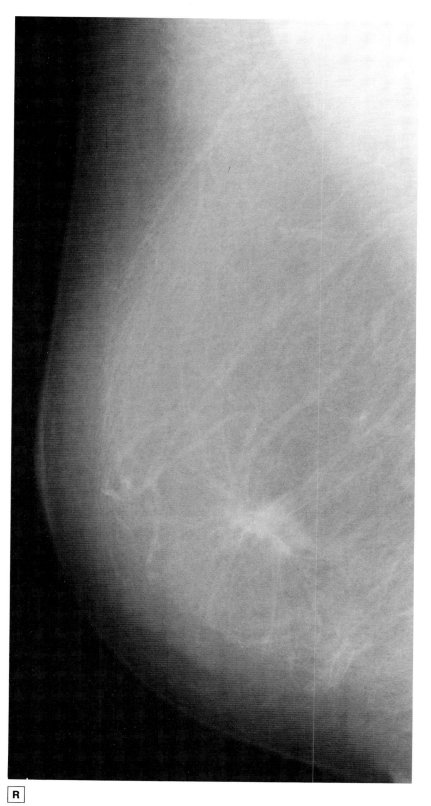

R

Fig. 6.1   70-year-old woman presenting with a right-sided breast lump.
Mammogram shows a 2 cm mass with extensive radiating spicules.
Pathology: invasive ductal carcinoma.

Spiculation may allow the identification of a lesion too small to be appreciated otherwise, particularly in a dense breast, where the linear lucencies between the fine strands may be considerably more obvious than the radiating fibres themselves (Figs 6.2, 6.3). The presence of a central density raises the index of suspicion for malignancy as opposed to radial scar or a postoperative scar (Fig. 7.32, p. 152; Fig. 7.31, p. 150).

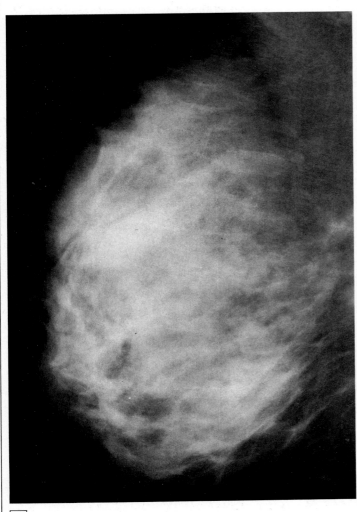

Fig. 6.2a

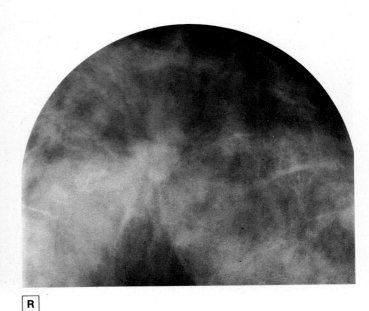

Fig. 6.2b

Fig. 6.2   Radiating tumour strands. *a* Lateral oblique view shows radiating lucent strands superior to the nipple. *b* Coned compression view demonstrates a small central mass. Pathology: ductal carcinoma.

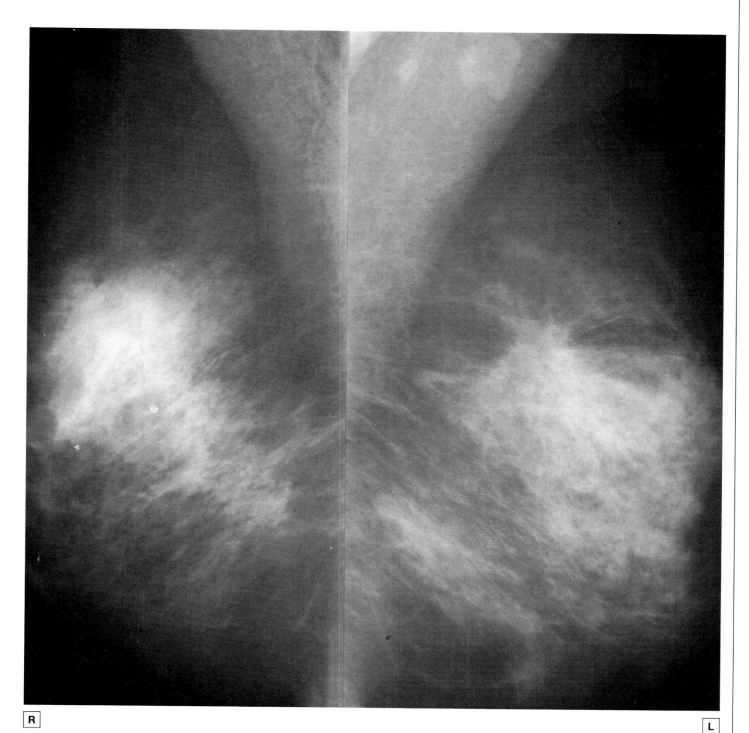

R L

Fig. 6.3 Spiculated mass in dense parenchyma. Cytology: malignant cells.

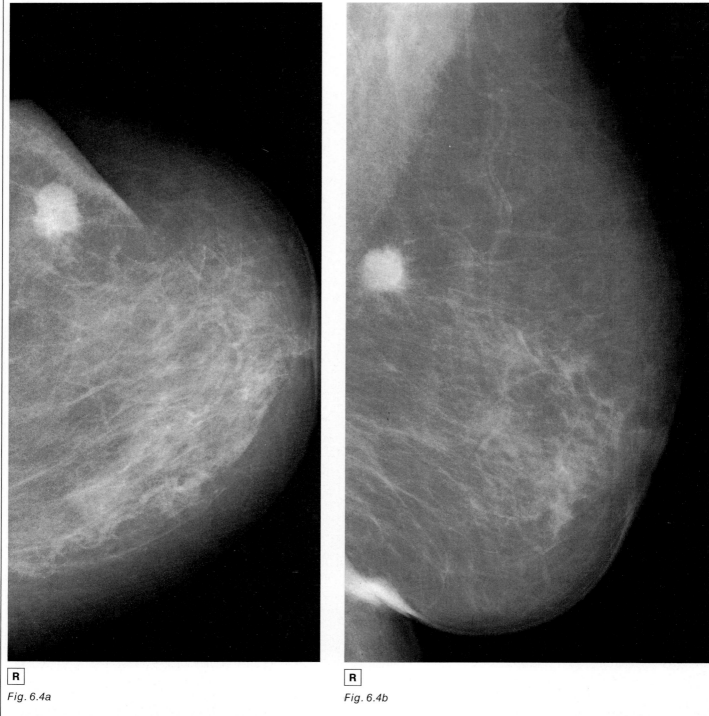

Fig. 6.4a

R

Fig. 6.4b

R

Fig. 6.4a & b   Mass with spiculated margin. Pathology: invasive ductal carcinoma: *a* shows craniocaudal view, *b* shows oblique view.

A mass with a spiculated ill-defined margin has a very high probability of being malignant (Figs 6.4, 6.5) (Andersson 1986). True spiculation of the margins of a mass should be distinguished from apparent spiculation caused by overlapping trabeculae. Coned compression and additional angled views are usually helpful (Fig. 6.6). Zuckerman (1986) has also stated that radiating tumour extensions are widest where they arise

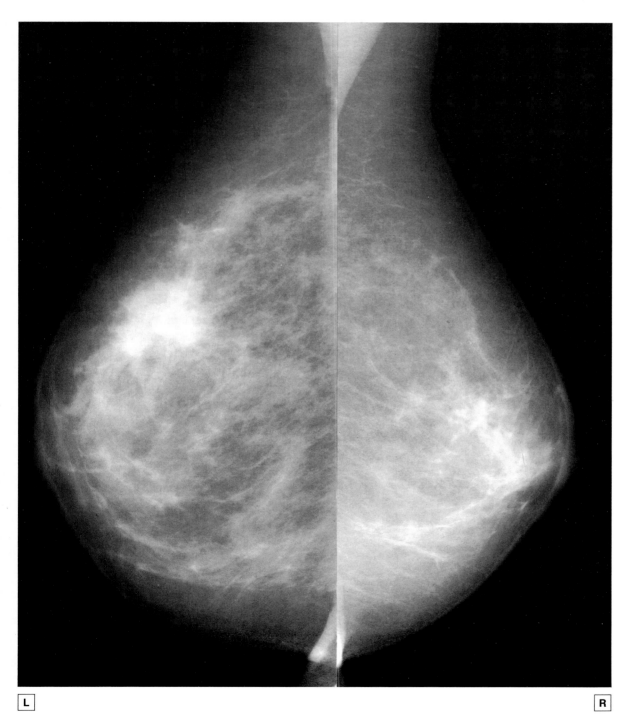

L

R

Fig. 6.5 Irregular dense mass. Pathology: invasive ductal carcinoma.

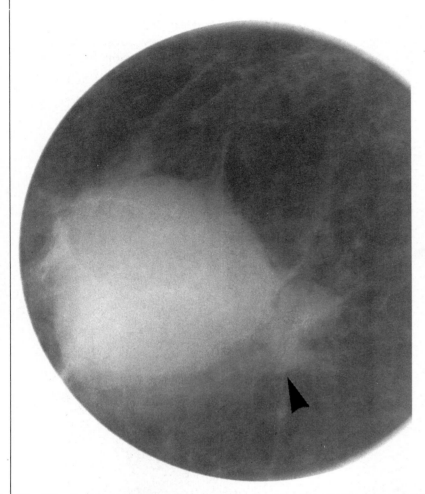

Fig. 6.6   Cysts with an adjacent carcinoma. Coned compression view showing two cysts adjacent to a small spiculate mass (arrowed). Pathology: two cysts and a small ductal carcinoma.

from the tumour margin and taper distally, unlike trabeculae which remain of the same diameter. Such trabeculae can be seen traversing a benign mass such as a cyst, rather than arising from the margin.

Differential diagnosis of a stellate lesion. A malignant stellate lesion has to be distinguished from a postoperative scar, radial scar, fat necrosis, or rarely resolving haematoma or abscess. These conditions are discussed in Chap. 7. On follow-up mammography, a postoperative scar should show either no change or regression, although after treatment with radiotherapy, some scars increase in density for at least 1 year.

Calcification

The accurate detection and assessment of microcalcifications is essential, as this is the only mammographic abnormality in up to 31% of screen-detected carcinomas (Andersson 1986). Mammographically detectable microcalcification is related to the uneven dystrophic calcification of necrotic intraductal debris (Barth 1979) and the active secretion of calcium particles into the duct lumen (Murphy & DeSchryver-Keckemeti 1978). There is considerable overlap in the histological appearance of the calcification seen in intraductal carcinoma and that in benign lesions (Rosen 1987). The use of magnification techniques is advocated by some (Sickles 1980) to assess the number and morphology of the microcalcifications.

Malignant calcifications have been shown to range from microscopic up to 2 mm in length (Sigfusson et al 1983), although microcalcification is defined as less than 1 mm in size. The conglomeration of microcalcifications can rarely produce the appearance of macrocalcification (Egan 1988). Malignant calcifications are often innumerable, irregular, tiny dot-like calcifications resembling grains of salt (Tabar & Dean 1985) (Figs 6.7–6.9).

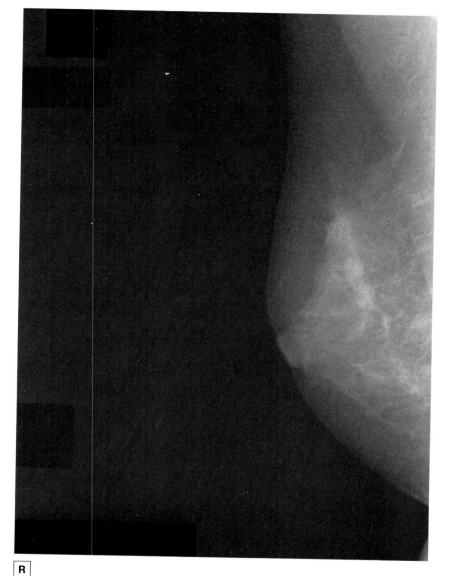

R

Fig. 6.7 Malignant punctate microcalcifications associated with a mass. Oblique view showing a 1 cm stellate mass in the right upper quadrant, with clustered punctate microcalcifications of irregular shape and density. Pathology: invasive ductal carcinoma.

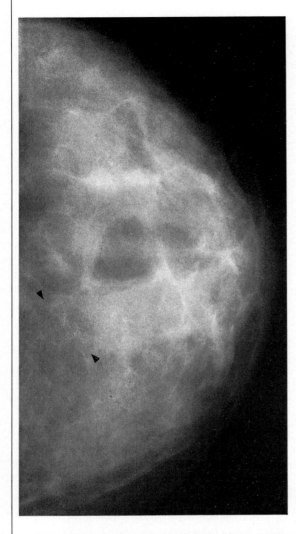

L

Fig. 6.8   Very fine punctate malignant microcalcifications (arrowed). Pathology: intraductal carcinoma.

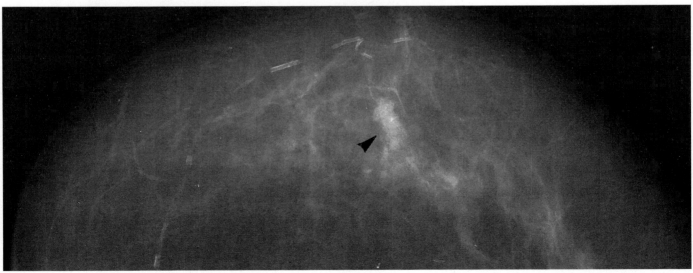

L

Fig. 6.9   Small mass with punctate calcifications (arrow). Note arterial calcification. Pathology: intraductal carcinoma.

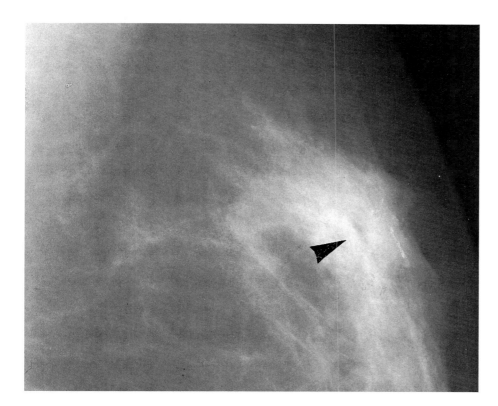

Other types are rod-like and linear or branching, forming casts of the duct lumen (Fig. 6.10). Branching is very suspicious for malignancy (Fig. 6.11).

L

Fig. 6.10 Clustered rod-shaped calcifications (arrow). Pathology: intraductal carcinoma.

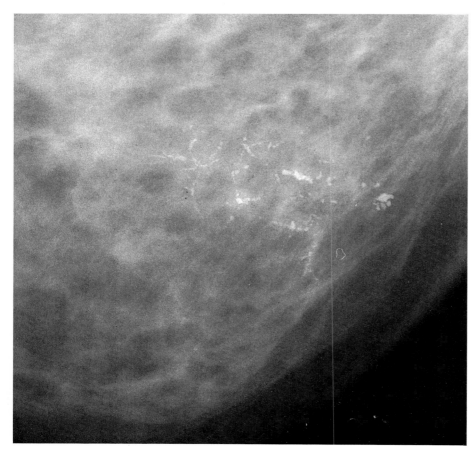

R

Fig. 6.11 Branching and rod-shaped calcifications. Pathology: intraductal comedo carcinoma.

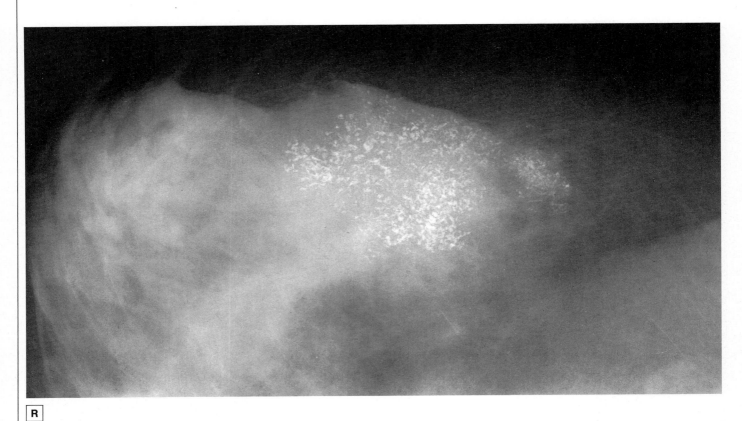

R

Fig. 6.12   Extensive branching and coalescent microcalcification. Extended craniocaudal view shows widespread casting calcification. Pathology: comedo carcinoma.

Number of calcifications. Most authorities require a minimum cluster of 5–10 microcalcifications before malignancy is suspected, although Homer (1985) has shown that as few as three grouped calcifications may be the only finding in some malignant lesions. Single specks of microcalcification, scattered widely throughout the breast, are often seen in benign conditions, and are not indicative of malignancy. However, carcinoma with minimal clinical signs can present as an extensive area of inumerable microcalcifications, sometimes occupying a whole segment or even more of the breast (Fig. 6.12). Extensive intraductal or comedo carcinoma may demonstrate a reticular pattern (Fig. 6.13). Freundlich et al (1989) noted that the probability of a malignancy increased with the number and proximity of particles within a cluster (Fig. 6.14). Multiple clusters of microcalcification are seen in multicentric carcinoma, both in-situ and invasive.

Configuration of calcium particles. Lanyi (1985) describes a triangular or trapezoid configuration for 65% of clusters of malignant microcalcifications, with the apex of the triangle directed towards the nipple. This is more obvious with larger clusters of calcifications. The triangle is not specific for carcinoma, and may be seen also in mammary duct ectasia. It is thought that the triangular shape results from a cast of the lactiferous ducts.

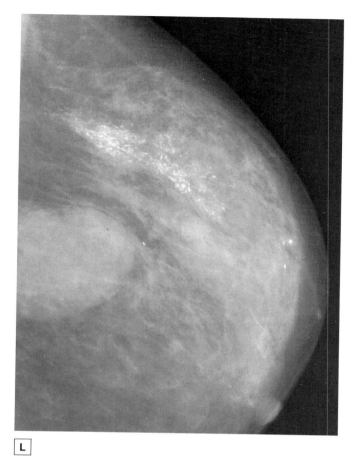

L

Fig. 6.13 Reticular calcification. Note large well-circumscribed mass posteriorly which is a cyst. Pathology: cyst and intraductal carcinoma.

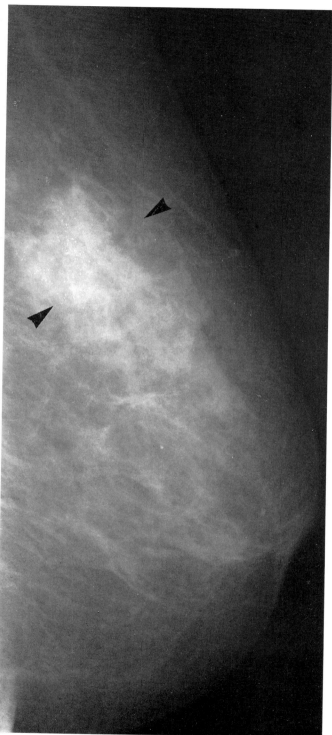

L

Fig. 6.14 Extensive fine punctate malignant microcalcification with an increase in parenchymal density (arrows). Cytology: malignant cells.

Associated mass. Fine irregular granular and duct casting microcalcifications are considered highly suspicious for malignancy if they are associated with a mass (Fig. 6.15). A purely intraductal in-situ tumour will not produce any mammographic abnormality except calcification or occasionally irregularly dilated ducts and lobules, and the presence of a mass on mammography implies an *invasive* component. A benign appearance to the mass is irrelevant if the calcification is suspicious of malignancy, as carcinomas may rarely arise in a fibroadenoma (Tabar & Dean 1985) and a ductal carcinoma may have a circumscribed appearance. Calcification within a fibroadenoma is usually larger than 0.4 mm; malignant calcifications tend to show a more asymmetric location within circumscribed nodules than in fibroadenomas (Mitnick et al 1989). The calcification may be within the mass or in an adjacent intraductal site (Fig. 6.16). Carcinoma and fibroadenoma may well occur synchronously.

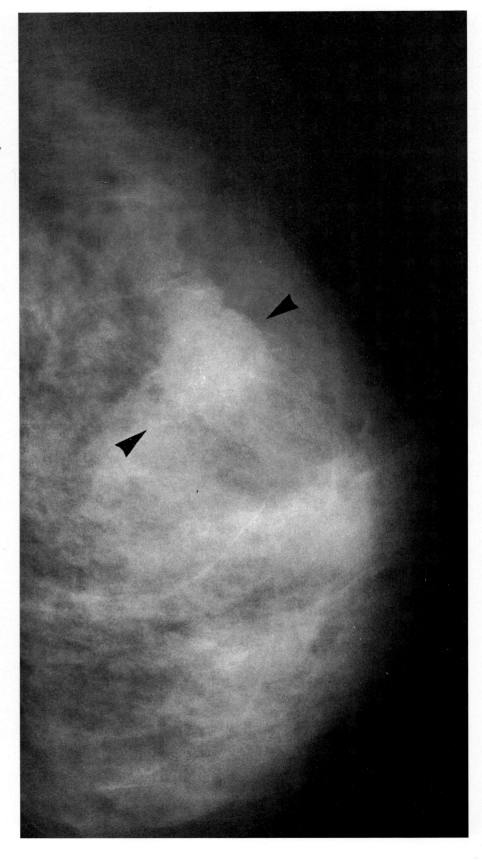

L

Fig. 6.15 Punctate and rod-like microcalcification in an irregular mass, against a background of dense stroma (arrows). Pathology: invasive ductal carcinoma.

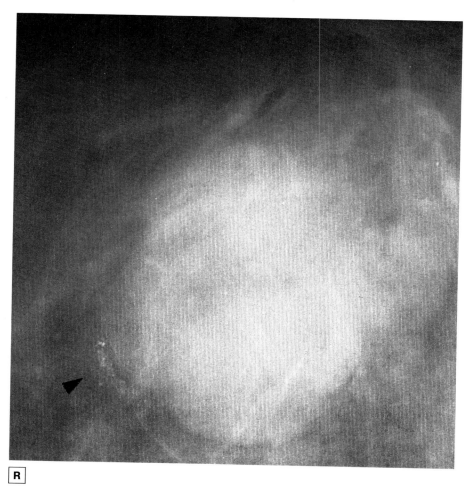

R

Fig. 6.16 Calcification separate from a malignant mass. Well-circumscribed lobulate mass with a partial thin 'halo'. Intraductal calcification (arrow) is adjacent but separate from the mass. Cytology: malignant cells.

Architectural distortion

The cicatrizing nature of breast carcinomas is related to their elastic tissue component, and tumours at the margin of dense fibroglandular tissue may be detected by infolding or 'tenting' (Tabar & Dean 1985) of the parenchymal/fat interface (Fig. 6.17). The tumour itself may be obscured by the density of the adjacent fibroglandular tissue. Progression of this fibroelastic retraction leads to skin puckering, nipple inversion, and in advanced cases the whole breast may become smaller.

Straightening or divergence of fibrous trabeculae may be the only sign of a desmoplastic process associated with a malignant tumour. These trabeculae arise from the deep layer of the enveloping fascia and normally arc forward to converge on the nipple.

Parenchymal asymmetry

Asymmetrical density of the breast parenchyma is best appreciated by comparison with the contralateral breast (Figs 6.18, 6.19). Asymmetry in the axillary region may occur as a normal variant (Fig. 5.11, p. 78), but is suspicious if associated with a palpable abnormality (Martin et al 1979) and if the area is of increased or variable density (Paulus 1987).

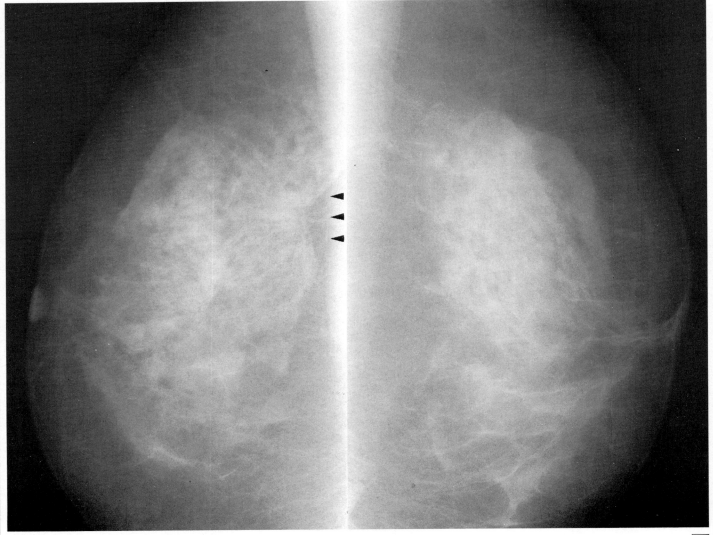

R   L

Fig. 6.17   Indrawing of parenchyma (arrowed). The indrawing overlies a 1 cm mass. Pathology: ductal carcinoma.

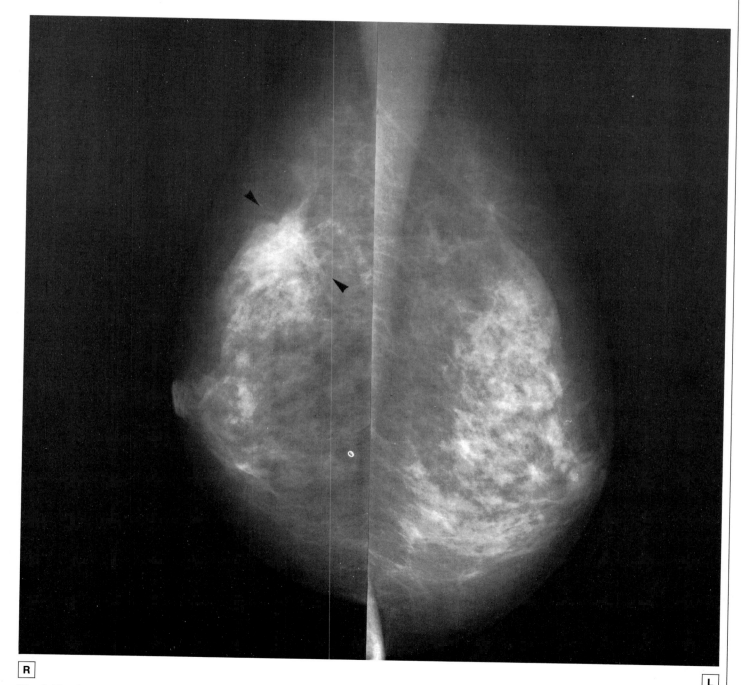

R   L

Fig. 6.18   Asymmetry of density. There is a dense irregular mass at the superior aspect of the fibroglandular tissue of the right breast (arrowed). Pathology: invasive ductal carcinoma.

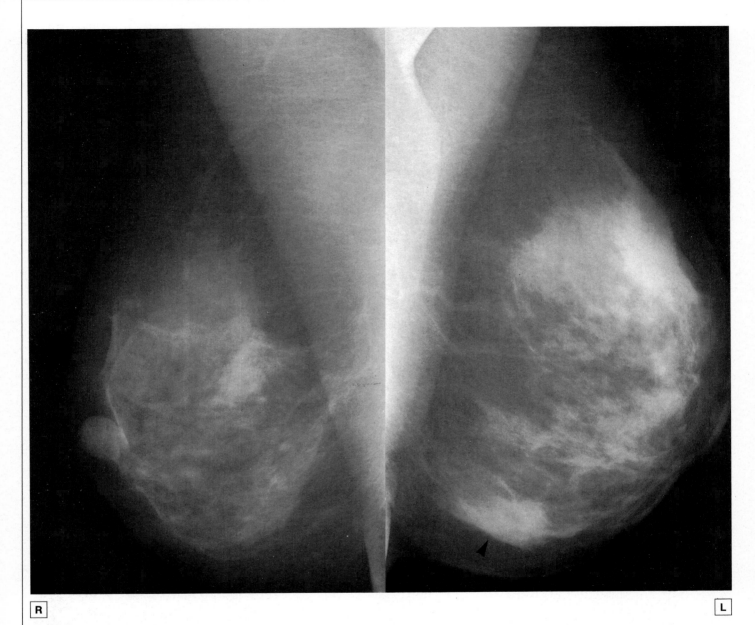

R   L

Fig. 6.19a

Fig. 6.19   Parenchymal asymmetry. *a* In the left breast inferiorly, there is an area of asymmetrically increased density with a straight margin (arrow). *b* Craniocaudal views reveal a 3 cm relatively well-circumscribed mass medially in the left breast (arrowed). Pathology: invasive ductal carcinoma with foci of in-situ ductal carcinoma in an area of sclerosing adenosis.

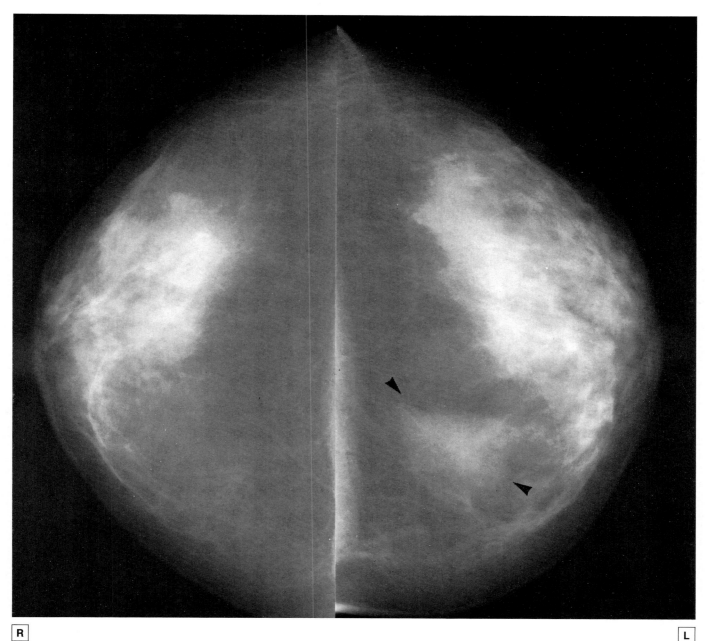

R L

Fig. 6.19b

Ducts

Dilatation of retroareolar ducts is most frequently due to mammary duct ectasia. A solitary enlarged duct or lobe of ducts is an unusual appearance and may be due to obstruction by a papilloma (Fig. 7.29, p. 148; Fig. 7.30, p. 149) or, rarely, by an intraduct carcinoma (Sadowsky & Kopans 1983). Occasionally, a localized segment of duct dilatation may be a sign of malignant disease (Fig. 6.20).

Rarely, a prominent duct pattern in one breast with a normal pattern in the contralateral breast may be associated with carcinoma.

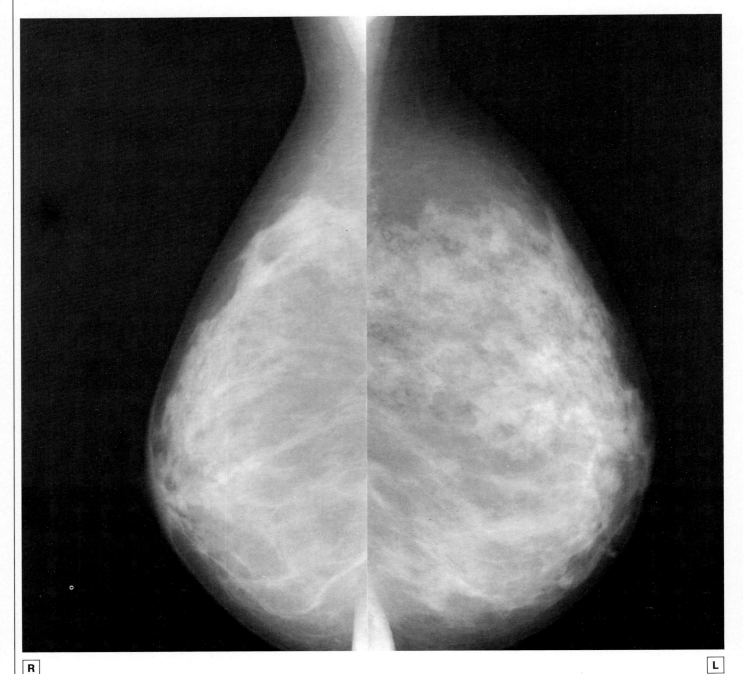

R   L

Fig. 6.20   Asymmetry of ductal pattern. Extensive abnormal ductal pattern superiorly in the left breast. Pathology: extensive intraductal carcinoma.

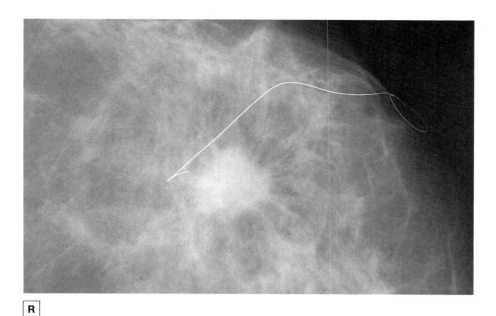

R

Fig. 6.21a

Peritumoral corona

Malignant lesions may show a broad indistinct 'pseudolipomatous' (Gravelle 1980) radiolucent zone at the margin of the tumour, associated with contraction of the malignant tumour mass (Fig. 6.21). This 'corona' is seen only when fat surrounds the tumour, and may reflect a similar type of optical illusion to the Mach effect (Gordenne & Malchair 1988). This peritumoral corona is quite different from the narrow band of lucency or 'halo' that may be seen around very well-defined, predominantly benign, lesions (Fig. 7.4, p. 124).

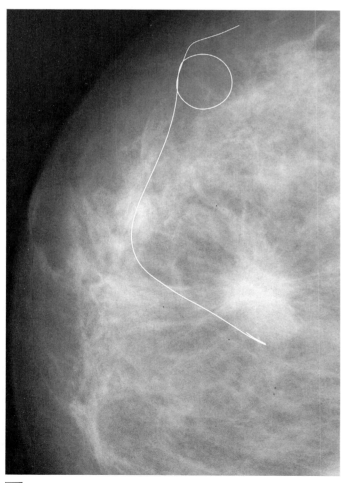

R

Fig. 6.21b

Fig. 6.21a & b Peritumoral corona.
A 4.5 cm impalpable carcinoma showing typical spiculation and a wide corona of fat. Localization wire present prior to excision. Pathology: invasive ductal carcinoma.

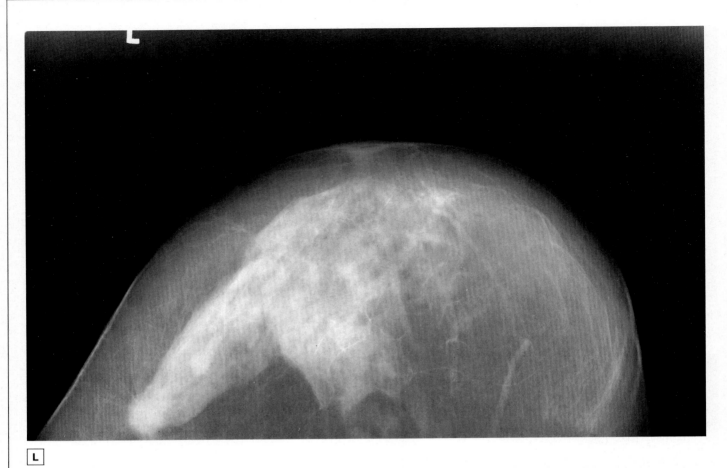

Fig. 6.22   Localized skin thickening ('drawing pin' sign). A 1.5 cm spiculate mass with stranding to thickened skin. Cytology: malignant cells.

Skin changes

The skin is usually less than 1.5 mm thick, with the maximal thickness at the inframammary fold (Gold et al 1987). Localized skin retraction and thickening of fibrous strands may be seen with the scirrhous type of carcinoma (Fig. 6.22), producing the 'drawing pin' sign (Baclesse & Willemin 1967). High-intensity illumination may be required to demonstrate this secondary sign of malignancy. Skin thickening or retraction not seen tangentially on the mammogram will appear as a band of increased density similar to a fold of skin (Fig. 6.23).

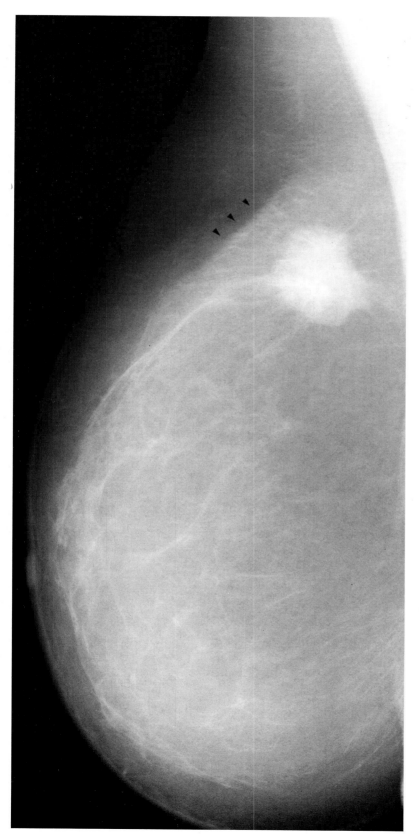

R

Fig. 6.23 Band of skin thickening. There is a 2.5 cm spiculate mass with an overlying band shadow of folded retracted skin (arrows) in the right axillary tail region. Pathology: ductal carcinoma.

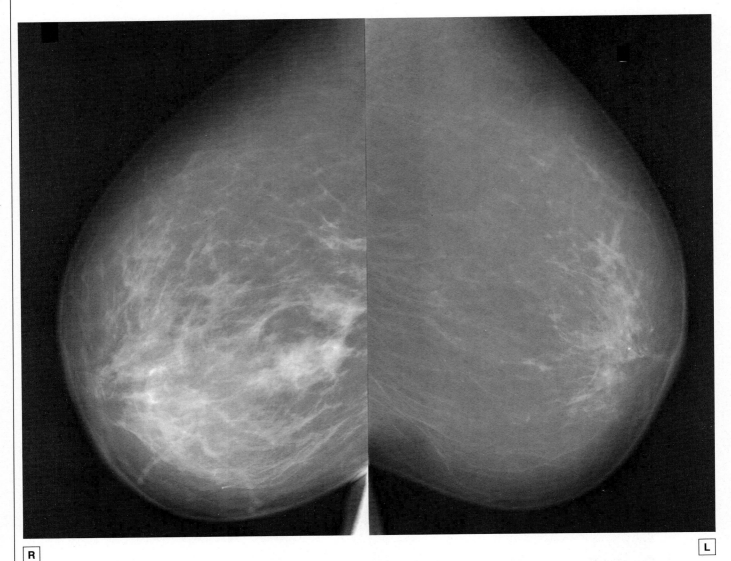

R

L

Fig. 6.24   Generalized skin thickening. There is an irregular mass deep in the right breast with skin thickening and thickened trabeculae. Pathology: ductal carcinoma.

Cross-lymphatic metastasis from a malignancy in the contralateral breast is another cause of localized skin thickening. This is the commonest type of metastasis to the breast, and occurs via peristernal lymphatics particularly when the primary lesion is extensive, ulcerated or inflammatory in nature. The earliest sign is of skin thickening on the medial aspect of the breast, best seen on the craniocaudal view (Paulus & Libshitz 1982). Diffuse skin thickening may be seen with oedema and extensive tumour infiltration (Fig. 6.24). Distended subcutaneous lymphatics may be apparent (Fig. 6.25).

Inflammatory carcinoma. In this condition there is diffuse lymphoedema due to extensive lymphatic obstruction and infiltration with tumour cells (Burstein 1983, Rosen 1987). It is not specific for any one tumour type, but is seen most commonly in poorly differentiated infiltrating ductal carcinomas (Rosen 1987). The clinical presentation mimics that of acute inflammation, and the tumour is often difficult to palpate although it is commonly larger than 4 cm and multifocal. Mammographically the tumour mass is frequently obscured by the generalized increase in density. This will be best appreciated by comparison with the contralateral breast.

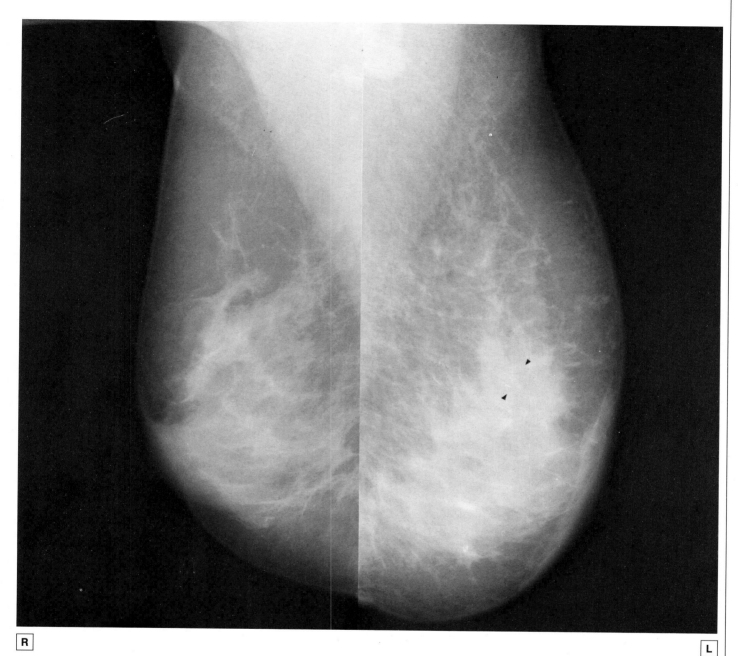

R

L

Fig. 6.25 Generalized skin thickening. A 75-year-old woman presenting with a swollen breast. There is enlargement of the left breast with skin thickening and extensive oedema of the trabeculae. Note oedema of the lymphatics in the subcutaneous fat, and malignant microcalcification (arrow) superior to the left nipple. Pathology: ductal carcinoma.

Other causes of generalized skin thickening in the breast include postradiotherapy change (Dershaw et al 1987), axillary lymphatic obstruction, obstruction to the venous return from the breast, and heart failure (Kaufman 1984). Lymphoma of the breast can also cause skin thickening, and infections such as tuberculosis must be considered.

Nipple changes

Nipple retraction may be due to traction on the nipple by an underlying carcinoma. However, congenital nipple inversion is common particularly in women with large pendulous breasts (Rothenberg 1986). Acquired nipple retraction is most commonly related to benign conditions such as mammary duct ectasia (Love et al 1987) (Fig. 7.39, p. 161; Fig. 7.41, p. 164). Enlargement of the nipple may be seen in Paget's disease, basal cell carcinoma and squamous carcinoma of the nipple and areola (Haagensen 1986). There may be associated ulceration and calcification. In some cases of Paget's disease the underlying ductal carcinoma may be demonstrated mammographically.

Malignant disorders rarely cause a nipple discharge (Devitt 1986). Haagensen (1986) states that the discharge associated with a ductal carcinoma is usually blood-stained, although clear and serosanguinous discharges have been described. If mammography is normal, the investigation of a persistent blood-stained discharge should include ultrasound and possibly galactography.

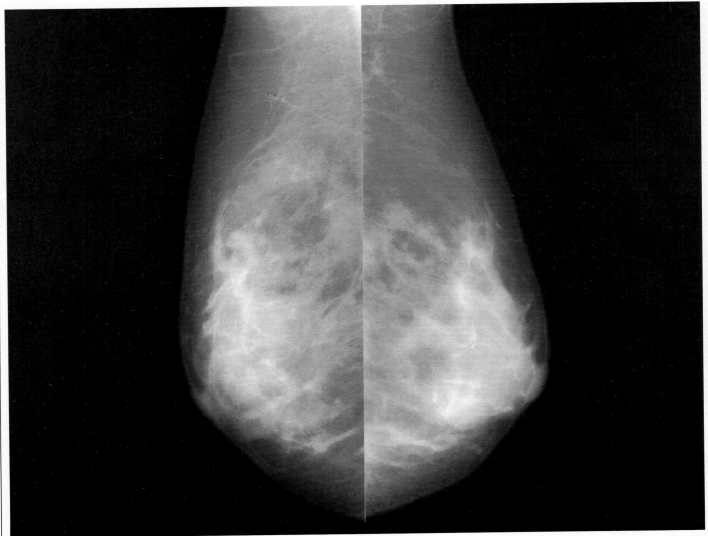

R   L

Fig. 6.26a

Fig. 6.26 Lobular carcinoma. *a* Architectural distortion in the upper half of the right breast with associated straightening of the trabeculae and early skin thickening. *b* Craniocaudal views show irregular poorly defined mass (arrow) deep in the right breast centrally. Note the large vessel inferiorly and medially in the right breast, representing a 'look again' sign. Pathology: invasive lobular carcinoma.

Axillary nodes

Axillary nodes may be considered suspicious of metastatic involvement in the presence of other mammographic abnormalities if they are greater than 2.5 cm in diameter, round and dense. Enlarged nodes are a non-specific finding commonly associated with infection, dermatological conditions and rheumatoid arthritis. Axillary nodes may enlarge in medullary carcinoma as a reactive phenomenon, without nodal metastases, which may lead to confusion in clinical staging (Rosen 1987). The presence of mammographically normal lymph nodes showing fatty replacement does not exclude their involvement with tumour.

Vascularity

Asymmetry of the veins has no diagnostic significance (Mitnick et al 1989) since the degree of venous distension varies with the menstrual cycle and the amount of compression applied. However, it does represent a 'look again' sign and should be noted in conjunction with other findings (Fig. 6.26).

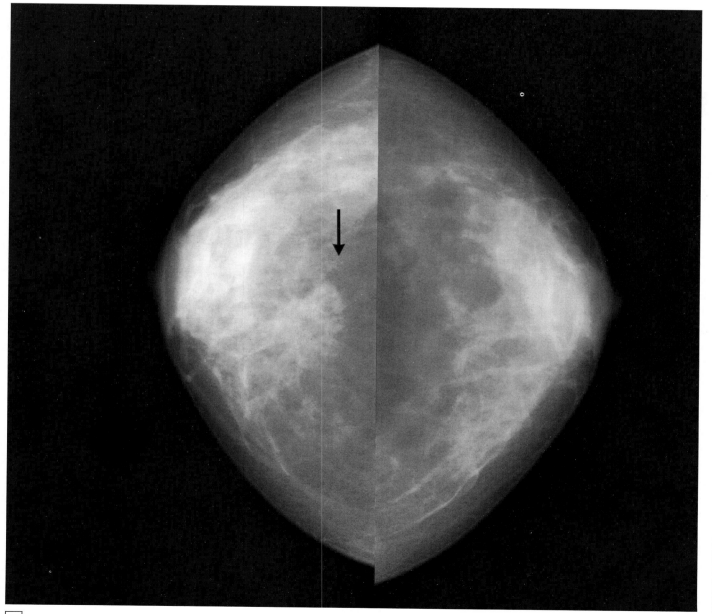

R   L

Fig. 6.26b

The following mammographic features of a mass may be of help in distinguishing a malignant from a benign lesion, but are not in themselves discriminatory.

Location of the mass. Approximately 50% of malignant lesions occur in the upper outer quadrant and may be obscured by delayed involution of the glandular parenchyma in this area (Zuckermann 1986). An extended craniocaudal view may be required to include the entire area on the film. Approximately one-quarter of malignant tumours occur in the central or subareolar region, and only 5% in the lower inner quadrant (O'Higgins 1984).

Outline and density of the mass. The more lobulated the mass, the more suspicious of malignancy. Malignant masses may appear too dense for their size (Moskowitz 1983).

Size of the mass. The size of a lesion is non-discriminatory between benign and malignant, except that the desmoplastic reaction around many carcinomas results in a tumour which feels much larger than it is mammographically (Zuckermann 1986).

Age of patient. Malignant disease increases wih age (Forrest 1986) and even well-circumscribed masses must be considered suspicious in the postmenopausal population. However, benign disease is still more common than malignant disease up to the age of 75 (Devitt 1986) and tissue diagnosis is as important in this age group as in others.

Multiple lesions. In the presence of multiple lesions, each must be considered on its own merit, as carcinomas do occur in the presence of multicystic disease and other, obviously benign, conditions (Fig. 6.6, p. 88; Fig. 7.19, p. 137).

TYPES OF BREAST MALIGNANCY

Ductal carcinoma-in-situ. 60% of intraductal carcinomas will contain calcification (Egan 1988). This tumour is rarely palpable and therefore dependent on mammographically visible microcalcifications for detection. Occasionally extensive tumour may cause a palpable ridge of breast thickening. Pathologically the lesion begins as an atypical epithelial proliferation that progresses to distend the duct with tumour cells (Robbins 1984). The epithelial cells may grow in a comedo, cribriform or papillary fashion (Teng 1986). The tumour may extend to fill a quadrant or more of the breast without evidence of invasion, as in comedo carcinoma. Invasive intraductal carcinoma occurs when the basement membrane is breached by tumour cells, and metastases may occur.

Lobular carcinoma-in-situ. The detection of lobular carcinoma-in-situ is incidental to the biopsy of another benign or malignant process (Martin et al 1979, Pope et al 1988). It is responsible for 1–6% of all carcinomas (Rosen 1987) and 30% of non-invasive carcinomas. The tumour develops in small and dispersed lobules, does not show any mammographic or clinical abnormality, and is frequently multifocal. There is an increased incidence of invasive ductal and lobular carcinoma, and vigilant follow-up is essential as there is a six- to ninefold increase in either breast (Haagensen 1986).

Invasive ductal carcinoma, not otherwise specified. At least 75% of breast carcinomas are of this type (Teng 1986). The epithelial : stromal ratio is very variable, although the stroma is usually extensive. The peak age of incidence is in the late 50s. The neoplastic epithelial cells form cords of cells and structures similar to glands and tubules which grow in a fibrous and elastic stroma. It is this fibrous stroma that causes the desmoplastic clinical and mammographic signs characteristic of these tumours, regardless of their histological type. Calcification is detected in up to 60% of tumours, representing dystrophic calcification in necrotic cellular debris, and cellular secretion of calcium particles (Ahmed 1975). Frequently the fibrotic mass is so radiographically dense that the microcalcifications are obscured and are only detected on the specimen radiograph (Egan 1988). Calcification will be much less likely to show in underpenetrated films.

Tubular carcinoma. This is a rare tumour, accounting for 2% of all breast carcinomas. Tubular carcinomas are small tumours with a mean size of 0.95 cm, presenting as a small stellate tumour or as clustered microcalcification (Feig et al 1978). Histologically the tumour is composed of well-differentiated neoplastic elements resembling tubules and ductules (Rosen 1987). The tumour tubules are dispersed irregularly in a dense collagenous and elastic stroma to produce an ill-defined infiltrating margin. Up to 60% contain mammographically detectable microcalcifications in the neoplastic tubules.

Invasive lobular carcinoma. The mean age at diagnosis is 57 years, which is similar to that for women with invasive ductal carcinoma (Rosen 1987). Invasive lobular carcinoma is frequently seen as an asymmetric increased density without distinct borders (Fig. 6.26). There is a range of mammographic abnormalities from indistinct architectural distortions and densities (Gold et al 1987) to more dense confluent tumour deposits with ill-defined or 'wispy' borders (Mendelson et al 1989). The ill-defined outline reflects the infiltrative behaviour of the tumour cells, which are widely dispersed in the tumour stroma. Lines of tumour cells permeate the breast parenchyma without forming a central tumour nidus. There are no specific mammographic signs to distinguish categorically between these various histological types, and there is considerable overlap in the mammographic appearances.

Circumscribed carcinomas

Masses with a sharply defined margin will have an approximately 2% chance of being malignant (Moskowitz 1983, Ciatto et al 1987). Only 0.7% of breast cancers are completely smooth, and 15% are partially smooth (Barth 1979). Fig. 6.27 shows a well-circumscribed mass representing an invasive ductal carcinoma. Careful inspection of the margins may reveal small fine hair-like projections from the tumour mass into the surrounding tissue (Fig. 6.28). Coned compression and magnification views may assist in

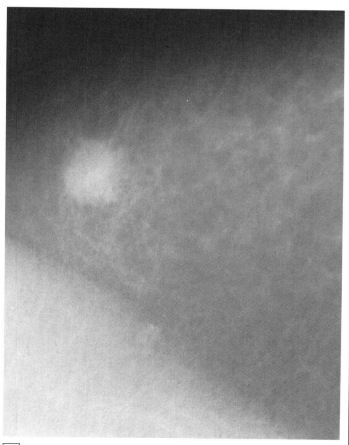

L

Fig. 6.28 Fine tumour projections. Extended craniocaudal view showing fine irregular margin to a 1.5 cm relatively well-circumscribed mass in the axillary tail. Pathology: invasive ductal carcinoma.

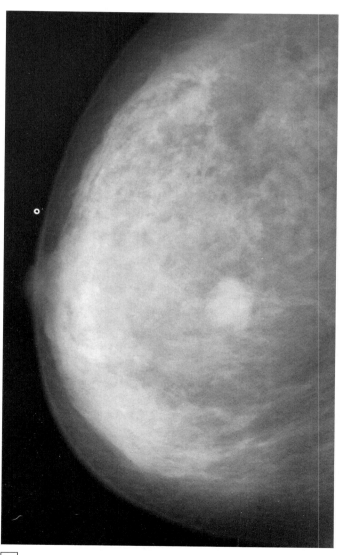

R

Fig. 6.27 Well-circumscribed carcinoma. Pathology: invasive ductal carcinoma.

differentiating these tumour 'comet tails' (Tabar & Dean 1985) from overlapping parenchyma (Sickles 1980). Cellular tumours such as medullary and mucinous carcinomas, and a small proportion of simple invasive ductal tumours, have little stroma and grow in a nodular fashion, displacing the surrounding parenchyma to give an apparently smooth outline on mammography (Barth 1979, Feig 1986).

Medullary carcinoma. Medullary carcinoma constitutes less than 5% of malignancies, and occurs more frequently in the younger age group than ductal carcinoma, accounting for 11% of lesions in women aged 35 or less (Meyer et al 1989). Mammographically these lesions are most often round or oval, often with lobulated margins, uncalcified and homogeneous in density (Fig. 6.29). A partial or complete 'halo sign' may be present (Swann et al 1987, Meyer et al 1989).

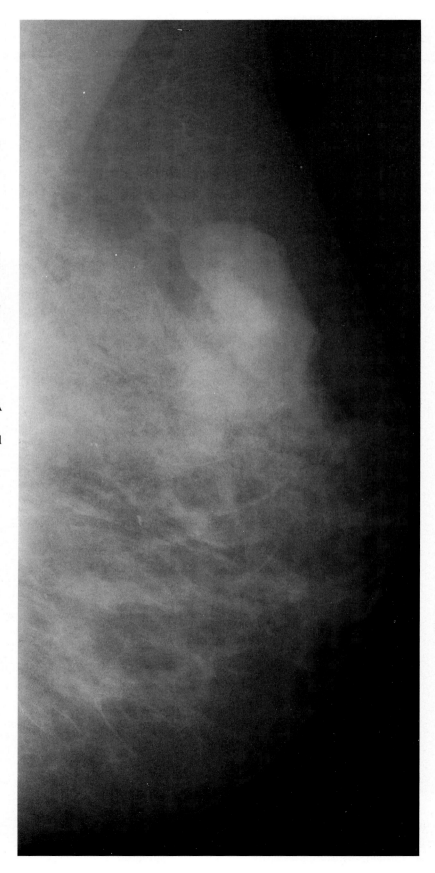

L

Fig. 6.29 Medullary carcinoma. Very well-defined 3 cm mass with surrounding partial lucent halo.

Mucinous carcinoma. This tumour constitutes 1–4% of all breast carcinomas and is seen more frequently in older patients (Haagensen 1986). Clinically the tumour is often soft and ill-defined, and mammographically it appears relatively well-defined, usually without calcification or evidence of a desmoplastic response (Sadowsky & Kopans 1983). Pathologically the tumour consists of groups of carcinoma cells surrounded by abundant mucin (Teng 1986).

Carcinoma in benign lesions. Carcinomas, particularly lobular carcinoma-in-situ (see p. 108), may develop in ductal and lobular tissue which has previously undergone some benign change such as sclerosing adenosis, radial scar, fibroadenosis or cyst formation. This is a very rare occurrence, with carcinoma being reported in less than 0.5% of fibroadenomas (Rosen 1987).

Intracystic carcinoma. A rare occurrence, intracystic carcinoma derives from an intraductal malignancy when it obstructs its duct of origin to form a cyst (Rosen 1987). Repeated haemorrhage and haemosiderin deposition may cause the cyst to appear mammographically denser than expected for its size. The density of the blood-stained cyst contents often prevents the mammographic detection of the associated microcalcifications which are seen pathologically (Egan 1988). Such tumours may reach a large size while remaining confined to the cyst wall. Extracystic extension with invasion of the adjacent tissues must be suspected if the cyst wall is flattened, lobulated or shows an irregular margin (Sadowsky & Kopans 1983).

Lymphoma (Fig. 6.30). Primary non-Hodgkin lymphoma of the breast accounts for 0.5% of breast malignancy (Paulus & Libshitz 1982). Lymphomatous and leukaemic breast deposits most commonly arise as part of a disseminated or multicentric disease process (Meyer et al 1980), but rarely they may present as a primary breast lesion, constituting approximately 0.25% of all breast tumours (Ariel & Caron 1986). Mammography reveals increased stromal density, skin thickening (which may be pronounced), circumscribed nodular masses, and enlarged axillary lymph nodes in 50% of patients (Millis et al 1976, Paulus & Libshitz 1982).

Fig. 6.30 Lymphoma of the breast. A 50-year-old woman with left breast mass and axillary lymphadenopathy. *a* Oblique view: there is a 4 cm oval mass superior to the left nipple, with increased density of the breast parenchyma and blurring of the stroma suggesting the presence of generalized oedema. *b* Axial CT scan: bilateral axillary lymph node enlargement. *c* Axial CT scan 3 cm inferior to *b*: large mass in the left breast and axillary lymph node enlargement. Pathology: non-Hodgkin lymphoma.

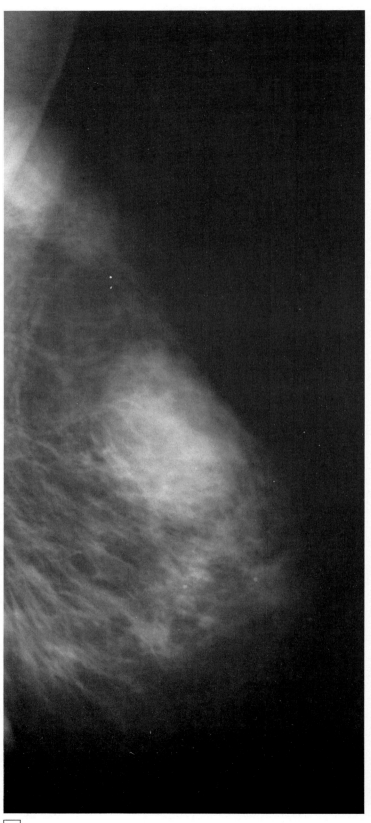

L

Fig. 6.30a

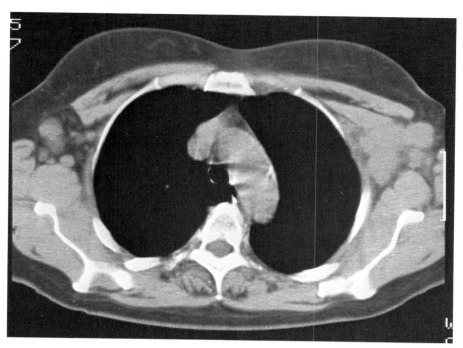

Fig. 6.30b

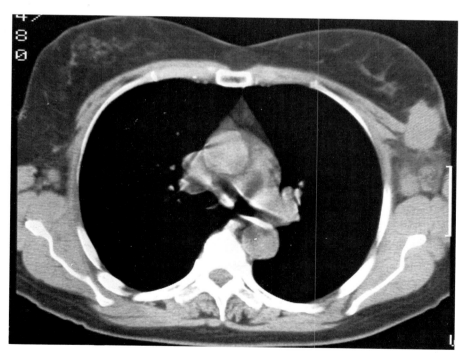

Fig. 6.30c

Second primary lesions. The reported incidence of bilateral primary carcinomas is 7.9–12% of all breast cancer patients (Cody & Urban 1986), with synchronous bilateral carcinoma in 1–2.9% of patients at presentation. Follow-up screening of the contralateral breast of a patient with a known breast carcinoma is advisable because a developing suspicious mass or calcifications are much more likely to represent a second primary lesion than a metastasis.

Metaplastic carcinoma. Squamous and sarcomatous metaplasia may be seen in invasive ductal carcinoma, primary breast sarcoma, and some phylloides tumours. It is often associated with poorly diferentiated tumours (Rosen 1987) and therefore the presence of bone and cartilage elements on histology or mammography may indicate a less favourable outcome. Usually this is a purely histological finding, but occasionally coarse and amorphous calcifications may be detected mammographically (Thompson & Machin 1989), emphasizing the fact that the presence of benign-looking calcification in association with a suspicious mass mammographically or clinically does not exclude malignancy. Metaplastic carcinoma constitutes 0.2% of breast carcinomas (Thompson & Machin 1989).

Sarcoma. Fibrosarcomas are the most common primary breast sarcomas, accounting for approximately 1% of breast malignancies (D'Orsi et al 1983). These tumours produce masses similar to fibroadenomas, which rapidly increase in size and which may show poorly defined margins consistent with areas of local infiltration (Millis et al 1976).

Male breast carcinoma. Carcinoma of the male breast constitutes approximately 1% of breast carcinomas (Crichlow & Evans 1986). The peak age of incidence is in the fifth and sixth decades, and therefore it is unlikely to be mistaken for the transitory benign gynaecomastia often encountered in the adolescent male. Mammographically these tumours present all the signs of malignancy previously described. The tumour is often at an advanced stage by the time of presentation due to diagnostic delay and the small volume of breast tissue which is rapidly infiltrated (Crichlow & Evans 1986). The differential diagnosis includes benign idiopathic gynaecomastia, and drug-related breast enlargement, particularly associated with chronic digitalis administration and oestrogen-related compounds in the treatment of prostatic carcinoma (Zuckerman 1986).

Multiple lesions. Occasionally multiple well-defined masses in the breast represent metastases from primary malignant lesions elsewhere in the body (D'Orsi et al 1983). In one-third of these patients this may be the first manifestation of an otherwise occult extramammary malignant tumour, most commonly melanoma (Ariel & Caron 1986) or bronchial carcinoma (Fig. 6.31).

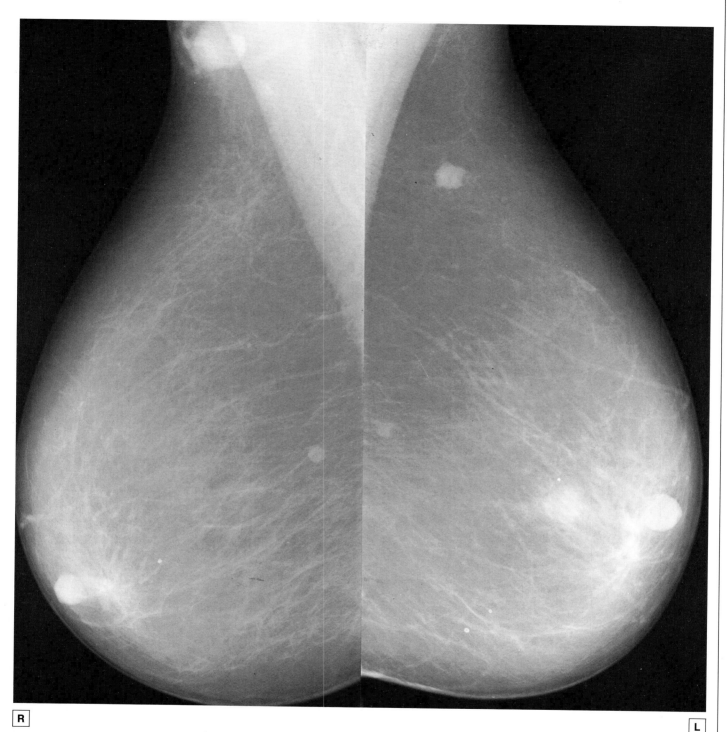

R

L

Fig. 6.31 Metastases to the breast. Bilateral rounded intramammary masses. Note the nipples are not in profile, but this should not cause diagnostic confusion. Autopsy: bronchial carcinoma with widespread metastases including those in the breast.

Multicentric carcinoma. This is a well-recognized phenomenon, and is seen particularly in screening programmes. Up to 10 small (less than 1 cm diameter) spiculate masses may be seen. These masses are usually of similar size, and each represents invasive disease. Multiple small clusters of microcalcification may be another manifestation of multicentric carcinoma (Fig. 6.32), and may occupy either a segment or sometimes the whole of the breast. This may represent invasive or in-situ ductal carcinoma, or a combination of the two. The cluster formation is important in the differentiation from benign microcalcification.

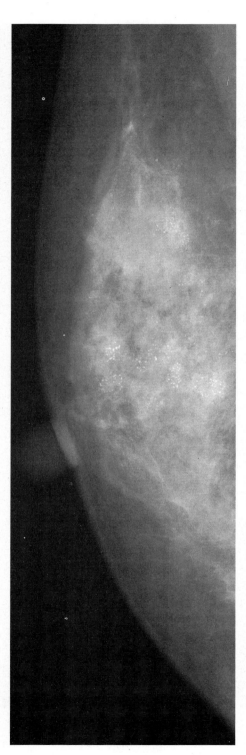

L

Fig. 6.32 Multicentric carcinoma. Chinese woman of 42 presenting with breast pain, presumably coincidental. Mammogram shows multiple small clusters of microcalcification. The clusters are unusually round, but the particles within each are irregular. Pathology: invasive and in-situ ductal carcinoma.

Multifocal disease. This is not uncommon, and is an important factor in the consideration of localized resection. Small foci of carcinoma can occur up to 3 cm from the presenting tumour mass. These may be microscopic, but may well show as small irregular masses, sometimes connected to the primary mass by fine strands (Fig. 6.33). Traces of microcalcification may also be seen, extending in the lines of ducts from the primary tumour.

PROGNOSTIC FACTORS

The most important factor in the prognosis of breast carcinoma is the metastatic potential of the tumour and the involvement of the axillary nodes, neither of which can be determined from the mammogram. Circumscribed tumours have a better outcome than infiltrating, scirrhous or inflammatory tumours (Burstein 1983). Multiplicity of sites and histological types is associated with a poorer prognosis (Egan 1988). The size of the tumour on pathology is generally considered a significant prognostic variable (Burstein 1983), but must be interrelated with histological type and differentiation. Medullary and mucinous carcinomas may reach a diameter of 5 cm without significantly worsening prognosis.

Acknowledgements
We wish to thank Dr John Sloane for his advice, and Dr Kate Walmesley for her permission to include Figures.

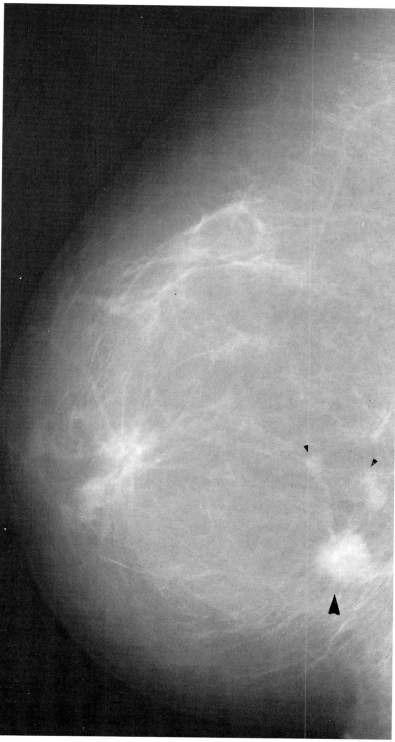

R

Fig. 6.33 Multifocal carcinoma. A typical spiculate opacity (large arrow), but surrounded by several small irregular opacities (small arrows), with some stranding to the main mass. Pathology: carcinoma with multiple foci of invasive disease.

REFERENCES

Ahmed A 1975 Calcification in human breast carcinomas: ultrastructural observations. Journal of Pathology 117: 247–251

Andersson I 1981 Radiographic screening for breast carcinoma III: Appearance of carcinoma and number of projections to be used at screening. Acta Radiologica Diagnosis 22: 407–420

Andersson I 1986 Medical radiography and photography 62 (2), Kodak publication, pp 1–39

Ariel I M, Caron A S 1986 Sarcomas and other unusual cancers of the breast. In: Ariel I M, Cleary J B (eds) Breast cancer diagnosis and treatment. McGraw-Hill, New York

Baclesse F, Willemin A 1967 Atlas of mammography. Libraire de Facultes, Paris

Barth V 1979 Atlas of diseases of the breast. Georg Thieme, Stuttgart

Burstein N A 1983 Pathology of breast cancer. In: D'Orsi C J, Wilson R E (eds) Carcinoma of the breast: diagnosis and treatment. Little, Brown & Co, Boston

Ciatto S, Cataliotti L, Distante V 1987 Nonpalpable lesions detected with mammography: review of 512 consecutive cases. Radiology 165: 99–102

Cody H S, Urban J A 1986 The opposite breast. In: Ariel I M, Cleary J B (eds) Breast cancer diagnosis and treatment. McGraw-Hill, New York

Crichlow R W, Evans D B 1986 Cancer in the male breast. In: Ariel I, Cleary J B (eds) Breast cancer diagnosis and treatment. McGraw-Hill, New York

Dershaw D D, Shank B, Reisinger S 1987 Mammographic findings after breast cancer treatment with local excision and definitive irradiation. Radiology 164: 455–461

Devitt J E 1986 Benign breast lesions in older women. Surgery, Gynecology and Obstetrics 162: 340–342

D'Orsi C J, Feldhaus L, Sonnenfeld M 1983 Unusual lesions of the breast. Radiologic Clinics of North America 21(1): 67–80

Egan R L 1988 Breast Imaging: Diagnosis and morphology of breast disease. W B Saunders, Philadelphia

Feig S A, Shaber G S, Patchefsky A S et al 1978 Tubular carcinoma of the breast. Radiology 129: 311–314

Feig S A 1986 The Breast. In: Grainger R, Allison D (eds) Diagnostic radiology: an Anglo-American textbook of imaging. Churchill Livingstone, Edinburgh, pp 1631–1668

Forrest P 1986 In: Breast cancer screening. Report to the Health Ministers of England, Wales, Scotland and Northern Ireland by a working group chaired by Professor Sir Patrick Forrest. Her Majesty's Stationary Office, London

Freundlich I M, Hunter T B, Seeley G W et al 1989 Computer-assisted analysis of mammographic clustered calcifications. Clinical Radiology 40: 295–298

Gold R H, Bassett L W, Coulson W F 1987 Mammographic features of malignant and benign disease. In: Bassett L W, Gold R H (eds) Breast cancer detection. Grune & Stratton, Orlando, pp 15–51

Gordenne W H, Malchair F L 1988 Mach bands in mammography. Radiology 169: 55–58

Gravelle H 1980 Mammography. In: Sutton D (ed) A textbook of radiology and imaging. Churchill Livingstone, Edinburgh, pp 1396–1410

Haagensen C D 1986 Diseases of the breast. W B Saunders, Philadelphia

Homer M J 1985 Breast imaging: pitfalls, controversies and some practical thoughts. Radiologic Clinics of North America 23(3): 459–472

Kaufman S A 1984 Nursing home breast. Annals of Surgery 119: 615

Lanyi M 1985 Morphologic analysis of microcalcifications; a valuable differential diagnostic system for early detection of breast carcinomas and reduction of superfluous exploratory excisions. In: Zander J, Baltzer J (eds) Early breast carcinoma. Springer-Verlag, Berlin

Love S M, Schnitt S J, Connolly J L, Shirley R L 1987 Benign breast disorders. In: Harris J R, Hellman S, Henderson I C, Kinne D W (eds) Breast diseases. J B Lippincott, Philadelphia

Martin J E, Moskowitz M, Milbrath J R 1979 Breast cancer missed by mammography. American Journal of Roentgenology 132: 737–739

Mendelson E B, Harris K M, Doshi N, Tobon H 1989 American Journal of Roentgenology 153: 265–271

Meyer J E, Kopans D B, Long J C 1980 Mammographic appearance of malignant lymphoma of the breast. Radiology 135: 623–626

Meyer J E, Amin E, Lindfor K K, Lipman J C, Stomper P C, Genest D 1989 Medullary carcinoma of the breast: mammographic and ultrasonic appearances. Radiology 170: 79–82

Millis R R, Atkinson M K, Tonge K A 1976 The xeroradiographic appearances of some uncommon malignant mammary neoplasms. Clinical Radiology 27: 463–471

Mitnick J S, Roses D F, Harris M N, Fiener H D 1989 Circumscribed intraductal carcinoma of the breast. Radiology 170: 423–425

Moskowitz M 1983 Minimal breast cancer redux. Radiologic Clinics of North America 21(1): 93–113

Murphy W A, DeSchryver-Keckemeti K 1978 Isolated clustered microcalcifications in the breast: radiologic-pathologic correlation. Radiology 127: 335–341

O'Higgins N 1984 In: Taylor S, Chisholm G D, O'Higgins N, Shields R (eds) Surgical management. Heinemann, London, p 609

Paulus D D, Libshitz H I 1982 Metastasis to the breast. Radiologic Clinics of North America 20(3): 561–568

Paulus D D 1987 Imaging in breast cancer. Ca-A journal for clinicians 37(3): 133–150

Pope T L, Fecher R E, Wilhelm M C, Wanebo H J, de Paredes E S 1988 Lobular carcinoma in situ of the breast: mammographic features. Radiology 168: 63–66

Robbins S L, Cotran R S, Kumar V 1984 The Breast. In: Robbins S L, Cotran R S, Kumar V (eds) Pathologic basis of disease, 3rd ed. W B Saunders, Philadelphia, pp 1161–1190

Rosen P R 1987 The pathology of breast carcinoma. In: Harris J R, Henderson I C, Hellman S, Kinne D W (eds) Breast diseases. J B Lippincott, Philadelphia, ch 7

Rothenberg R E 1986 The nipple. In: Ariel I, Cleary J B (eds) Breast cancer diagnosis and treatment. McGraw-Hill, New York

Sadowsky N, Kopans D B 1983 Breast cancer. Radiologic Clinics of North America 21(1): 51–65

Sickles E A 1980 Further experience with microfocal spot magnification mammography in the assessment of clustered breast microcalcification. Radiology 137: 9–14

Sigfusson B F, Andersson I, Aspegren K, Janzon L, Linell F, Ljungberg O 1983 Clustered microcalcifications. Acta Radiologica Diagnosis 24: 273–281

Swann C A, Kopans D B, Koerner F C, McCarthy K A, White G, Hall D A 1987 The halo sign and malignant breast lesions. American Journal of Roentgenology 149: 1145–1147

Tabar L, Dean P B 1985 Teaching atlas of mammography. Stuttgart, Thieme, New York

Teng P K 1986 Pathology of breast cancer. In: Ariel I, Cleary J B (eds) Breast cancer diagnosis and treatment. McGraw-Hill, New York

Thompson A J, Machin L 1989 A case of breast carcinoma with sarcomatous metaplastia. Clinical Radiology 40: 98–100

Zuckerman H C 1986 The role of mammography in the diagnosis of breast cancer. In Ariel I, Cleary J B (eds) Breast cancer diagnosis and treatment. McGraw-Hill, New York

CHAPTER 7

Benign diseases of the breast

Yin Y. Ng

INTRODUCTION

The term 'benign breast change' (Breast Group of the Royal College of Radiologists 1989) refers to a spectrum of mammographic and pathological change ranging from normal physiological responses through variants of normal to frank pathological change. This includes changes with breast development, cyclical changes, changes with pregnancy and involution. Synonymous terms are aberrations of normal development and involution (ANDI; Hughes et al 1987), fibrocystic disease and benign mammary dysplasia.

PATHOLOGY

The histological spectrum of benign breast change includes lesions that produce microcalcifications such as cysts, sclerosing adenosis and blunt duct adenosis, and irregular mammographic densities mimicking cancer, e.g. sclerosing adenosis, radial scars and fibrocystic change. None of these have malignant potential unless associated with epithelial hyperplasia (epitheliosis or papillomatosis). Regular epithelial hyperplasia is believed to be associated with a slightly increased risk of developing carcinoma. Atypical epithelial hyperplasia carries an intermediate risk of malignancy. Regular and atypical hyperplasia cannot be recognized cytologically. False negatives can never be eliminated as benign breast change may coexist with cancer (Herbert 1989). It is often difficult to differentiate histologically between some intraductal hyperplastic lesions (papillomatosis, epitheliosis) and proliferative fibrocystic disease from intraductal carcinoma of the breast (Fisher et al 1979).

Radiological correlates are changes in density with or without nodularity, disturbance of trabeculation, ductal prominence, calcification and/or microcalcifications, and mass lesions. These appearances result from changes in the lobular, ductal and stromal components of the breast (Breast Group of the Royal College of Radiologists 1989). The radiographic densities of lobules, ducts and stroma are all similar when measured by contact microradiography (Pye 1989), but it is the relative proportions of these tissues within the breast which cause the variations in radiographic density observed with different parenchymal patterns.

MAMMOGRAPHIC FEATURES OF BENIGN LESIONS

One of the most important contributions of a radiologist to the management of the patient with breast symptoms is the ability to recognize benign change, and thereby to reduce the anxiety and excess workload associated with a high false-positive rate and unnecessary breast biopsy for benign change. On the other hand it is also desirable to minimize the false-negative rate.

As has already been mentioned in Chap. 6, it is not always possible to distinguish benign from malignant lesions on the basis of the mammographic features alone. Characteristics of a mass, and of calcification, which would favour a benign rather than malignant pathology, will be further discussed. The radiographic signs include the outline, shape, density, and change of the mass with time.

Mass lesions

Patients are often referred for mammography because of a palpable mass. Mammography may fail to detect 10% of clinically suspicious abnormalities (Homer 1985). This will apply particularly to breasts with dense stroma, and to masses on the chest wall which may be difficult to include on the film for technical reasons.

Outline and shape

A mass which is well-defined has a high probability of being benign. Overlapping trabeculae may obscure the margin of a benign mass, but good compression, and views in varying degrees of obliquity will help to distinguish this from a malignant lesion. Well-defined masses are usually fibroadenomata in young women (Figs 7.1–7.3), or cysts in perimenopausal women (Figs 7.4, 7.5). A few malignant tumours, such as medullary, mucoid or invasive ductal carcinoma, have been reported with well-defined outlines (Mitnick et al 1989); see Fig. 6.29, p. 110. It has also been stated that a well-circumscribed border does not differentiate intraductal from microinvasive carcinoma (Homer, 1989).

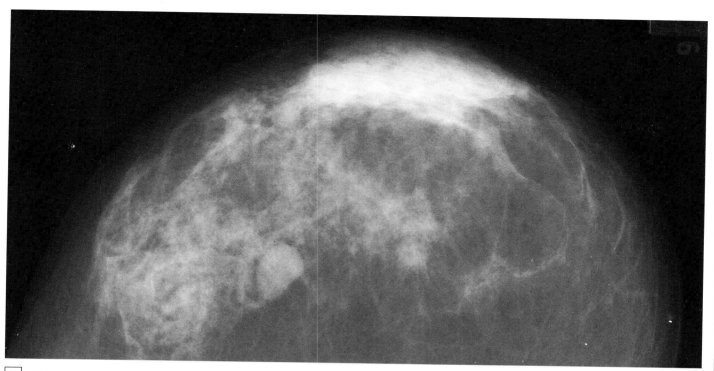

R   **Fig. 7.1**   Fibroadenoma. Craniocaudal view showing well-defined, slightly lobulated margin.

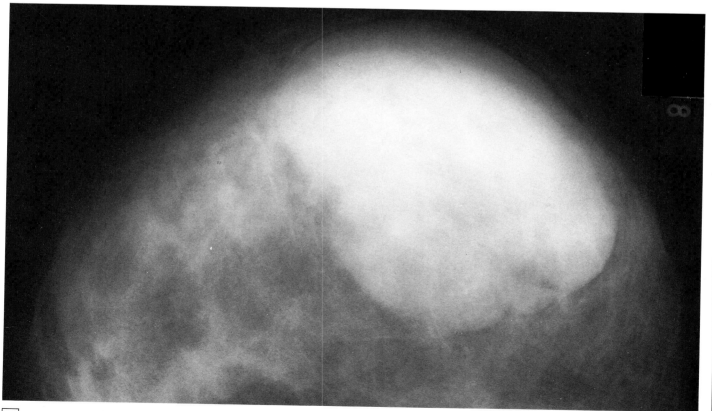

R   **Fig. 7.2**   Giant fibroadenoma in a 17-year-old girl. Note lobulated margin.

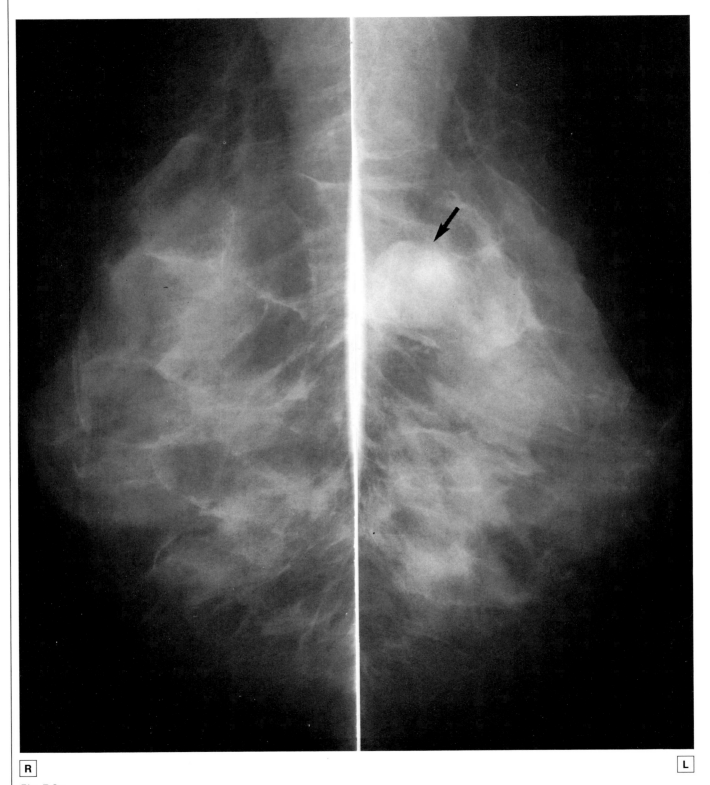

R

L

Fig. 7.3a

Fig. 7.3 Fibroadenoma in left breast (arrow). *a* Mammogram: lateral-oblique views show a mass with less well-defined margins than in the previous examples, and ultrasound was performed to elucidate the nature of the mass. *b* Ultrasound: shows a solid mass of homogeneous echogenicity, associated with posterior acoustic enhancement, consistent with a fibroadenoma.

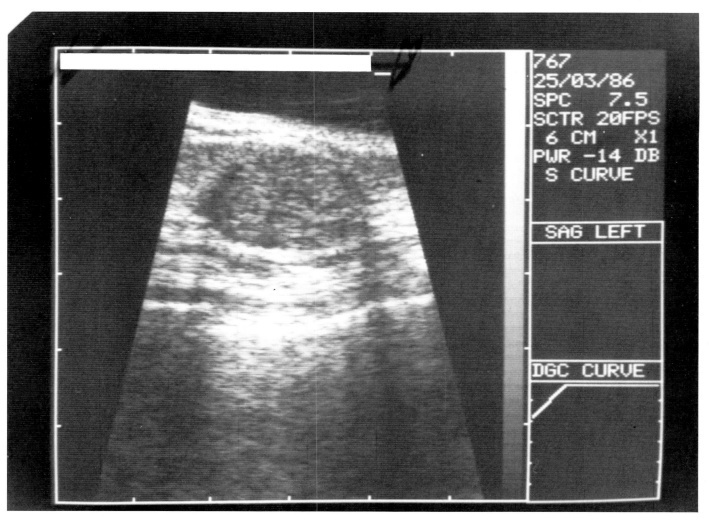

Fig. 7.3b

'Halo sign'. This is described as a complete or partial radiolucent ring surrounding the periphery of a breast mass (Fig. 7.4). It is most frequently seen with cysts and fibroadenomata, and is thought by some to represent compressed fat adjacent to the mass (Wolfe 1983). More probably it is due to the Mach effect (Lane et al 1976, Swann et al 1987, Gordenne & Malchair 1988). Tabar & Dean (1985) state that, with the rare exception of papillary carcinoma, intracystic carcinoma and carcinoma arising in a fibroadenoma, the halo sign is diagnostic of a benign process. However, Swann et al (1987) reported 25 malignant breast lesions in 19 women showing a partial or complete halo sign. None of these were medullary carcinomas: 11 were infiltrating ductal carcinomas, four were lymphoma, and there was one case each of the following: metastatic melanoma, cystosarcoma phylloides, malignant fibrous histiocytoma, and breast carcinoma metastatic to intramammary lymph nodes. The size of the lesions ranged from 1 to 7.2 cm (mean 2.4 cm). The authors state that although the mammographic margins appeared smooth and a thin radiolucent halo was present, the histological margins showed infiltration. They were able to simulate a halo by immersing a round water-filled latex sphere in fat with surrounding air excluded. The halo could be eliminated by obscuring the round density. They were unable to show objectively a change in density across the zone by densitometry, supporting their view that the 'halo sign' is an optical illusion due to the Mach effect. The Mach effect is a retino-optical phenomenon which occurs when viewing an edge: contiguous cones in the retina suppress the adjacent receptors,

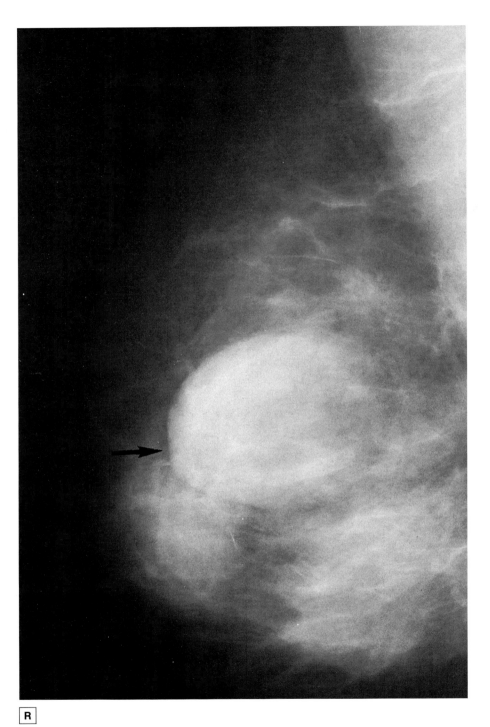

R

Fig. 7.4 Cyst showing the 'halo' sign (arrow).

resulting in a reduced signal to the brain, and producing the optical illusion of a darker zone.

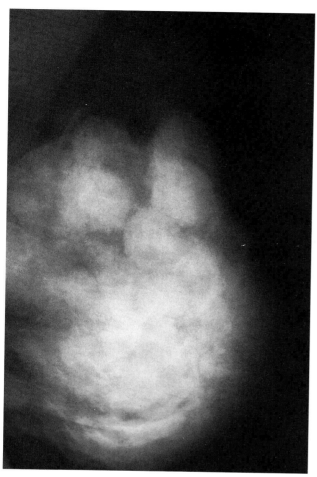

Fig. 7.5a

Fig. 7.5   Multiple cysts. Note rounded, well-defined masses of relatively low density. *a* Lateral-oblique view. *b* Craniocaudal view.

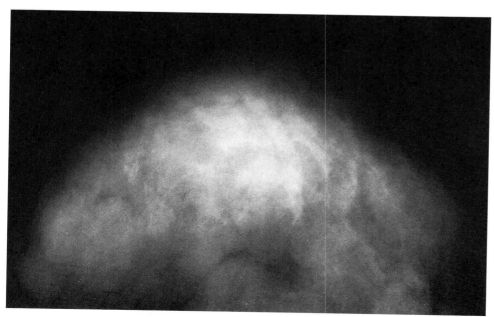

Fig. 7.5b

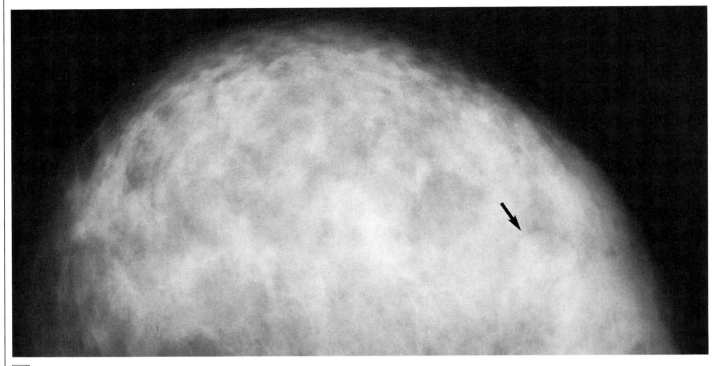

R

Fig. 7.6   Skin mole (arrow).

Skin lesions such as moles, warts, sebaceous cysts and neurofibromata (Figs 7.6–7.9) may be distinguished by the conventional radiological characteristics of extreme clarity of a margin which is outlined by the adjacent air. Tangential views would also help to elucidate.

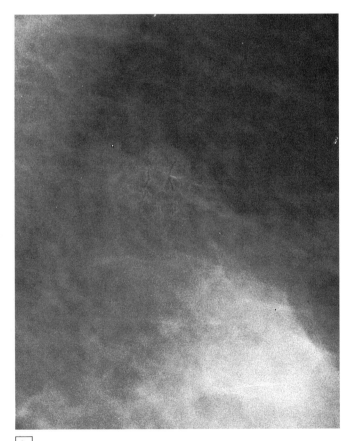

L

Fig. 7.7   Skin wart, localized view.

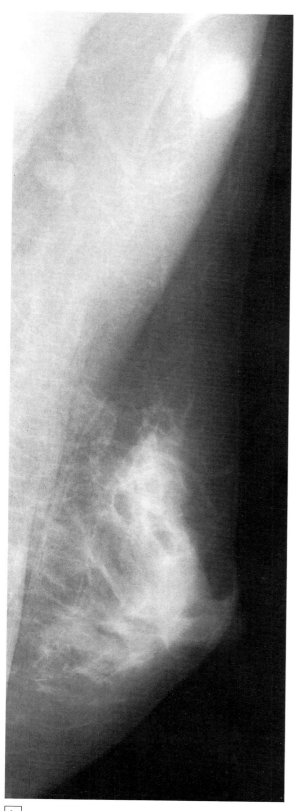

L

Fig. 7.8a

Fig. 7.8 Sebaceous cyst. *a* Lateral-oblique view showing a well-defined 2 cm mass in the left axilla. *b* Localized view from an extended craniocaudal projection showing the cutaneous location of the mass; appearances consistent with a sebaceous cyst.

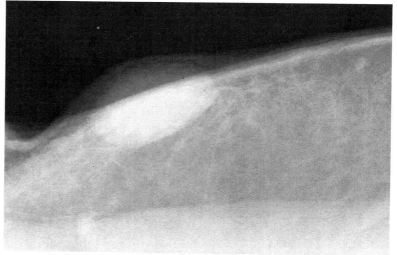

L

Fig. 7.8b

Fig. 7.9   Cutaneous neurofibromata.
a Lateral oblique view showing several
well-defined masses inferior to the nipple.
The extreme clarity of their margins
suggests a superficial location. These
were obvious clinically. *b* Craniocaudal
view.

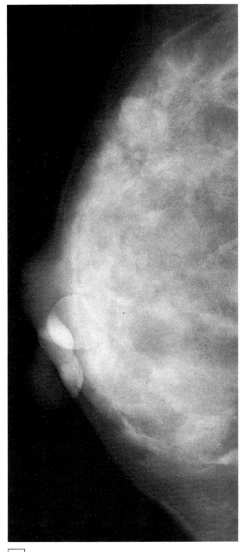

R   *Fig. 7.9a*

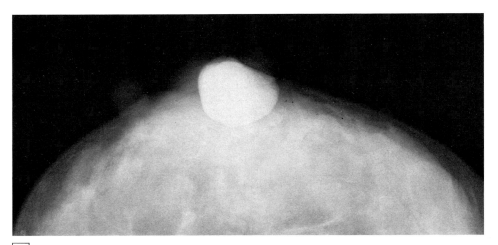

R   *Fig. 7.9b*

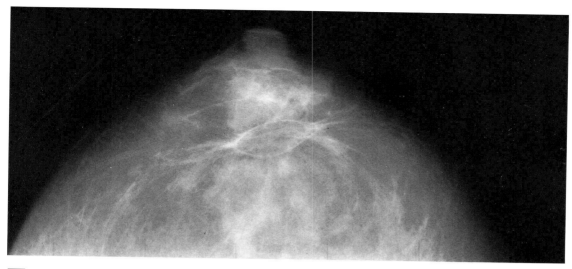

L

Fig. 7.10 Fat necrosis following horsebite.

Radiographic density of the lesion
A lesion containing material of fat
density has a high probability of being
benign. It may represent a variety of
pathologies including a traumatic oil
cyst (Fig. 7.10), lipoma (Figs 7.11,
7.12), intramammary lymph node
(Fig. 5.3, p. 71) galactocele, or rarely a
fibroadenolipoma (Figs 7.13, 7.14).

Benign masses of soft tissue density
include cysts, fibroadenomas, and
haematomas. In general, benign
masses tend to be of low density and
overlapping trabeculae, and vessels
may be seen through the mass;
whereas malignant masses are often
denser than the adjacent parenchyma
and may appear too dense for their size
(Moskowitz 1983).

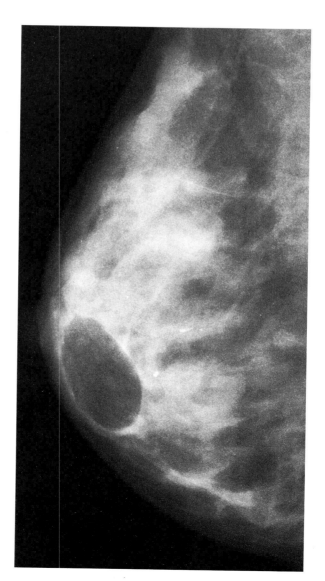

R

Fig. 7.11 Lipoma: well-defined
mass of fat density.

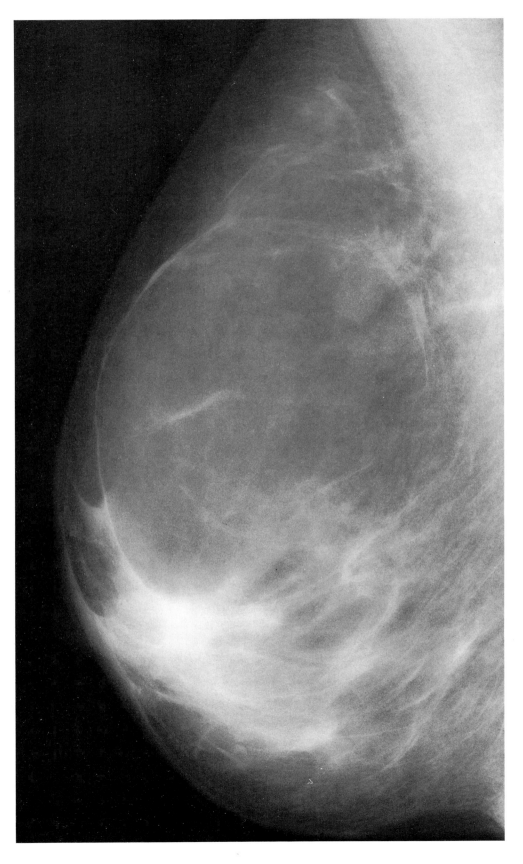

R

Fig. 7.12   Large lipoma.

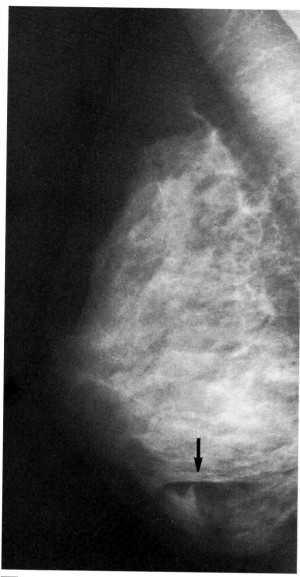

Fig. 7.13a

Fig. 7.13 Fibroadenolipoma. *a* Lateral-oblique view showing a well-defined mass (arrow) of mixed fat and soft-tissue density in the inferior half of the breast. *b* Craniocaudal view.

R | *Fig. 7.13b (below)*

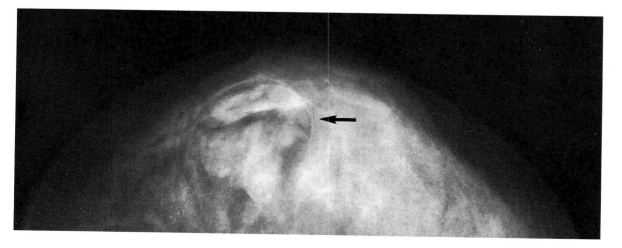

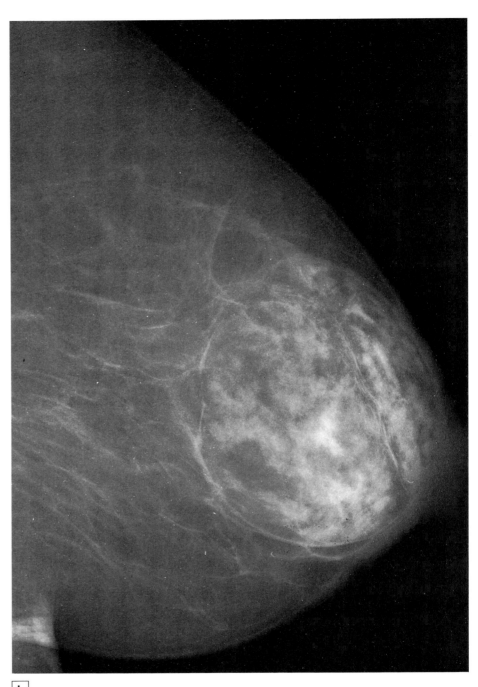

L

Fig. 7.14   Large fibroadenolipoma.
a Lateral view. b Craniocaudal view.

Fig. 7.14a

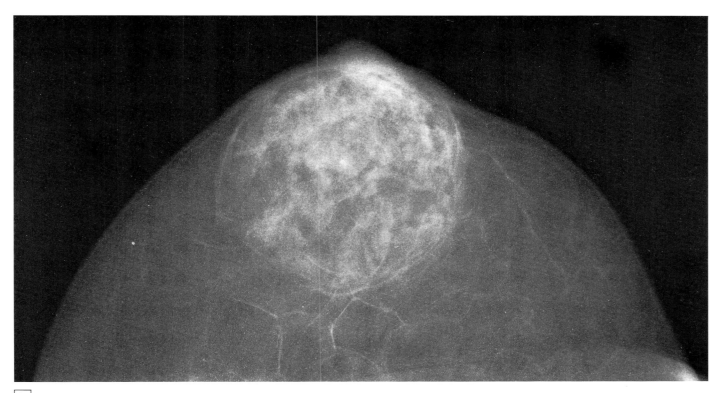

L

Fig. 7.14b

Change with time

A mammographically detectable mass which changes little in size and shape over several years is most likely to be benign, although there have been reports of carcinomas which have not increased in size over 2–4 years (Meyer & Kopans 1981). If there is associated microcalcification, an increase in the amount of calcification in itself is not necessarily an indication for biopsy, unless the nature of the new calcification is significantly different and suspicious of malignant-type calcification. Any benign-looking mass which increases in size with time, especially in a postmenopausal woman, should be regarded with suspicion.

Fibroadenoma

This is the most common benign tumour of the breast in women under 25 years of age (Haagensen 1986); the mean age of incidence in his series was 34 years. Physical examination reveals a firm mobile mass. The tumour appears encapsulated as it is usually sharply delineated from the surrounding breast tissue, although there is no true capsule. Histologically, the tumour is composed of various amounts of connective tissue and glandular elements and often has epithelium-lined clefts.

On mammography, a fibroadenoma may be seen as a well-circumscribed mass which is round or oval and may be lobulated (Fig. 7.1). Fibroadenomata are multiple in 15–20% of patients, and are frequently bilateral, rarely exceeding 3 cm in size. They regress with age, and necrosis within the tumour results in coarse nodular calcification seen on mammography (Figs 7.15–7.18). The peripheral distribution of such calcification is characteristic.

Ultimately the soft tissue components may disappear completely so that only calcification remains. This does not usually present a diagnostic problem because the calcification is often large and nodular.

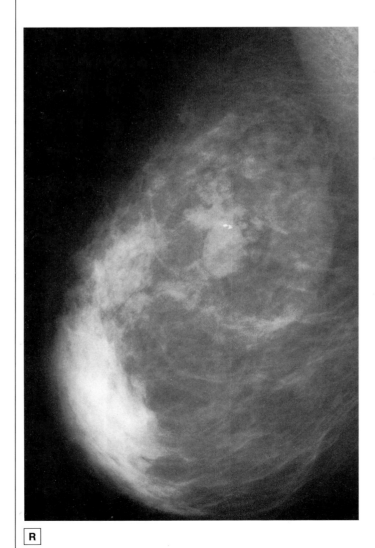

R

Fig. 7.15   Early calcification in a fibroadenoma.

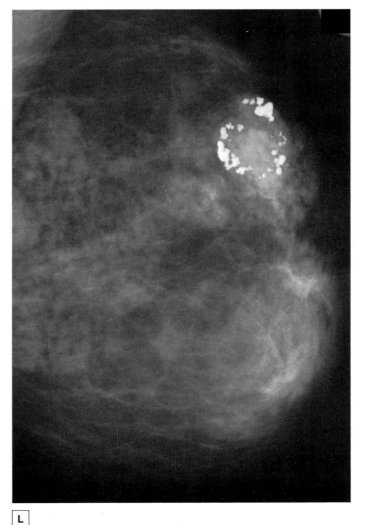

L

Fig. 7.16   More advanced nodular calcification, peripherally distributed, in a fibroadenoma.

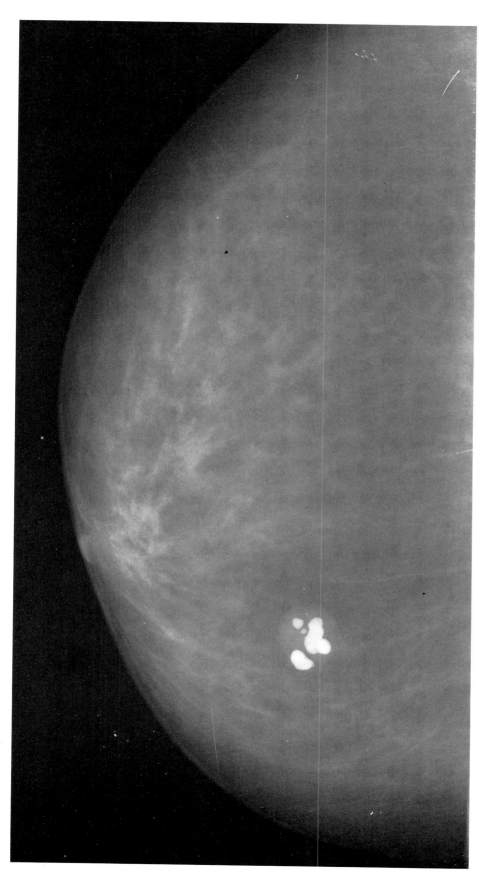

R

Fig. 7.17 Central nodular calcification in fibroadenoma.

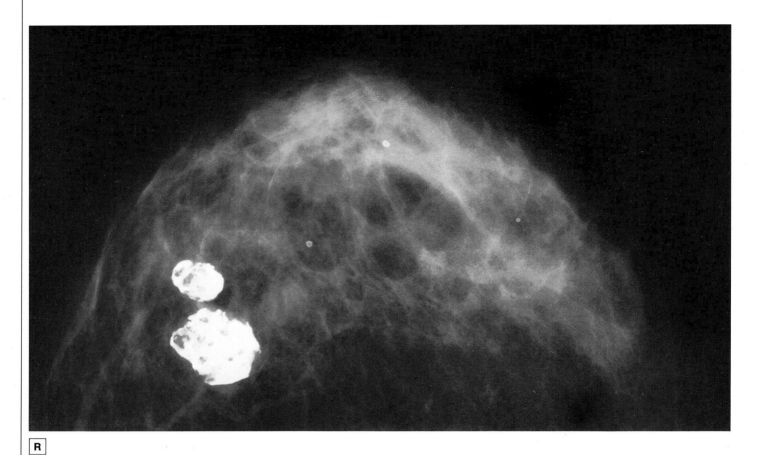

R

Fig. 7.18   Dense nodular calcification in a fibroadenoma. The soft tissue mass of the fibroadenoma can just be discerned at the periphery of the area of calcification.

The ultrasonic appearances of fibroadenomata will be discussed in Chap. 9. The question of carcinoma arising in a fibroadenoma is difficult to resolve unless a large amount of the surrounding breast parenchyma is removed and carcinoma is found only within the fibroadenoma. The cases described to date have been lobular carcinoma-in-situ; Haagensen (1986) has 14 such cases, followed up for a maximum of 18 years, in whom there has been no evidence of malignant progression of disease or of metastasis. Malignant change in a fibroadenoma is extremely rare, but fibroadenoma and carcinoma may coexist (Fig. 7.19).

Giant fibroadenoma
This tumour is defined as a fibroadenoma which exceeds 6 cm in diameter. It is always benign, and is seen most commonly in adolescent and young black women (Fig. 7.2).

Phylloides tumour
A rare tumour of fibroepithelial origin. The mean age of the patients in one series was 40.5 years (Haagensen 1986). The term 'cystosarcoma phylloides' is a misnomer because most of these tumours are benign, and the name was originally used to emphasize the leaf-like growth pattern rather than a statement of prognostic significance (D'Orsi et al 1983).

Macroscopically these tumours are well-circumscribed without a true capsule. The stromal pattern varies considerably, from that of a fibroadenoma at one end of the spectrum to a highly cellular pattern resembling anaplasia at the other end. A striking feature of most phylloides tumours is the very long branching clefts lined by one or several layers of bland epithelium (Haagensen 1986).

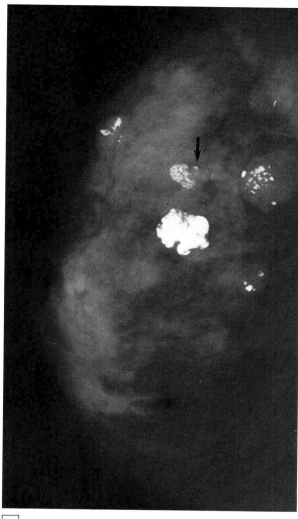

Fig. 7.19 Carcinoma (arrows) coexisting with fibroadenomata. Note the different characteristics of the malignant microcalcifications. *a* Lateral oblique view. *b* Craniocaudal view.

▽ R Fig. 7.19b

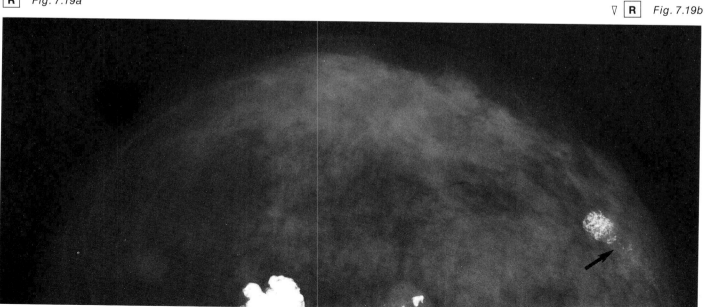

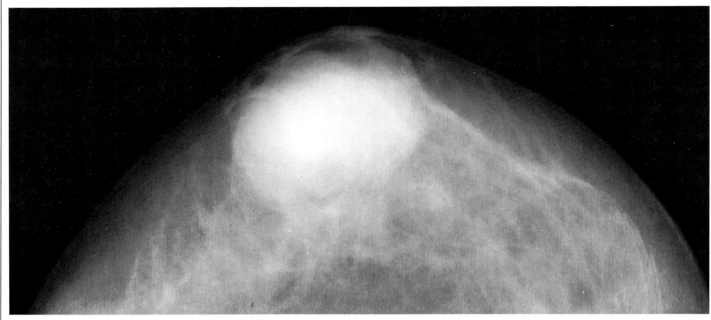

L

Fig. 7.20 Phylloides tumour. The mass is not very dense for its size, and has an irregular margin, particularly posteriorly.

Mammographically the tumour resembles a large lobulated fibroadenoma (Fig. 7.20); some of the margins may be irregular, suggesting local breast invasion, and if not completely excised the tumour may recur. Cole-Beuglet et al (1983) observed in eight patients that malignancy is suggested histologically by an increase in the number of mitoses, stromal pleomorphism and invasive borders. Approximately 27% of all phylloides tumours will show one of these three malignant characteristics, but only 12% will metastasize, usually to lung or bone; malignant change is almost always confined to the stromal component.

Cyst

Breast cysts develop when the lumina of the ducts and acini become dilated and lined by atrophic epithelium. They may evolve from duct ectasia, fat necrosis, or they may be induced by oestrogen administration. Rarely they may be associated with an intraduct papilloma.

Cysts may be divided into 'microcysts', which are less than 3 mm in diameter, and 'gross cysts', which are 3 mm or more in diameter (Haagensen 1986). Gross cysts originate from blunt ducts and microcysts. Gross cystic change is the most frequent benign change seen in the breast. The peak age of incidence is 40–49 years (Haagensen 1986). Cysts frequently disappear or subside following the menopause, so that any increase in size of a mass during this period should raise the index of suspicion for malignancy. Clinically, cysts may vary in size with the menstrual cycle. Symptoms of pain and tenderness relate to fluid tension within the cysts.

On mammography, cysts may be indistinguishable from non-calcified fibroadenomas. Although fibroadenomas are often lobulated in outline, a multiloculated cyst or a cluster of several cysts may also be lobulated. The shape of cysts is variable depending on the amount of

contained fluid: a tense cyst is round, whereas a lax cyst may be of any shape, and vary according to the amount of compression applied. Cysts are also frequently multiple and bilateral. The presence of multiple rounded masses bilaterally would favour a benign process such as cystic change (Fig. 7.5) but malignancy must be searched for diligently in such a breast (Fig. 6.6, p. 88), and may very occasionally be multifocal and bilateral (Fig. 6.33, p. 117).

Calcification is infrequent, occurring mostly in cysts less than 10 mm in diameter, but when present may be seen as a thin peripheral rim, quite distinct from that of a fibroadenoma. Rarely, microcysts may contain milk of calcium fluid, which on an erect lateral mammogram layers out on the floor of the cyst, forming the so-called 'tea-cup' calcification (Figs 7.21, 7.22).

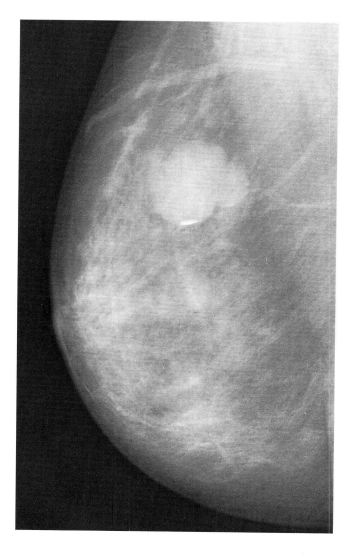

Fig. 7.21 'Tea-cup' calcification in the wall of a cyst. *a* Lateral-oblique view showing linear calcification at the inferior margin of the cyst. *b* Craniocaudal view showing rounded calcification anteriorly. The change in shape of the calcification may be attributed to change in its orientation relative to the incident X-ray beam.

◁ R *Fig. 7.21a*

▽ R *Fig. 7.21b*

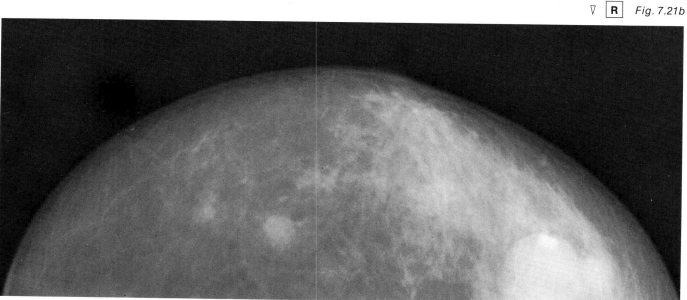

Fig. 7.22 Multiple 'tea-cup' calcifications. *a* Lateral view. *b* Craniocaudal view, confirming the benign origin of these calcifications.

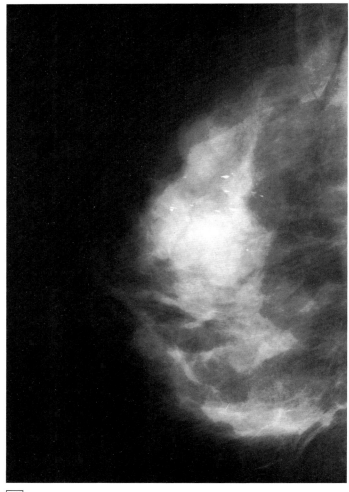

R   *Fig. 7.22a*

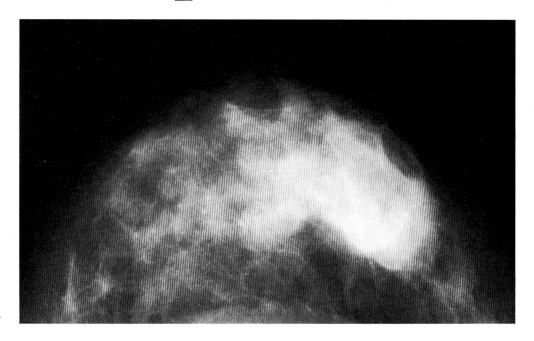

R   *Fig. 7.22b*

Galactoceles are cysts containing inspissated milk. They occur in lactating women in whom breast-feeding is terminated more or less abruptly. The usual site is the central breast area, and the mass has all the clinical and mammographic appearances of a benign lesion (Fig. 7.23).

Gross cystic change is associated with an increased risk of breast carcinoma, but the fact that the carcinomas do not develop within the cysts suggests a common predisposing factor for the two conditions, rather than a causative role for cystic change (Haagensen 1986).

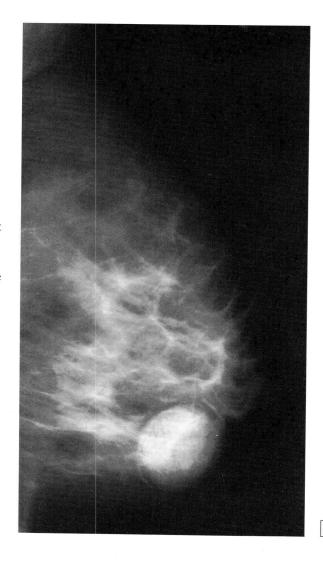

Fig. 7.23 Galactocele in lower inner quadrant of the breast. *a* Lateral-oblique view. *b* Craniocaudal view.

L *Fig. 7.23a*

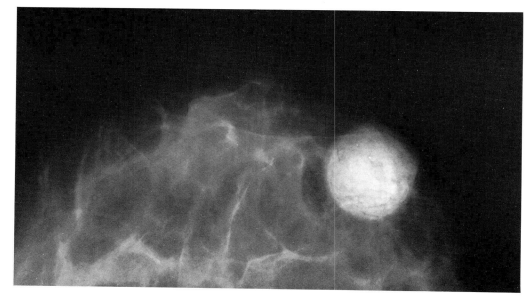

L *Fig. 7.23b*

Lymph nodes

Axillary lymph nodes are usually oval-shaped opacities with a fatty hilum (Fig. 7.24). Round densely homogeneous axillary nodes which are more than 2.5 cm in diameter should be regarded as suspicious for metastatic involvement (Parsons 1983).

Intramammary lymph nodes are typically well-circumscribed lobulated densities less than 1 cm in diameter, with a hilar notch and lucent centre if fatty replacement has occurred (Fig. 7.25). The typical location is in the upper outer quadrant posteriorly (Lindfors et al 1986). Enlarged (> 1 cm diameter) intramammary lymph nodes of homogeneous density which lack the characteristic lucent centre or hilar notch are suspicious for metastatic involvement, providing that local dermatitis or mastitis has been excluded clinically. A lymph node which appears normal on the mammogram is not necessarily free of tumour.

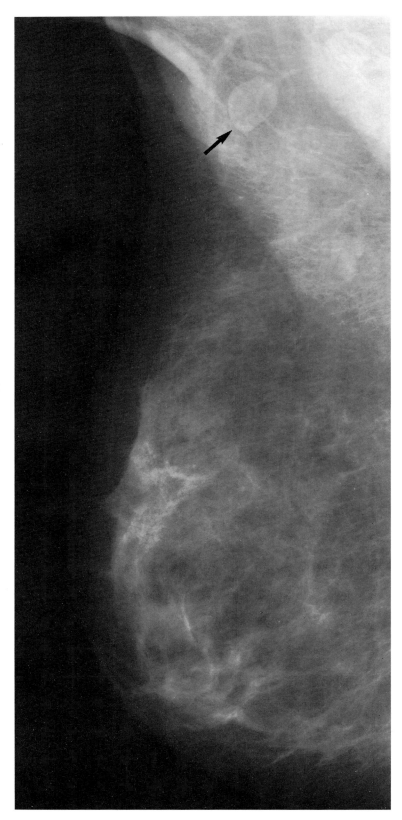

R

Fig. 7.24 Fatty replacement of a lymph node (arrow) in the right axilla.

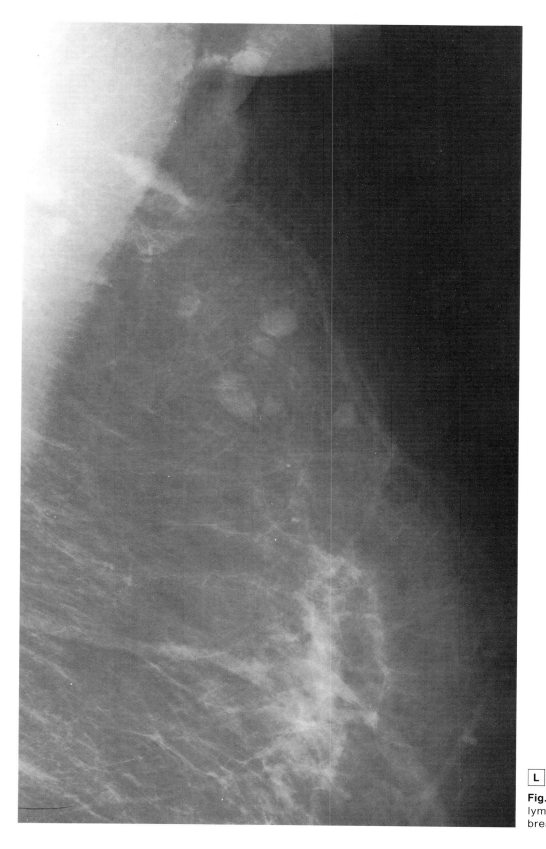

L

Fig. 7.25 Multiple intramammary lymph nodes in the upper half of the breast.

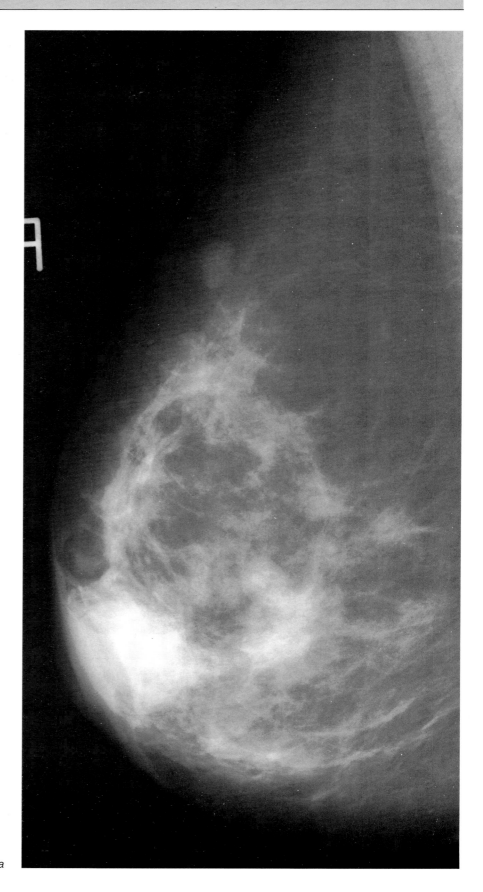

Fig. 7.26   Breast abscess. Note typical subareolar location (and two 1 cm diameter intramammary lymph nodes). *a* Lateral-oblique view. *b* Craniocaudal view.

R   *Fig. 7.26a*

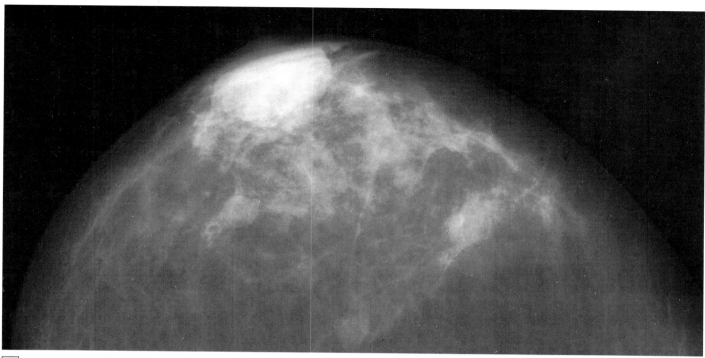

R   *Fig. 7.26b*

Haematoma

Trauma to the breast may result in haematoma formation, which may present clinically and mammographically as an ill-defined mass mimicking a carcinoma. However, the history is usually helpful, and follow-up should reveal regression of the oedema and the mass. Occasionally the late sequela of a haematoma may resemble a carcinoma with microcalcification and architectural distortion. Attempted aspiration of a suspected cyst within 2 weeks prior to mammography may also lead to diagnostic confusion due to associated haematoma formation (Sickles et al 1983). This situation may be avoided by the use of mammography before any interventional diagnostic procedure.

Abscess

Breast abscesses are most commonly encountered during lactation, although they may occur in non-lactating women where they may be sterile abscesses associated with mammary duct ectasia. Abscesses usually occur in a central or subareolar location producing an irregular density (Fig. 7.26) often associated with trabecular, skin and/or nipple distortion. The diagnosis is often obvious clinically in the presence of a hot, red, painful mass.

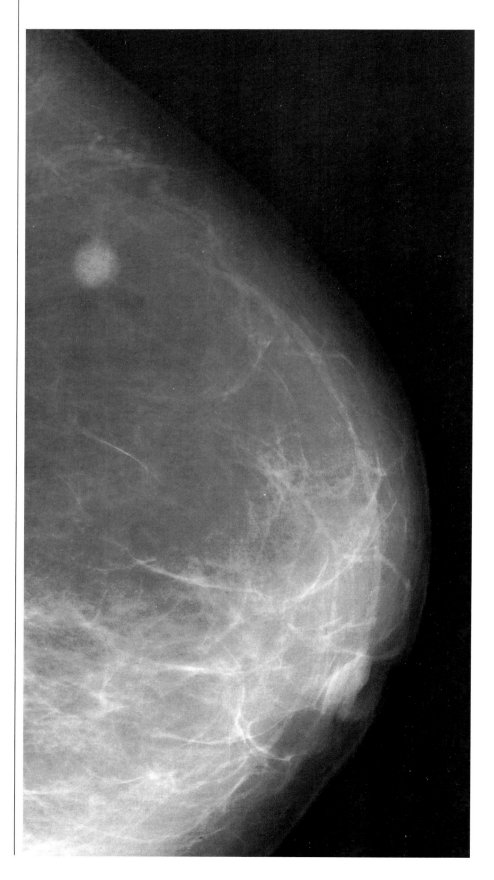

Granular cell tumour

This is an extremely rare benign lesion probably of Schwann cell origin (Demay & Kay 1984). The tumour usually occurs in the tongue or subcutaneous tissue, with 6% occurring in the breast. It is most frequently seen in the 20–59 year age group, and is more common in black races (Elias et al 1970, Greenberg 1967). The tumour has a fibrous stroma and infiltrative margin mimicking scirrhous carcinoma clinically and mammographically (Fig. 7.27).

Infections and infestations

Tuberculosis of the breast is very rare in the United Kingdom, but may be seen in Africa and Asia. It is most often seen in women between the ages of 20 and 50, and young pregnant women are predisposed to the disease. It is rarely bilateral, and may coexist with carcinoma (Smith & Mason 1926). The infection has to be distinguished mammographically from carcinoma, whether in its nodular, diffuse or sclerosing form. In the nodular form, a dense mass with irregular margins is seen on mammography; in the diffuse form, the associated skin thickening and surrounding oedema mimic an inflammatory carcinoma, and the sclerosing type results in fibrosis and uniformly increased density of one breast.

L

Fig. 7.27 Granular cell tumour. This benign tumour could easily be mistaken for a malignant tumour because of its density relative to its size and its spiculated margins.

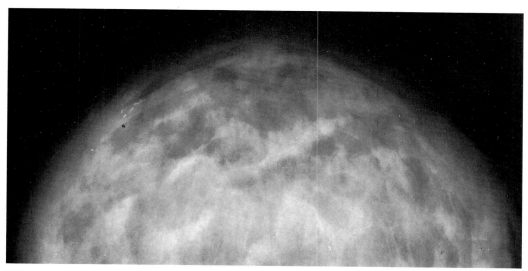

R   *Fig. 7.28a*

Filariasis of the breast presenting as a mass is rare, with only about 20 cases reported, most from Sri Lanka (Chandrasoma & Mendis 1978). As with tuberculosis, a solitary inflammatory mass surrounding the filarial worms may mimic a carcinoma both clinically and radiologically. However, calcified worms are not infrequently seen on mammograms of women attending for other reasons (Fig. 7.28).

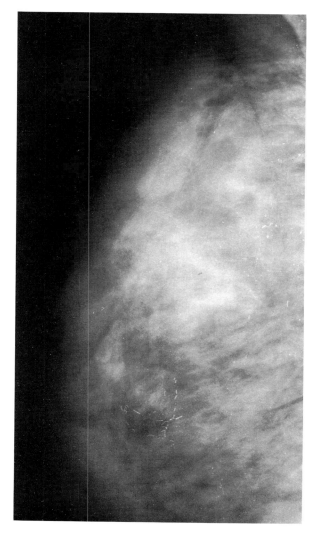

Fig. 7.28   Calcified loa loa. *a* Lateral-oblique view. *b* Craniocaudal view showing cutaneous location of the calcified parasites.

R   *Fig. 7.28b*

Ducts

Normal ducts appear as symmetrical retroareolar tubular densities which taper as they extend away from the nipple. A solitary enlarged duct (Fig. 5.7, p. 74) or lobe of ducts is an unusual appearance and may be due to obstruction by inspissated duct material, an intraductal papilloma (Figs 7.29, 7.30) or rarely by an intraduct carcinoma (Sadowsky & Kopans 1983).

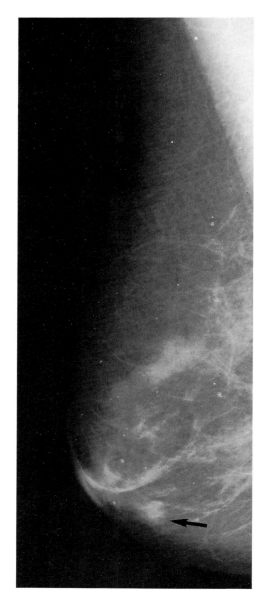

Fig. 7.29 Intraduct papilloma (arrow). Note also scattered dermal calcification.
a Lateral-oblique view.
b Craniocaudal view.

R   *Fig. 7.29a* ▷

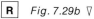

R   *Fig. 7.29b* ▽

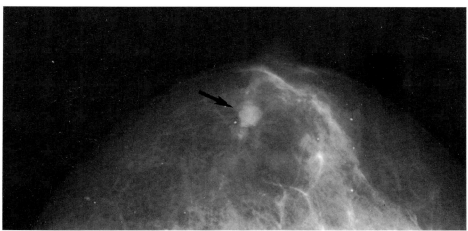

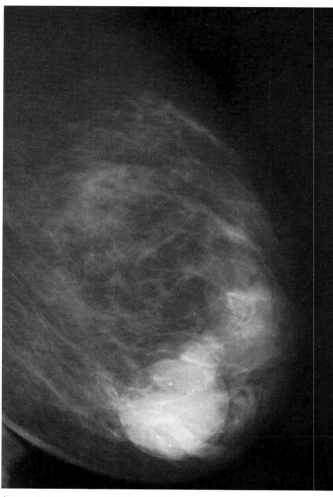

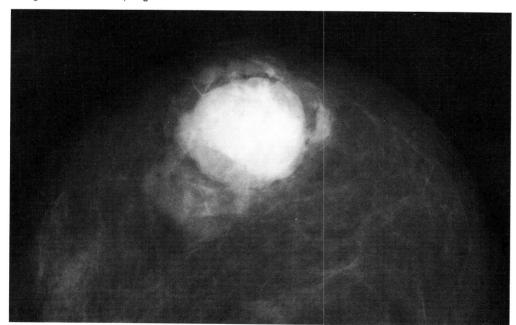

Fig. 7.30 Large intraduct papilloma. The mass is lobulated with a 'halo', and is associated with benign-looking calcification. *a* Lateral view. *b* Craniocaudal view.

△ *Fig. 7.30a*   ▽ *Fig. 7.30b*

Stellate lesions

The two most common benign lesions which may cause diagnostic difficulty because of their shape are the radial scar and fat necrosis. Previous surgery causing distortion of the parenchyma may also present a diagnostic problem (Fig. 7.31) (Sickles & Herzog 1980). However, Mitnick et al (1988) claim that the presence of a central radiolucency will distinguish a postoperative scar from a malignant tumour, the latter showing increased density centrally. In their experience, the only situation in which this rule did not apply is in the presence of a hypertrophic scar or keloid contiguous with the underlying mammary scar. Postoperative scarring may vary in appearance with different projections, e.g. a true lateral or the opposite 45° oblique view, and on follow-up mammography should show either no change or regression with time (Sickles & Herzog 1990).

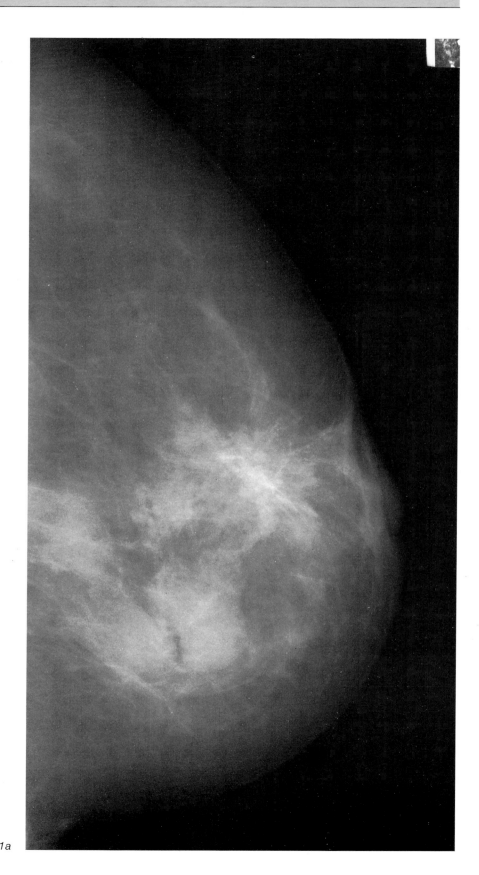

Fig. 7.31 Postoperative scar mimicking carcinoma. Note multiple cysts, indicating the reason for previous biopsy. *a* Lateral view showing stellate opacity behind the nipple with associated skin thickening and distortion. *b* Craniocaudal view. The stellate opacity is again noted (single arrows) representing the operative scar. At least two cysts (double arrows) are well demonstrated on this view.

L *Fig. 7.31a*

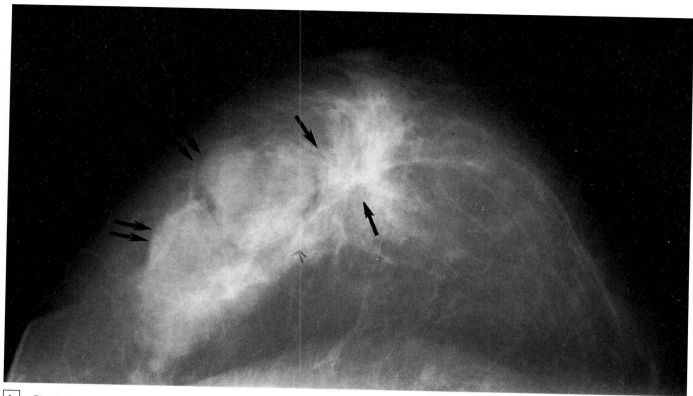

L *Fig. 7.31b*

Radial scar

Also known as 'sclerosing duct hyperplasia' (Tabar & Dean 1985), and 'non-encapsulated sclerosing lesion' (Fisher et al 1979). Radial scar is now thought to be a variant of sclerosing adenosis and part of the spectrum of benign breast change. Pathologically, this tubular lesion has a stellate configuration in which the tubular structures are disposed in a central sclerotic core. Ducts in the peripheral areas show papillomatosis as well as other features of non-proliferative fibrocystic disease such as sclerosing adenosis and apocrine change (Fenoglio & Lattes 1974). The association between radial scar and breast carcinoma, in particular tubular carcinoma, is a subject for debate. Fisher et al (1979) noted the morphological similarities between these two conditions and postulated that radial scars represent incipient tubular carcinomas. However, both conditions would be treated by local excision only, and follow-up of their 15 patients with radial scar showed no evidence of recurrence or development of overt cancer. Other studies have shown no relation between radial scar and breast malignancy (Rickert et al 1981, Andersen & Gram 1984, Nielsen et al 1987). Andersen and Gram followed up 32 patients with radial scar for a mean of 20 years and failed to reveal any increased incidence of carcinoma. In almost all cases, radial scar was found in breasts with features of benign breast change, and in 93% papillomatosis and/or benign epithelial hyperplasia was associated. In 63% of cases, there were small uniform microcalculi.

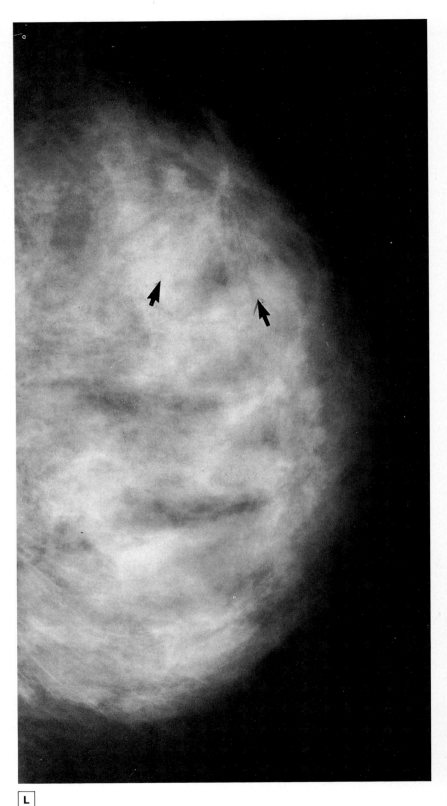

L

Fig. 7.32a

Fig. 7.32 Radial scar (arrows). Coned compression view (*b*) demonstrates more clearly the central radiolucency (cf. Fig. 6.2, p. 84; Fig. 6.13, p. 93).

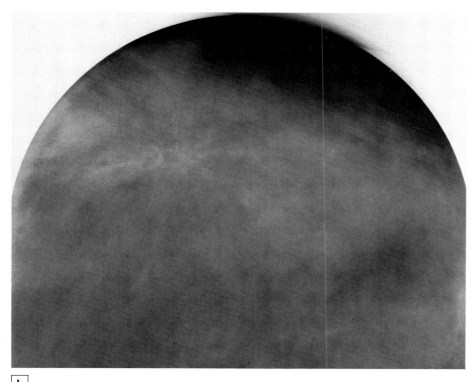

L

Fig. 7.32b

Tabar & Dean (1985) observed a prevalence of radial scar in 0.9 per 1000 women screened. Mammographic features distinguishing a radial scar from a malignant scirrhous tumour include a central radiolucency or several tiny oval lucencies (Fig. 7.32). This central radiolucency has been attributed to a hypertrophic fibroelastic core surrounded by stellate proliferations of the duct system (Fenoglio & Lattes 1974). In general, radial scars are impalpable and, unlike carcinoma, are not associated with skin retraction or nipple inversion. However, microcalcification may occur along the radiating strands of a radial scar, leading to further diagnostic confusion with malignancy. These signs—the central radiolucency, lack of skin or nipple changes—are not sufficiently specific to obviate the need for biopsy in the presence of a clinically suspicious mass.

The aetiology of radial scar is unknown, although several hypotheses exist. It has been postulated to relate to duct ectasia in its obliterative form (Hamperl 1975), to obliterative changes in blood vessels (Fisher et al 1983), or to a chronic inflammatory response (Anderson & Battersby 1985).

Fat necrosis

The clinical importance of fat necrosis of the breast was first emphasized by Lee & Adair (1920) who described two cases of fat necrosis misdiagnosed as carcinoma. However Haagensen (1986) states that in his experience fat necrosis producing a breast tumour which is detected clinically is not common, being seen in only 54 patients over 37 years. The age range in his series was 27–80 years, with a mean of 52 years. Often there is no history of trauma—in his series only 32% gave a definite history of trauma. A strong point in favour of the traumatic origin of mammary fat necrosis is the frequency of gross or microscopic evidence of haemorrhage in these lesions. Harbitz (1935) found blood pigment in 15/17 examples of fat necrosis.

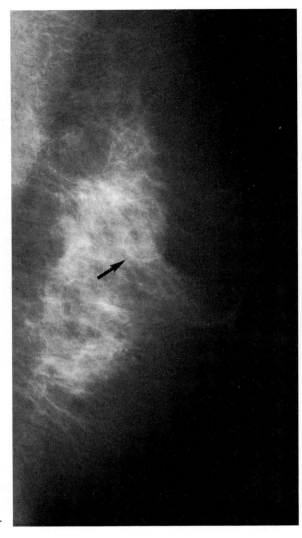

L   *Fig. 7.33a* ▷

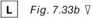

L   *Fig. 7.33b* ▽

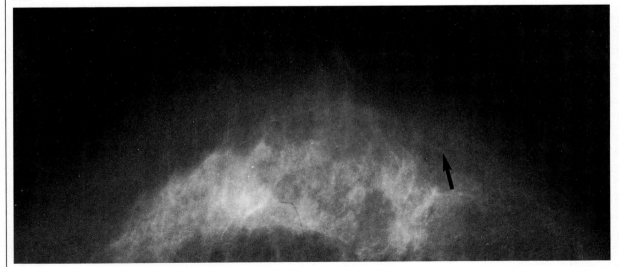

Fig. 7.33   Oil cyst (arrow). No history of trauma. *a* Lateral-oblique view. *b* Craniocaudal view. Note superficial location.

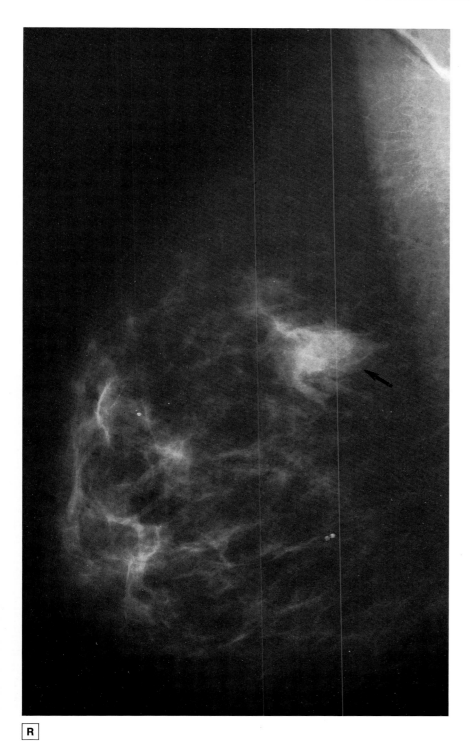

R

Fig. 7.34 Fat necrosis presenting as an ill-defined mass (arrow) suspicious of malignancy both clinically and mammographically. Biopsy-proven fat necrosis.

Pathologically the earliest change is of haemorrhage in an indurated area of fat. Three to four weeks later the lesion forms a rounded firm tumour containing liquefied fat and/or altered blood and necrotic material. Calcification of the walls of the cavity is common. Fibrosis predominates at the periphery of the lesion, and an excessive desmoplastic reaction may give rise to the spiculate mass sometimes seen on mammography (Bassett et al 1978).

Mammographically there is a wide spectrum of appearances ranging from well-defined superficial oil cysts which may show rim calcification (Fig. 7.33), through a spiculate mass resembling carcinoma (Fig. 7.34), to malignant-looking microcalcifications (Bassett et al 1978, Orson & Cigtay 1983). A characteristic feature of the lesion is its superficial location, the commonest site being in the areolar region (Haagensen 1986). The typical appearance is of ring-like calcific densities situated near the skin surface (Leborgne 1967).

In summary, the following benign masses may simulate carcinoma:

1. Postoperative scar (Fig. 7.31)
2. Fat necrosis (Fig. 7.34)
3. Haematoma
4. Radial scar (Fig. 7.32)
5. Abscess (Fig. 7.26)
6. Granular cell tumour (Fig. 7.27)
7. Tuberculosis
8. Filariasis

The following malignant lesions may simulate benign masses:

1.   Medullary carcinoma (Fig. 6.29, p. 110)
2.   Mucoid carcinoma
3.   Fibrosarcoma
4.   Lymphoma—primary or secondary (Fig. 6.30, p. 112)
5.   Pseudolymphoma
6.   Metastases, e.g. from malignant melanoma (Fig. 6.31)
7.   Metastatic involvement of intramammary lymph nodes

All may be single lesions, with smooth or lobulated well-defined margins and no associated microcalcification, and therefore may be mistaken for a cyst or fibroadenoma. Some of these lesions are very occasionally multiple.

Calcification

Breast calcifications may be categorized as benign, probably benign, and suggestive of malignancy (Sickles 1986), on the basis of size, shape, density and spatial characteristics of the particles. However, in the case of isolated microcalcifications not associated with a mass, it may be extremely difficult to distinguish benign from malignant pathologies (Egan et al 1980). Benign conditions such as sclerosing adenosis, intraductal hyperplasia and papillomatosis all produce microcalcification similar to that seen in malignant disease (Fig. 7.35). Price & Gibbs (1978) suggested that microcalcification is a product of increased cellular activity in the lobulo-ductal complex and may be extruded into the surrounding interstitial tissue, whether by malignant cells or by abnormal or preneoplastic cells in dysplastic breast epithelium. The origin and distribution of the calcifications appear to be the same in epitheliosis, non-invasive and invasive carcinoma.

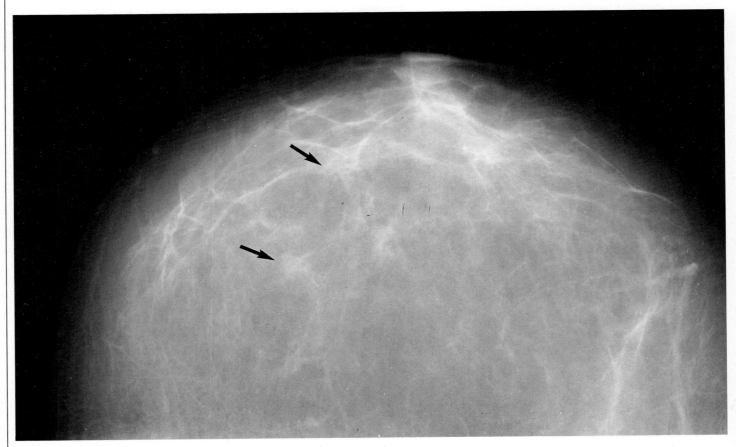

L

Fig. 7.35   Bilateral malignant-looking grouped microcalcification (arrows) misdiagnosed as carcinoma. Histological diagnosis = sclerosing adenosis only.

Spatial characteristics

Several groups have tried to analyse the spatial characteristics of benign versus malignant microcalcifications. Hansell et al (1988) analysed 21 cases in whom grouped microcalcification was the only xeromammographic abnormality, and found no difference in the spatial characteristics of benign versus malignant microcalcification, in terms of shape parameter, spatial frequency of the particles and neighbour-to-neighbour relations. However, Olson et al (1988), using an image digitizer to analyse 52 clusters of calcification from 48 cases, found that the average distance between the particles in malignant conditions was greater than in benign conditions, and that tissue region averages (reflecting local neighbourhood intensities) surrounding malignant calcifications were consistently higher than those for benign conditions. Freundlich et al (1989) analysed 127 isolated clusters of microcalcification, a cluster being 3 or more particles, and found that a group of less than 10 particles per cm² was associated with an 82% chance of being benign, whereas more than 10 particles per cm² had a 44% chance of being malignant. If the particles were more than 1 mm apart, there was a 92% chance of being benign, as compared with a 52% chance of being malignant if the particles were less than 1 mm apart. They confirmed the lack of specificity of clustered microcalcifications. However, Lanyi (1988) analysed 153 microcalcification clusters of malignant aetiology and found no rounded or oval clusters. He states that a triangular or trapezoid configuration is evident in over 50% of cases of malignant microcalcification.

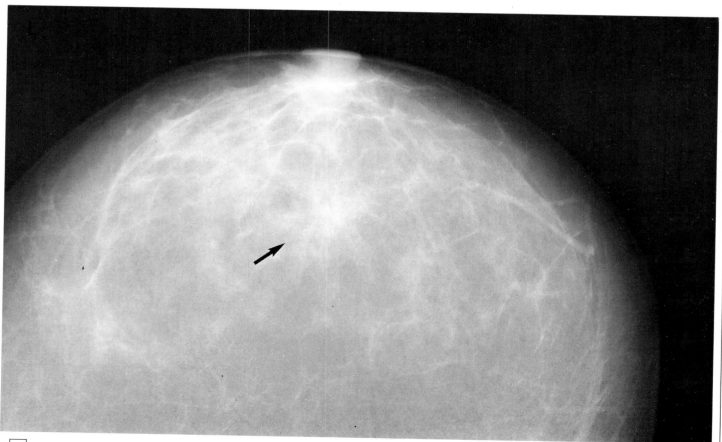

R

Characteristically benign calcifications will be discussed under the following headings (Sickles 1986):

1. Calcifications with radiolucent centres
2. Arterial calcification
3. Duct ectasia
4. Calcified fibroadenoma
5. Postsurgical calcification
6. Milk of calcium in tiny benign cysts
7. Foreign body injection granulomas.

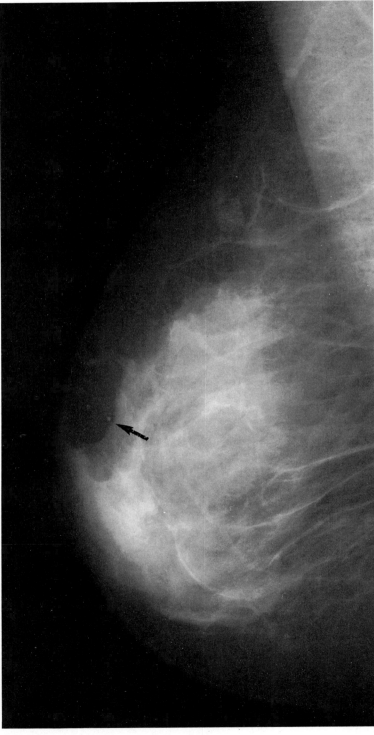

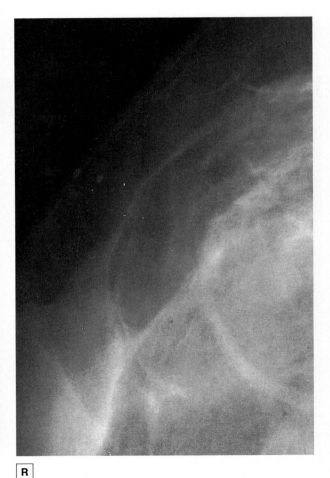

Fig. 7.36a   *Fig. 7.36b*

Fig. 7.36   Dermal calcification. *a* Lateral-oblique view showing ring calcification (arrow). *b* Localized view from a craniocaudal projection confirming their subcutaneous location.

Calcifications with radiolucent centres

These calcifications may be located within the breast parenchyma or the skin (Figs 7.36, 7.37). The entire circumference need not be calcified to present a typically benign appearance. The pathogenesis of these calcifications has not been fully clarified, and they may represent calcification in apocrine cysts or blunt duct adenosis (Barnard et al 1988). When such calcification is seen in one view only, it is most likely to represent dermal calcification.

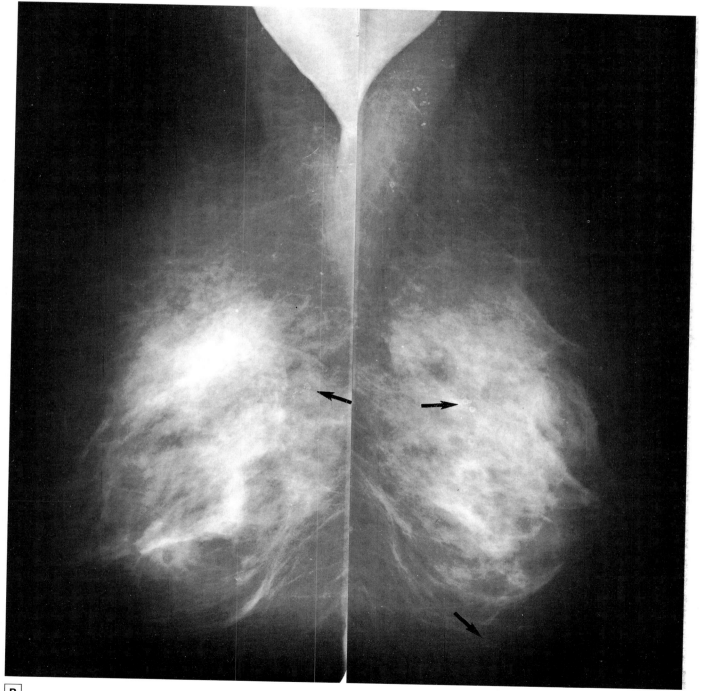

Fig. 7.37   Scattered faint dermal calcification (arrows indicate some groups of calcification).

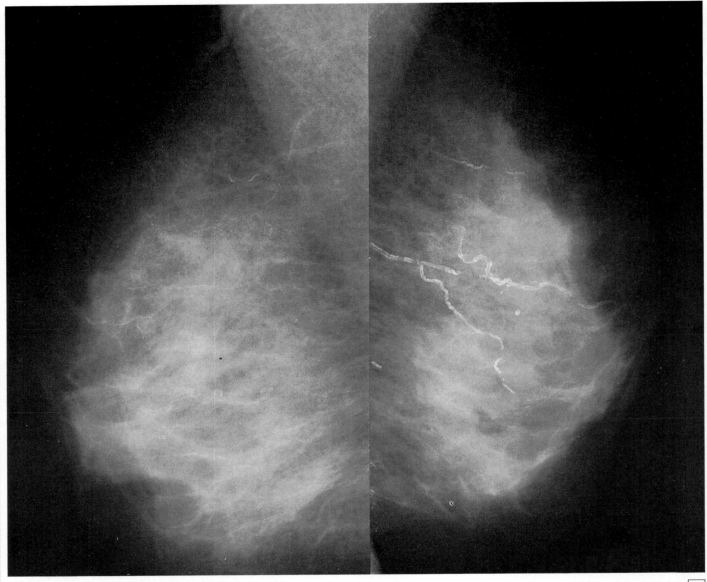

R   L

Fig. 7.38   Vascular calcification. Note asymmetry with less marked calcification in the right breast.

Arterial calcification

This does not usually present a diagnostic problem because the calcification occurs typically in two parallel lines, as elsewhere in the body. Both breasts are usually affected, although often asymmetrically (Fig. 7.38). Early arterial calcification may be difficult to distinguish from suspicious microcalcification, but the situation will usually be clarified on follow-up mammography.

Duct ectasia

This is usually associated with large calcifications, and therefore is not often confused with malignant-type microcalcification. The ipsilateral nipple may be retracted or inverted (Figs 7.39–7.41). The calcification is thought to occur in inspissated secretions within dilated benign ducts. In some cases, the calcifications are periductal rather than intraductal, and then they may have radiolucent centres which represent the non-calcified duct lumina. Thus it can be seen that the calcification of duct ectasia is linear with the long axis pointing towards the nipple, only very occasionally branching; it may be oval or round, often with radiolucent centres, and is usually bilateral and symmetrical in distribution. It is important to note that comedo carcinoma may present with very extensive ductal calcification, but in this case the calcifications tend to be variable in size and shape, with much branching (Fig. 6.12, p. 92). The distribution is often asymmetrical, with only one breast affected in this way.

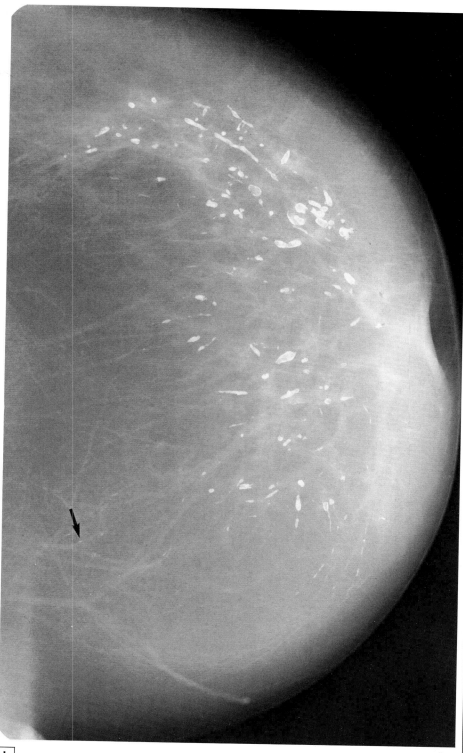

L

Fig. 7.39   Duct ectasia. Note typical ductal calcification and indrawn nipple. Arrow indicates early arterial calcification.

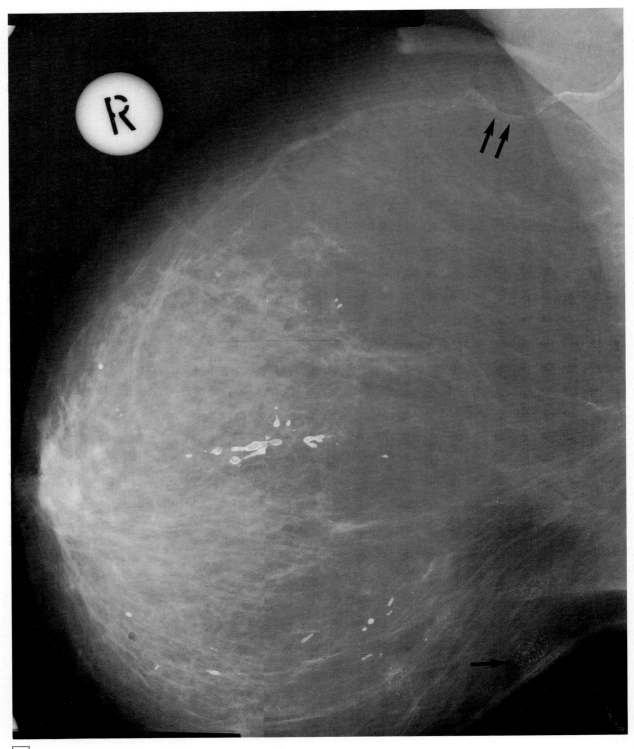

R

Fig. 7.40a

Fig. 7.40   Benign calcifications: ductal, skin warts (arrow), and vascular (double arrows).
a Lateral-oblique view. *b* Craniocaudal view.

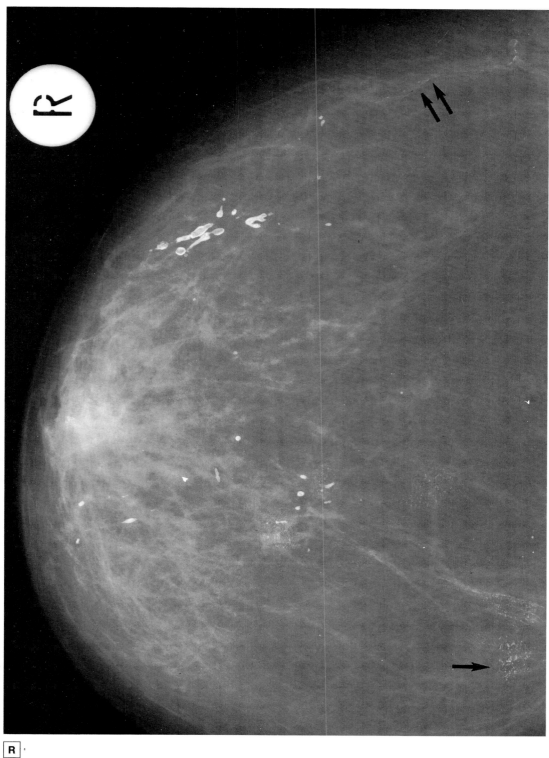

Fig. 7.40b

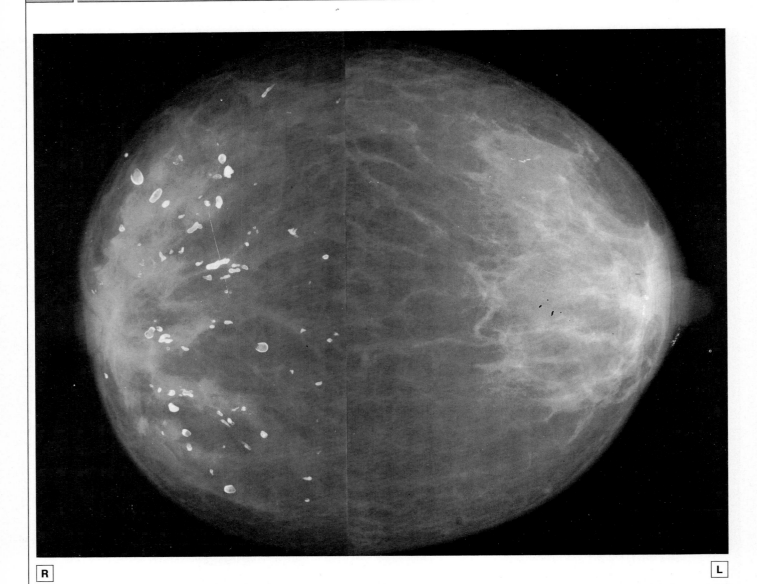

R   L

Fig. 7.41 Duct ectasia in right breast and probable calcified loa loa adjacent to left nipple. The asymmetry is unusual in duct ectasia. Note early nipple retraction on the right.

Calcified fibroadenoma

Many fibroadenomas calcify as they undergo myxoid degeneration. Again the calcification is usually large, and therefore not easily mistaken for malignant-type microcalcification. Early calcification usually occurs at the periphery of the mass (Figs 7.15, 7.16). Advanced calcification has a characteristic 'popcorn' appearance (Figs 7.17, 7.18), and may then be indistinguishable from a fully calcified haematoma or lipid cyst of fat necrosis.

Post surgical calcification

This may be seen following biopsy, with large amorphous streaks and clumps of calcification oriented along the plane of surgical incision. Occasionally calcified suture material may be identified as 5–10 mm-long linear calcification (Fig. 8.8, p. 177). Calcification may also be seen following radiotherapy, but this is not normally significant and will be discussed in more detail in Chap. 8. Localized microcalcification is occasionally seen following cyst aspiration, and lipid cysts of fat necrosis may occur postoperatively.

Milk of calcium in tiny benign cysts

These are usually small calcifications, of the order of 1–2 mm, and although commonly occurring as multiple scattered microcalcifications bilaterally, when confined to one breast and clustered in distribution they may present diagnostic difficulties. The characteristic feature of these calcifications is their change in shape with position: a lateral oblique view taken with a horizontal beam reveals a fluid-calcium level ('tea cup', Lanyi 1977) whereas on a craniocaudal view taken with a vertical beam they appear as poorly defined smudges (Figs 7.12, 7.13) (Sickles & Abele 1981).

Foreign body injection granulomas

Calcification has been described in relation to granulomas formed in reaction to injected foreign body material such as silicone, paraffin, and homologous fat transplants used for breast augmentation (Figs 8.14, 8.15, 8.21). Again these tend to be large calcifications, or to have radiolucent centres, and therefore are not a source of diagnostic confusion.

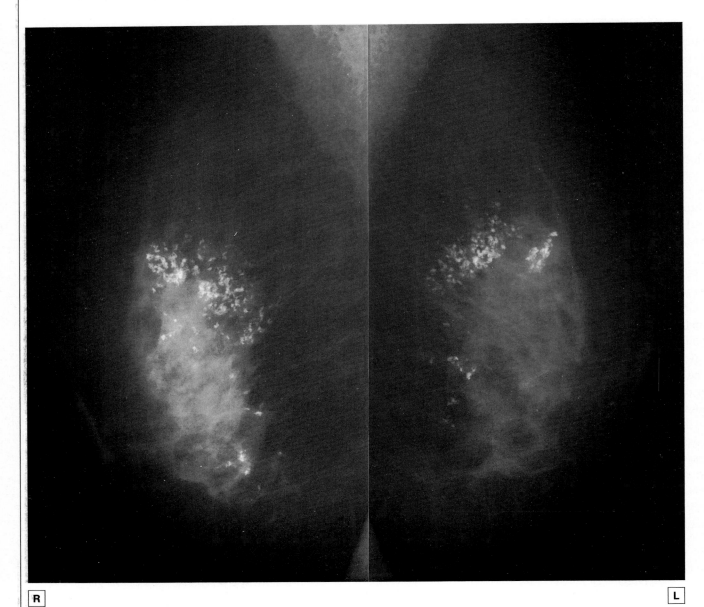

R

L

Fig. 7.42   Osseous metaplasia. Marked symmetrical benign-looking large calcifications. (Reproduced by courtesy of Mr. C. Royston.)

Osseous metaplasia (Fig. 7.42)
Osseous metaplasia is an unusual condition in which bone is laid down probably by fibroblasts in various tissues, commonly cartilage, scar tissue, muscle or in areas of dystrophic calcification (Walter & Israel 1987). Rarely this occurs in the breast. Osseous and cartilaginous components have been recognized in intraductal papilloma, phylloides tumours and stromal sarcoma (Smith & Taylor 1969). An et al (1983) describe a case of breast carcinoma with osseous metaplasia which they postulate has originated from stromal connective tissue rather than carcinoma cells.

In one series of 151 women, Sommer et al (1987) found that patients on haemodialysis for renal disease had significantly more breast calcification, in arteries, ducts and parenchyma, than patients with normal renal function. The calcifications were bilateral in all but one case and was easily distinguishable from that seen in malignant disease. The frequency of calcifications correlated with serum levels of parathyroid hormone.

MANAGEMENT OF IMPALPABLE LESIONS WHICH ARE PROBABLY BENIGN (Homer 1987)

There are two courses of action:

1. Biopsy or fine-needle aspiration, depending on the available pathology/ cytology services. Stereotactic methods of localization will be discussed in Chap. 10.

2. Follow-up within 6 months in the first instance, and for at least $2\frac{1}{2}$ to 3 years to ensure no change. Very few cancers do not show any mammographic change within 3 years (Meyer & Kopans 1981). One has to balance a low biopsy rate against a large number of patients being brought back for follow-up.

Acknowledgements
I wish to thank Dr Marigold Curling for her advice on the pathology; Dr Kate Walmesley for Figs 7.14, 7.20, 7.27; and Mr Christopher Royston for permission to use Fig. 7.42.

REFERENCES

An T, Grathwohl M, Frable W J 1983 Breast carcinoma with osseous metaplasia: an electron microscopic study. American Journal of Clinical Pathology 81: 127–132

Andersen J A, Gram J B 1984 Radial scar in the female breast. Cancer 53: 2557–2560

Anderson T J, Battersby S 1985 Radial scars of benign and malignant breasts: comparative features and significance. Journal of Pathology 147: 23–32

Barnard N J, George B D, Tucker A K, Gilmore O J 1988 Histopathology of benign non-palpable breasts lesions identified by mammography. Journal of Clinical Pathology 41(1): 26–30

Bassett L W, Gold R H, Cove H C 1978 Mammographic spectrum of traumatic fat necrosis. American Journal of Roentgenology 130: 119–122

Breast Group of the Royal College of Radiologists 1989 Radiological Nomenclature in Benign breast change. Clinical Radiology 49: 374–379

Chandrasoma P T, Mendis K N 1978 Filarial infection of the breast. American Journal of Tropical Medicine and Hygiene 27: 770–773

Cole-Beuglet C, Soriano R, Kurtz A B, Meyer J E, Kopans D B, Goldberg B B 1983 Ultrasound, X-ray mammography, and histopathology of cystosarcoma phylloides. Radiology 146(2): 481–486

Demay R M, Kay S 1984 Granular cell tumour of the breast. Pathology Annual 19 pt 2: 121–148

D'Orsi C J, Feldhaus L, Sonnenfeld M 1983 Unusual lesions of the breast. Radiologic Clinics of North America 21(1): 67–80

Egan R L, McSweeney M B, Sewell C W 1980 Intramammary calcifications without an associated mass in benign and malignant disease. Radiology 137: 1–7

Elias E G, Valenzuela L, Pickren J W 1970 Granular cell myoblastoma. Journal of Surgical Oncology 2: 33–43

Fenoglio C, Lattes R 1974 Sclerosing papillary proliferations in the female breast. A benign lesion often mistaken for carcinoma. Cancer 33: 691–700

Fisher E R, Palekar A S, Kotwal N, Lipana N 1979 A nonencapsulated sclerosing lesion of the breast. American

Journal of Clinical Pathology 71: 240–246

Fisher E R, Palekar A S, Sass R, Fisher B 1983 Scar cancers: pathologic findings from the National Surgical Adjuvant Breast Project (Protocol no 4): IX. Breast Cancer Research and Treatment 3: 39–59

Freundlich I M, Hunter T B, Seeley G W 1989 et al Computer-assisted analysis of mammographic clustered calcifications. Clinical Radiology 40: 295–298

Gordenne W H, Malchair F L 1988 Mach bands in mammography. Radiology 169(1): 55–58

Greenberg M W 1967 Granular cell myoblastoma of the breast. Archives of Surgery 94: 739–740

Haagensen C D 1986 Diseases of the breast. W B Saunders, Philadelphia

Hamperl H 1975 Strahlige narben und obliterierende mastopathie: Beitrage zur pathologischen histologie der mamma. Virchows Archiv [A], Pathological Anatomy and Histopathology 369: 55–68

Hansell D M, Cooke, J C, Parsons C A et al 1988 A quantitative analysis of the spatial relationships of grouped microcalcifications demonstrated on xeromammography in benign and malignant breast disease. British Journal of Radiology 61: 21–27

Harbitz H F 1935 Lipogranuloma-a foreign body inflammation often suggesting a tumour. Acta Chirurgica Scandinavica 76: 401

Herbert A 1989 Benign Breast Change: histology, cytology and terminology. Symposium Mammographicum, Abstract, p 20

Homer M J 1985 Breast imaging: Pitfalls, controversies and some practical thoughts. Radiologic Clinics of North America 23(3): 459–472

Homer M J 1987 Imaging features and management of characteristically benign and probably benign lesions. Radiologic Clinics of North America 25(5): 939–951

Homer M J 1989 Circumscribed intraductal carcinoma of the breast (Letter). Radiology 171(3): 877

Hughes L E, Mansell R E, Webster D J T 1987 Aberrations of normal development and involution (ANDI): A new perspective on pathogenesis and nomenclature of benign breast disorders. Lancet (ii): 1316–1319

Lane E J, Proto A V, Phillips T W 1976 Mach bands and density perception. Radiology 121: 9–17

Lanyi M 1977 Differential diagnose der Mikroverkalkungen. Die verkalkte mastopathische Mikrocyste. Radiologe 17: 217–218

Lanyi M 1988 Diagnosis and differential diagnosis of breast calcifications. Springer-Verlag, Berlin, pp 94–95

Leborgne R 1967 Esteatonecrosis quistica calcificada de la mamma. Torax 16: 172

Lee B J, Adair F E 1920 Traumatic fat necrosis of the female breast and its differentiation from carcinoma. Annals of Surgery 37: 189

Lindfors K K, Kopans D B, Googe P B, McCarthy K A, Koerner F C & Meyer J E 1986 Breast cancer metastasis to intramammary lymph nodes. American Journal of Roentgenology 146(1): 133–136; published erratum appears in AJR 146(3): 614

Meyer J E, Kopans D B 1981 Stability of a mammographic mass: a false sense of security. American Journal of Roentgenology 137: 595–598

Mitnick J, Roses D F & Harris M N 1988 Differentiation of postsurgical changes from carcinoma of the breast. Surgery, Gynecology and Obstetrics 166(6): 549–550

Mitnick J S, Roses D F, Harris M N, Feiner H D 1989 Circumscribed intraductal carcinoma of the breast. Radiology 170: 432–425

Moskowitz M 1983 Minimal breast cancer redux. Radiologic Clinics of North America 21(1): 93–113

Nielsen M, Christensen, L, Andersen J 1987 Radial scars in women with breast cancer. Cancer 59: 1019–1025

Olson S L, Fam B W, Winter P F, Scholz F J, Lee A K, Gordon S E 1988 Breast calcifications: analysis of imaging properties. Radiology 169: 329–322

Orson L W, Cigtay O S 1983 Fat necrosis of the breast: characteristic xeromammographic appearance. Radiology 146: 35–38

Parsons C A 1983 Diagnosis of breast disease. Chapman & Hall

Price J L, Gibbs N M 1978 The relationship between microcalcification and in-situ carcinoma of the breast. Clinical Radiology 29: 447–452

Pye J K 1989 Microradiography of the breast. Symposium Mammographium, Abstract, p 25

Rickert R R, Kalisher L, Hutter R V P 1981 Indurative mastopathy: a benign sclerosing lesion of breast with elastosis which may simulate carcinoma. Cancer 47: 561–571

Sadowsky N, Kopans D B 1983 Breast cancer. Radiologic Clinics of North America 21(1): 51–65

Sickles E A, Herzog K A 1980 Intramammary scar tissue: a mimic of the appearance of carcinoma. American Journal of Roentgenology 135: 345–352

Sickles E A, Abele J S 1981 Milk of calcium within tiny benign breast cysts. Radiology 141: 655–658

Sickles E A, Klein D L, Goodson W H, Hunt T K 1983 Mammography after needle aspiration of palpable breast masses. American Journal of Surgery 145(3): 395–397

Sickles E A 1986 Breast calcifications: mammographic evaluation. Radiology 160(2): 289–293

Smith B H, Taylor H B 1969 The occurrence of bone and cartilage in mammary tumours. American Journal of Clinical Pathology 51: 610–618

Smith L W, Mason R L 1926 The concurrence of tuberculosis and cancer of the breast. Surgery, Gynecology and Obstetrics 43: 70

Sommer G, Kopsa H, Zazgornik J, Salomonowitz E 1987 Breast calcifications in renal hyperparathyroidism. American Journal of Roentgenology 148: 855–857

Swann C A, Kopans D B, Koerner F C, McCarthy K A, White G, Hall D A 1987 The halo sign and malignant breast lesions. American Journal of Roentgenology 149(6): 1145–1147

Tabar L, Dean P B 1985 Teaching atlas of mammography. Thieme-Stratton, New York

Walter J B, Israel M S 1987 General pathology, 6th edn. Churchill Livingstone, Edinburgh

Wolfe J N 1983 Xeroradiography of the breast, 2nd edn. Charles C Thomas, Springfield

Wolfe J N 1976 Breast patterns as an index of risk for developing breast cancer. American Journal of Roentgenology 126: 1130–1139

Wolfe J N, Albert S, Belle S, Salane M 1983 Breast parenchymal patterns and their relationship to risk for having or developing carcinoma. Radiologic Clinics of North America 21(1): 127–136

CHAPTER 8

Iatrogenic appearances on mammography

N. M. Perry, R. Toye

INTRODUCTION

Many procedures will result in the alteration of normal mammographic patterns. Familiarity with the range of such appearances will assist in the interpretation of later mammograms, allow early detection of recurrence of significant pathology and reduce unnecessary recalls for assessment from screening programmes. The appearances described will relate primarily to film-screen mammography.

BREAST SURGERY

The commonest surgical procedures accounting for alteration of mammographic patterns will be excision biopsies and either augmentation or reduction mammoplasties. Many procedures, however, will show no obvious radiological sequelae on later mammograms.

Excision biopsy

Abnormal mammographic appearances have been reported following excision biopsy of breast lesions in up to 45% of patients (Sickles & Herzog 1981). The most common changes seen are skin thickening and deformity at the site of the scar, associated with retraction and loss of the normal rounded contour of the breast (Fig. 8.1).

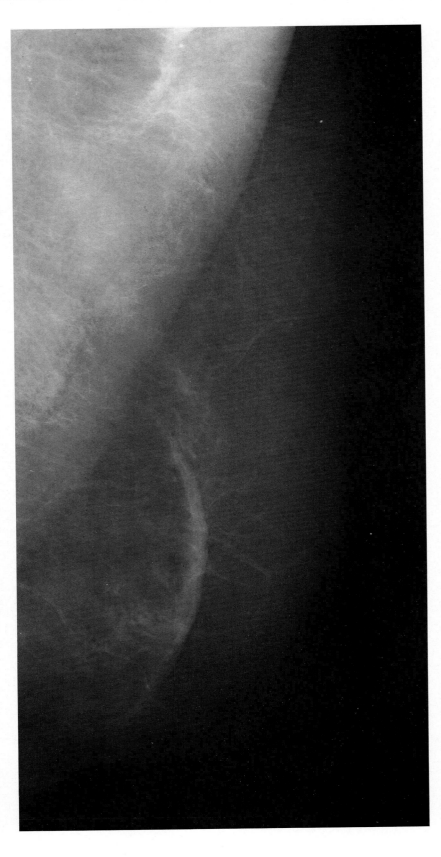

Fig. 8.1 7 years previously the patient had a segmental mastectomy with axillary node sampling. Skin thickening and retraction is noted at both incision sites with accompanying minor architectural distortion.

Skin thickening. Localized skin thickening is usually present early following biopsy, and is almost always seen by 6 months. It shows partial or complete resolution over the next 3 years (Fig. 8.2).

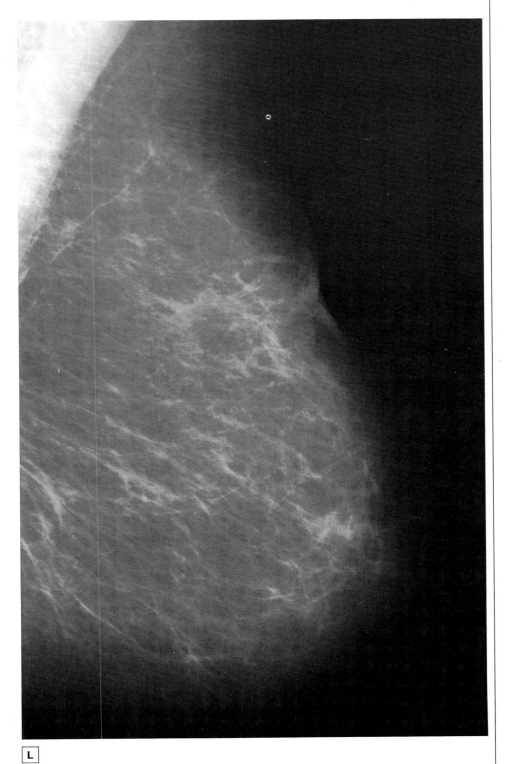

L

Fig. 8.2 Very localized skin thickening and retraction seen high in the breast 2 years following a benign biopsy.

Distortion. Architectural distortion may be seen due to local fibrous strand formation with resultant disturbance of the trabecular pattern (Fig. 8.3). Similarly there may be disruption of the normal interface between fat and glandular tissue. Asymmetry of the residual glandular tissue between the two breasts may be apparent depending upon the volume of tissue excised (Fig. 8.4).

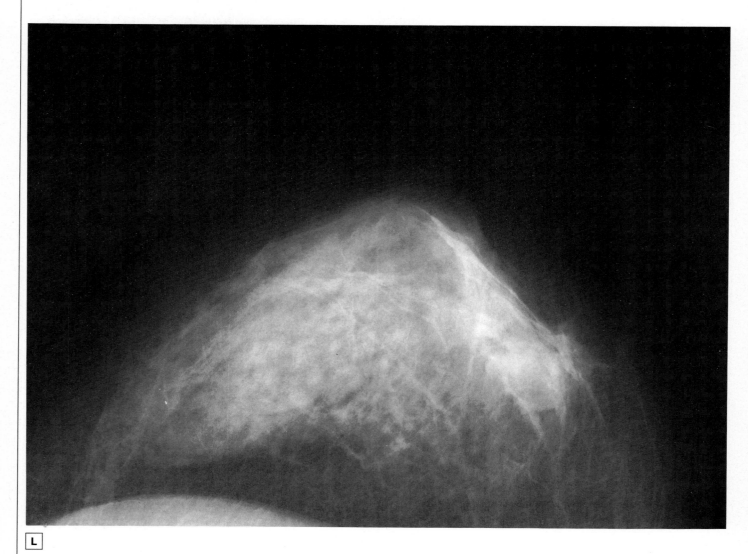

L

Fig. 8.3 Considerable architectural distortion is present medially in the breast 10 years following a benign biopsy. Localized thickening and linear scarring is also present.

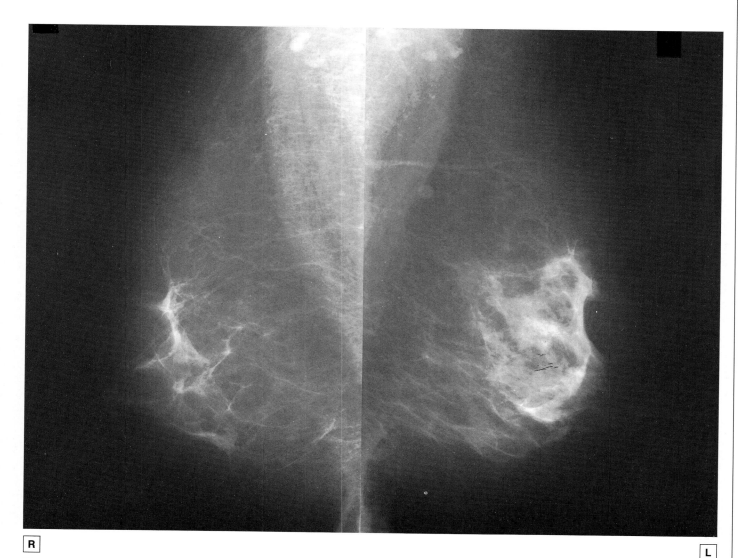

R

L

Fig. 8.4 10 years following a benign excision biopsy on the right side there is residual asymmetry of the glandular tissue between the two breasts.

Oedema. Oedema at the site of surgery causes increased density and trabecular thickening. It will be seen immediately after excision biopsy and in most cases has resolved within 4 weeks (Peters et al 1988).

Scarring. Sickles & Herzog (1980) have described parenchymal scar tissue being present in 7% of previously biopsied breasts. It may be seen as a fine linear parenchymal scar (Fig. 8.5), or appear as a mass up to several centimetres in diameter, either well or poorly-defined and occasionally spiculate. Local skin retraction may be found as an associated feature. Such appearances are thought to be due to a combination of haematoma formation with localized fibrous tissue response.

Differentiation of scar tissue from malignancy can be extremely difficult (Fig. 8.6). A central lucency suggests the presence of fat necrosis and usually indicates a benign nature (Mitnick et al 1988). Spicules of a benign parenchymal scar tend to be fine, long and may be discontinuous from localized skin retraction, in contrast to those of malignancy (Tabar & Dean 1985). Spicules from a benign scar are also more likely to be asymmetric and curvilinear (Fig. 8.7) as opposed to

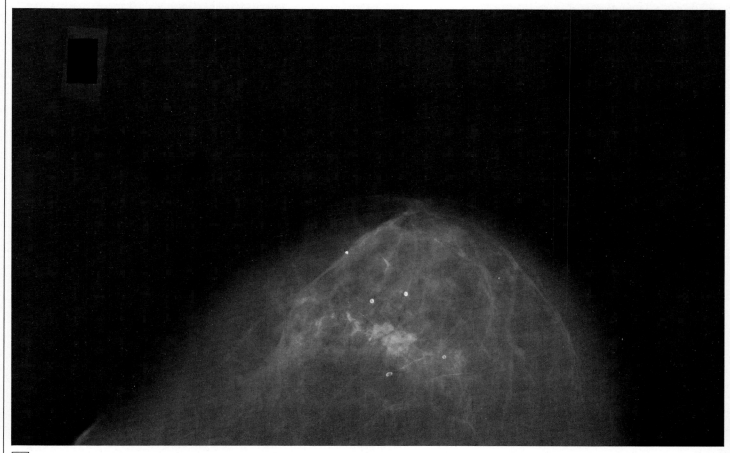

L

Fig. 8.5   A linear parenchymal scar is identified lateral to the nipple following benign biopsy 15 years earlier. Multiple rounded benign calcifications are also seen.

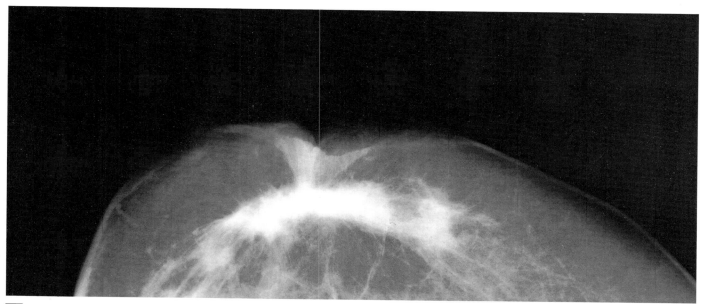

R | *Fig. 8.6a*

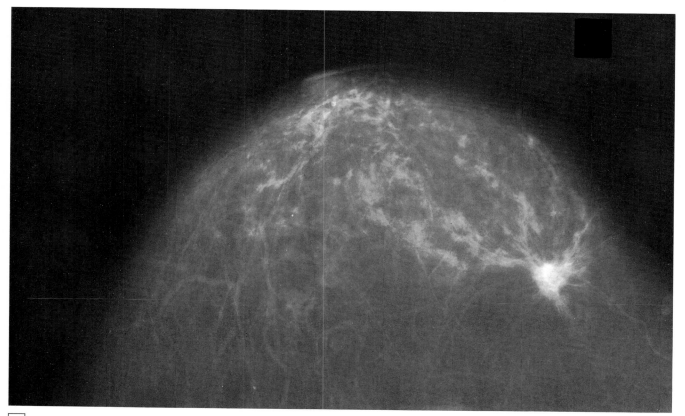

R | *Fig. 8.6b*

Fig. 8.6 *a* There is distortion of breast contour with widespread skin thickening, nipple retraction and a spiculate elongated subareolar mass. The patient had undergone abscess drainage 10 years previously and claimed the clinical deformity to be unchanged over the past 10 years. *b* There is a highly irregular 2 cm spiculate opacity placed laterally in the breast. Clinically a hard mass and skin dimpling was present at this site. The patient had undergone a benign biopsy here several years earlier. Histology: Lesion *a* showed widespread infiltrating malignancy. Lesion *b* showed only scar tissue.

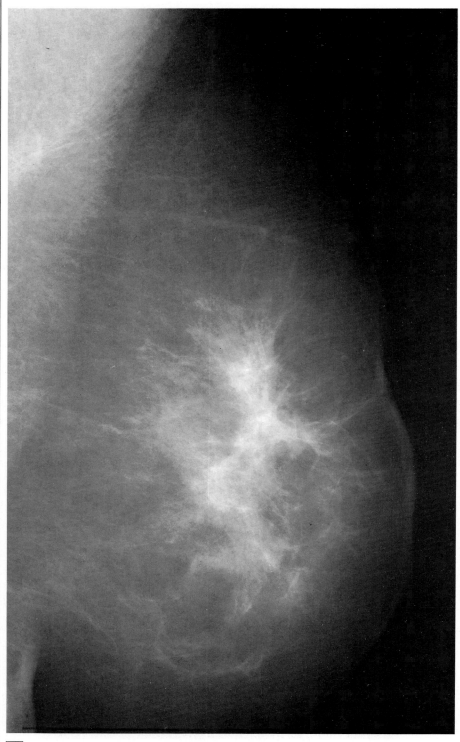

those of a carcinoma, which tend to be straight and symmetrical (Wolfe 1979). A mass which shows resolution over a period of time is generally benign. On palpation, the mass of a parenchymal scar is more likely to be equivalent in size with its mammographic appearance; conversely a carcinoma often feels larger than suggested by the mammogram (Sickles & Herzog 1980). None of these signs has been proven to be entirely reliable, and fine-needle aspiration cytology is useful if there is any doubt.

Routine baseline mammography is generally not warranted after surgery for benign lesions because only a small proportion of women develop scar tissue suspicious enough to require further investigation. A baseline mammogram however, can be recommended in patients who have a tendency to develop extensive post-surgical scarring, or who have previously required scar tissue biopsy (Sickles & Herzog 1981).

R

Fig. 8.7 2 years following excision biopsy there are post-surgical changes of localized skin thickening and considerable architectural distortion with fine curvilinear spiculations present.

Calcification. Calcification after surgery takes many different forms. Egg-shell calcification is associated with fat necrosis. Linear calcification may be seen along the incision line or can occur along a drain site (see Fig. 8.26) (Lanyi 1988). Large, irregular calcification is often due to dystrophic change pathologically. Small, irregular calcification may mimic malignancy but can be due to fibrous change or sclerosing adenosis. Dermal plaques of calcification are occasionally seen.

Calcification in the collagen of suture material has been described (Davis et al 1989), and may be knotted (Fig. 8.8), curvilinear (Fig. 8.9), horse-shoe-shaped or as a cluster of non-specific appearance.

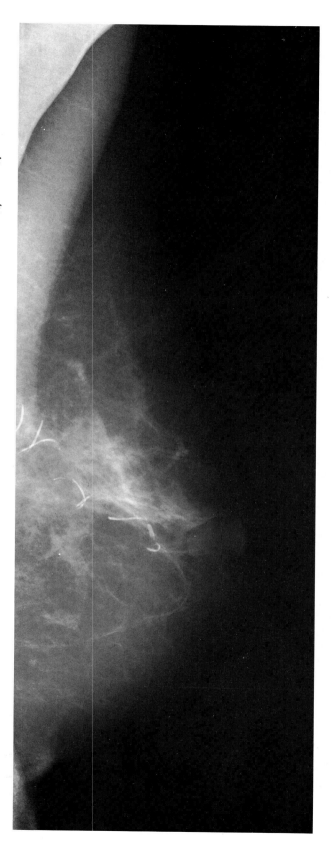

L

Fig. 8.8 Obvious suture calcification 3 years following surgery and radiotherapy.

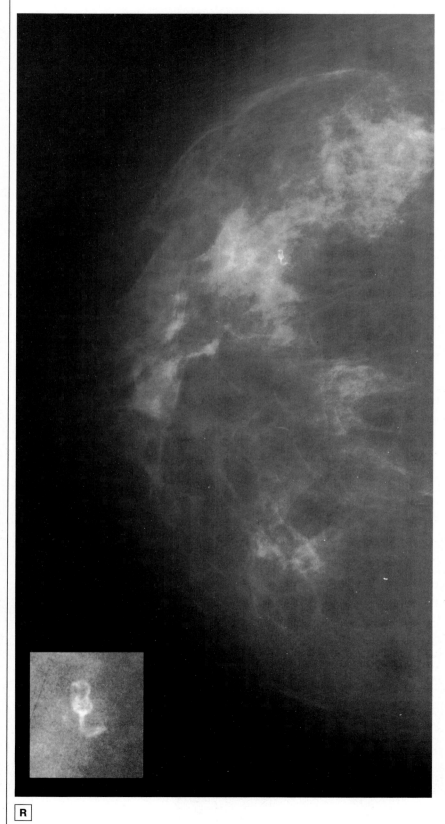

R

Fig. 8.9 Fine curvilinear and knotted suture calcification.

Fat necrosis. Manifestations of post-surgical fat necrosis range from entirely benign to lesions with appearances highly suspicious for malignancy. Clinical confusion with malignancy has long been recognized (Lee & Adair 1920). Apart from nipple and skin retraction, other clinical findings may include tenderness, a hard, possibly fixed, mass and ulceration through the skin (Hadfield 1930). If a mass is seen on the mammogram it is generally smaller than would be expected from the clinical examination, again erroneously suggestive of malignancy (Meyer et al 1978).

The features seen on mammography will depend upon the pathological stage of repair (Meyer et al 1978). Individual fat cells dissolve and fuse to form vacuoles which are subsequently surrounded by macrophages. Foreign body giant cells and plasma cells migrate into the lesion and a fibrous reaction takes place.

The result may be a well-defined rounded soft tissue density having benign features compatible with a fibroadenoma, but an irregular fibrotic response may result in a spiculate mass indistinguishable from infiltrating malignancy. While a mass associated with fat necrosis does not usually progress in size (Hadfield 1930), increasing size has been reported (Bassett et al 1978).

Skin thickening and retraction associated with fat necrosis and simulating carcinoma has been reported by Minagi & Youker (1968) and Coren & Libshitz (1974). Casting microcalcification suggestive of malignancy can occur, either with or without a mass, and irregular calcification may also be present in the regional draining axillary lymph nodes (Bassett et al 1978).

Formation of an oil cyst gives the characteristic appearance of a thin-walled lesion of fat density (Leborgne 1967). Subsequent development of curvilinear mural calcification in such a lesion is not uncommon (Fig. 8.10).

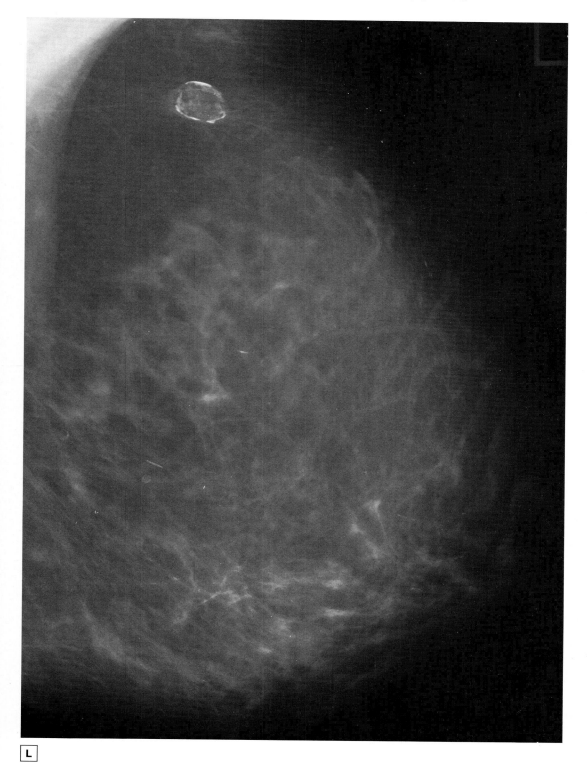

L

Fig. 8.10   A calcified oil cyst is seen high in the left breast many years following surgery.

After excision biopsy and radiotherapy both the number of oil cysts and the amount of calcification associated with them may increase over a period of several years (Fig. 8.11) (Bassett et al 1982). It is possible that radiotherapy promotes these post-surgical appearances. An opacity within the oil cyst itself has been reported (Andersson et al 1977), which is thought to represent material that has not yet liquefied. Microcalcification may also be associated with such an intracystic body (von Hoeffken & Lanyi 1973).

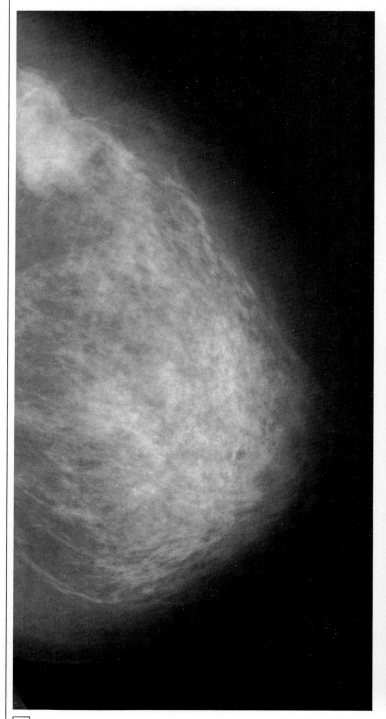

L   *Fig. 8.11a*

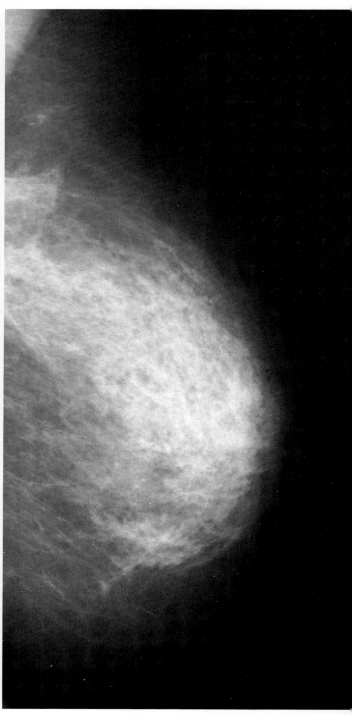

L   *Fig. 8.11b*

Other sequelae of fat necrosis include areas of stromal irregularity with or without coarse calcifications, lesions indistinguishable from benign breast change, markedly enlarged vessels, and almost any combination of the appearances described (Coren & Libshitz 1974, Minagi & Youker 1968).

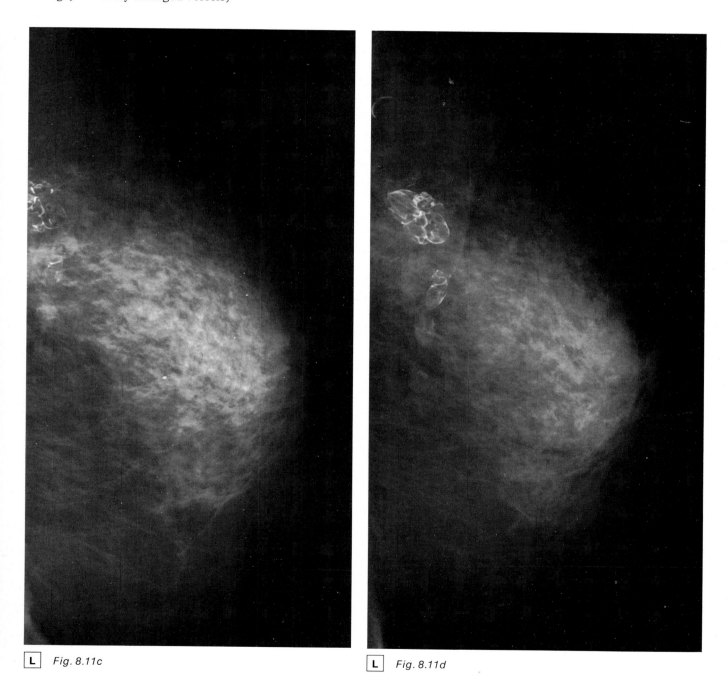

L   *Fig. 8.11c*   L   *Fig. 8.11d*

Fig. 8.11   *a* A 3 cm carcinoma is present high in the left breast. *b* 1 year following excision there are typical radiotherapy sequelae. *c* 1 year later there is some resolution of these appearances but note the development of typical fat necrotic areas with fine curvilinear calcification deep in the breast. *d* 3 years following treatment, there has been further increase in the calcification associated with these areas of fat necrosis.

Other findings. After biopsy there may be localized periareolar oedema due to lymphatic disruption. An axillary lymphocele, appearing as a well-defined dense mass with localized skin thickening, has been reported folowing axillary node sampling (Peters et al 1988).

Localized haematomata often appear as rounded and well-defined densities persisting for a month or more, but they may also be small and poorly-defined. Surgical emphysema may be visible on the rare occasions that mammography is performed very soon after biopsy.

Needle aspiration

Needle aspiration of solid or cystic masses is increasingly used for both symptomatic and screen detected breast lesions. In the short term needle aspiration can result in a haematoma or local oedema both resulting in loss of definition of any mass previously present. Aspiration of a cyst is not likely to cause diagnostic problems in subsequent mammography but aspiration of a solid lesion could well result in loss of features normally associated with benignity, particularly if multiple passes are performed (Sickles et al 1983). Any mammography within 2 weeks of aspiration should be interpreted with caution (Klein & Sickles 1982). It is therefore recommended practice to perform diagnostic mammography before needle aspiration has taken place.

Cosmetic surgery

Augmentation mammoplasty. Breast augmentation is performed on approximately 150 000 women every year in the USA and over the years many methods have been used. It was common particularly in the Far East and South America, to inject substances directly into the breast tissue. The degree of foreign body reaction depended upon the material used. Substances known to have caused granulomatous mastitis from injection include petroleum jelly, paraffin waxes, silicone wax and fluid, bees wax, putty and epoxy resin (Symmers 1968) (Fig. 8.12). The granulomatous reaction and ingestion of injected material by macrophages in regional lymph nodes often resulted in diffuse breast lumpiness, palpable and even visible masses, localized or generalized skin infiltration, abscess formation and axillary lymphadenopathy (Ortiz-Monasterio & Trigos 1972).

In more reputable centres from the 1950s paraffin was used for injection mammoplasty. Paraffin resulted in oval or rounded areas of low density possibly with surrounding thickening due to fibrosis (Wren & Crosbie 1968). Although paraffinomata are radiolucent and do not obscure underlying tissue, the pronounced skin thickening and tissue distortion that may arise after paraffin injection can make interpretation of mammograms difficult.

Silicone was used from the 1960s, silicone fluid injections being either in a pure form, or adulterated with small amounts of vegetable oil or fatty acid in an attempt to provide fibrosis, firmness and immobility. Problems arose from the formation of haematomata or of granulomata with tenderness and nodularity (Boo-Chai 1969). Migration of silicone gave rise to hard, poorly defined, tender subcutaneous masses not only in the breasts but also in axillae, upper arms, chest wall, anterior abdominal wall and inguinal canals (Delage et al 1973). It was not infrequent to see diminution of breast size after 2 years, possibly due to migration.

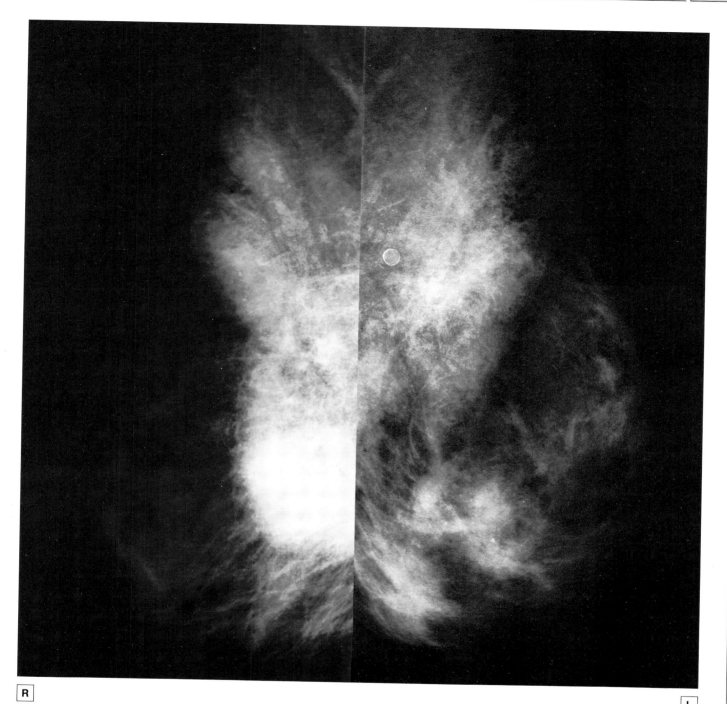

R

L

Fig. 8.12 A bizarre appearance due to granulomatous mastitis following injection mammoplasty with an unknown substance many years previously. Infiltration along the pectoral planes is noted and some benign calcification is also seen. The poorly defined mass in the right breast cannot be radiologically differentiated from malignancy.

Uncomplicated cases show a large homogeneous density after injection of pure silicone and small to moderate sized well-defined opacities, typical for benign lesions after injection of the adulterated form (Minagi et al 1968). On occasions, however, silicone opacities may be very irregular and difficult to differentiate from malignancy (Fig. 8.13).

Calcification due to injection mammoplasty has been observed in 75% of patients following paraffin injections and 29% of those treated with silicone (Koide & Katayama 1979). The calcification does not occur in the paraffin or silicone itself, neither of which saponifies, but in hyaline degeneration of the surrounding fibrous capsule. After paraffin injections numerous small annular or rounded calcifications are generally seen (Fig. 8.14), sometimes involving the lymph nodes. Larger, less numerous, more spherical calcifications are more typically seen after silicone injection, although small irregular calcification has been reported (Jensen & Mackey 1985).

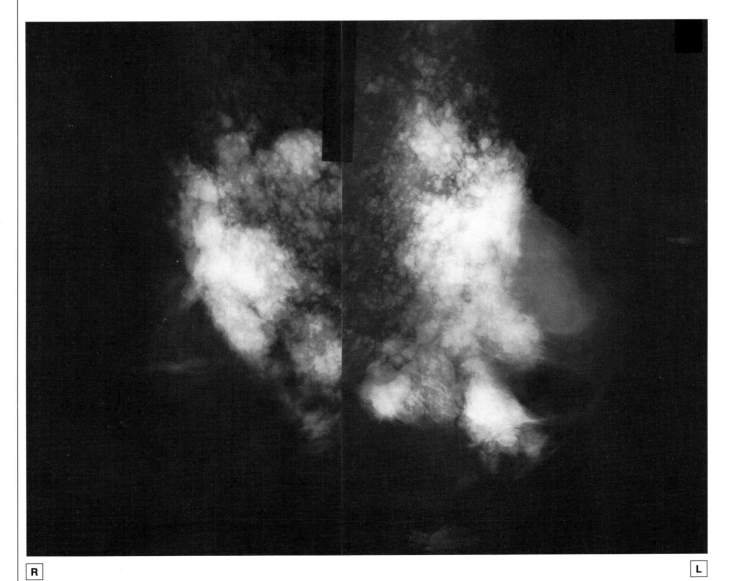

R   L

Fig. 8.13 A typical appearance following silicone injection mammoplasty. There are multiple small ovoid and rounded densities but also larger more irregular densities are present. There is outlining of an ectatic duct on the right side.

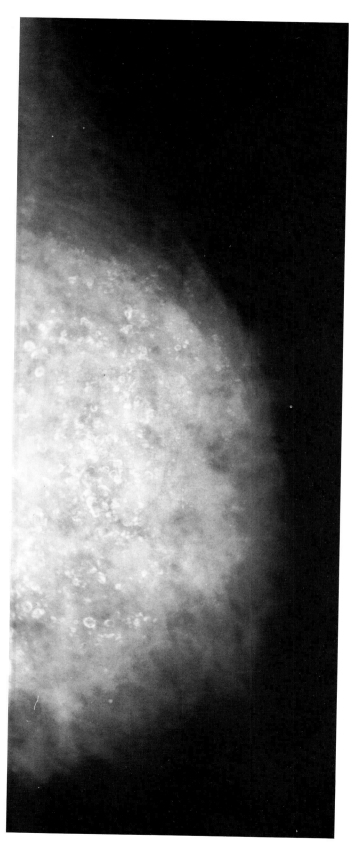

L

Fig. 8.14 Typical small ring and punctate
calcifications following paraffin injection
mammoplasty many years earlier.

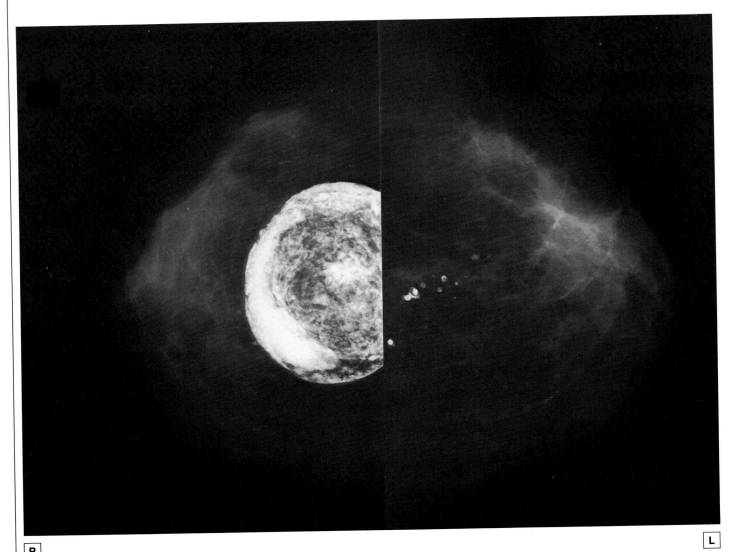

R   **L**

Fig. 8.15   Bilateral augmentation mammoplasty 20 years previously using autologous buttock fat. The left implant had previously been removed. The right implant shows considerable coarse calcification with fat necrosis.

Animal studies showed the possibility of the induction of breast carcinoma or sarcoma by injection of materials used for augmentation (Russell et al 1959, Ben-Hur & Neuman 1965). In the 1960s the practice of injection mammoplasty was largely abandoned to be replaced by autologous fat transplantation (Fig. 8.15), or silastic sacs filled with silicone or saline. Initially these were thick-walled, valved (Fig. 8.16) or Dacron-patched with a tear-drop shape. Subsequently thin-walled, valveless, patchless and rounded low-profile prostheses have been used. An implant may be placed subcutaneously if there has been a subcutaneous mastectomy performed previously, in the retromammary plane for standard augmentation purposes or subpectorally for more stability. Saline tends to leak more than silicone (Fig. 8.17) but has the advantage of not obscuring the underlying breast tissue on mammography. An observation of interest to environmentalists is that a silicone implant has been assessed as requiring approximately 500 000 years to biodegrade.

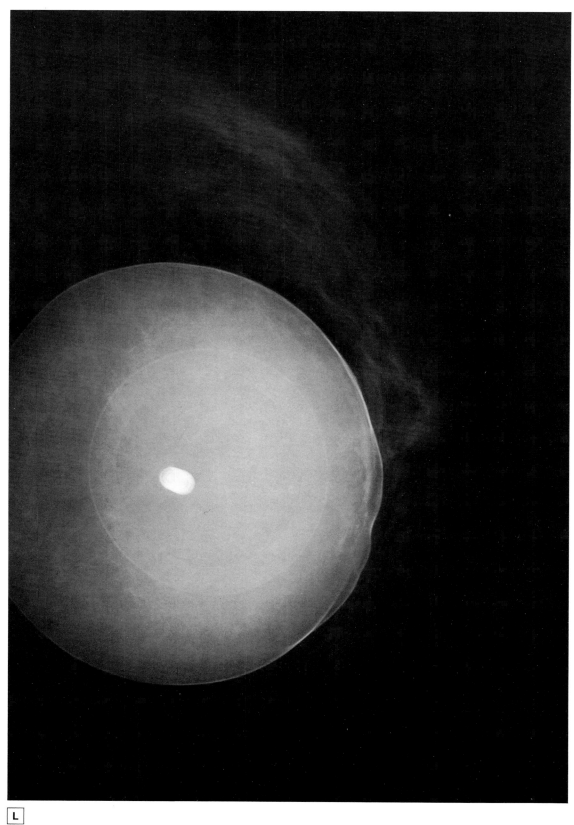

L

Fig. 8.16 A valved implant.

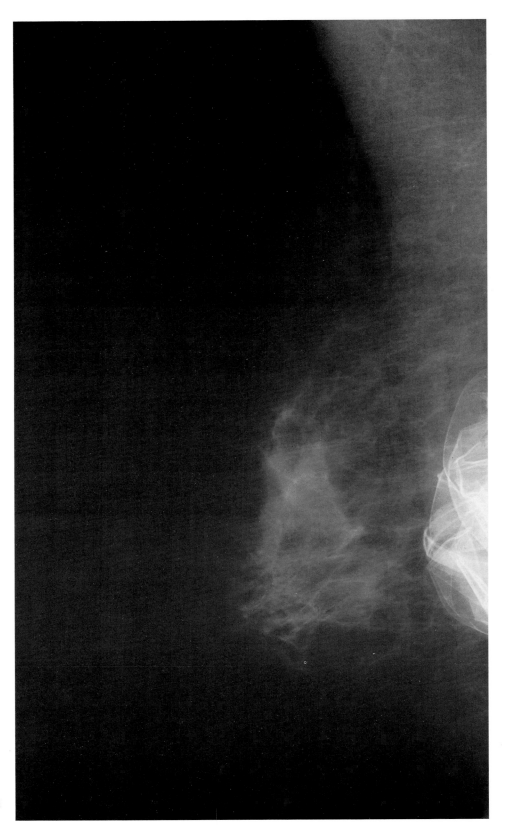

R

Fig. 8.17   A collapsed saline-filled implant is seen deep in the breast.

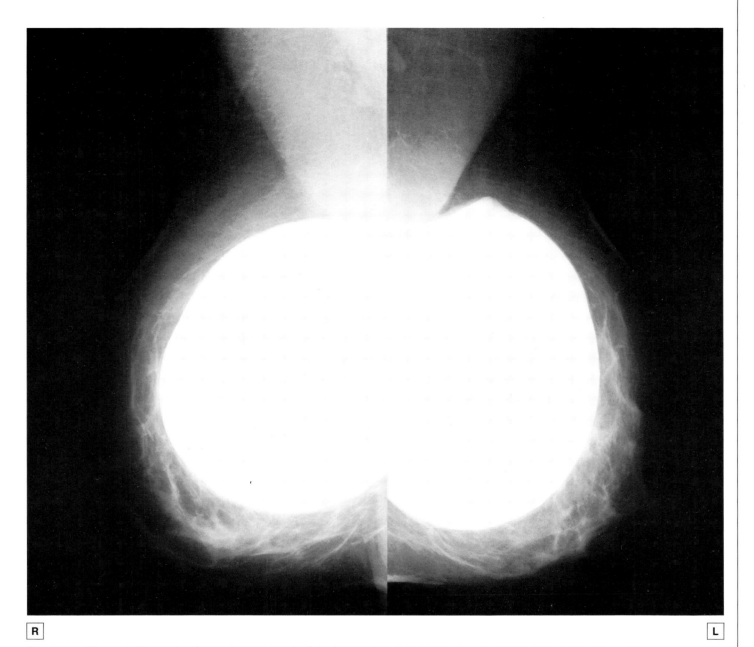

R   L

Fig. 8.18 Bilateral silicone implants obscure much of the breast tissue and it can be very difficult to obtain adequate exposure.

The percentage of breast tissue obscured by silicone implants varies from 22% to 83% (Fig. 8.18) (Hayes et al 1988). In addition the implants cause problems of exposure and compression. Multiple tangential views around an implant would allow imaging of more breast tissue, but would result in too high a radiation dose for routine use (Ecklund et al 1988). When reading mammograms of women with implants, it is helpful to employ a suitably shaped mask over the implant in order to reduce the transmitted light and thus obtain a better view of the surrounding breast tissue. There may be evidence of a fibrous capsule (Fig. 8.19) around the implant and capsular calcification (Fig. 8.20) can be seen (Dershaw & Chaglassian 1989). Special views and ultrasound play an important part in the full assessment of women with breast implants who develop masses (Leibman & Kruse 1990).

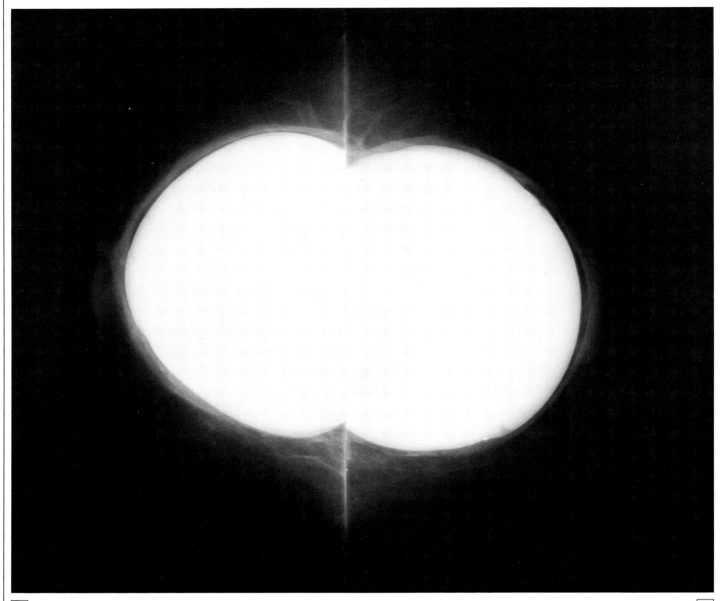

R

L

Fig. 8.19   A thick fibrous capsule can be made out surrounding these implants.

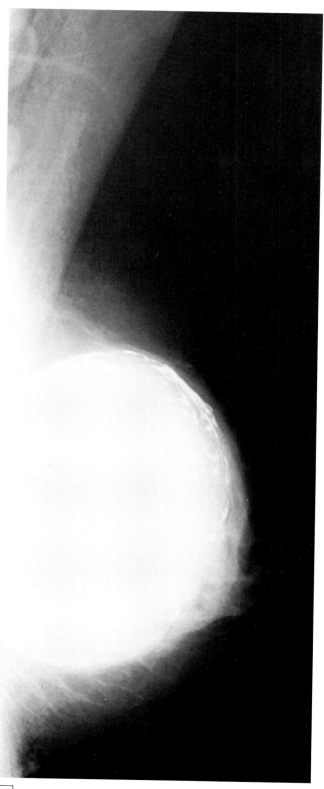

Clinical problems of implants include infection, haematomata requiring evacuation and formation of a thick fibrous capsule causing firmness and implant elevation (Biggs et al 1982). Deflation of inflatable prostheses has been described in up to 15% of patients and occurs from 24 hours to several years after surgery (Mckinney & Tresley 1983).

Rupture of an implant may occur apparently spontaneously (Wan 1987), following trauma (this could include over zealous compression at mammography) or closed manual compression for fibrous capsular contraction (Theophelis & Stevenson 1986). Leaked silicone may track through the tissue planes, or form multiple masses adjacent to, but separate from, an implant. A small collection of silicone adjacent to an implant may represent a diverticulum of the sac through the fibrous capsule rather than a localized leak (Smith 1985).

L

Fig. 8.20   Capsular calcification is identified surrounding this implant.

Failed prostheses may be removed and not replaced. The mammographic consequences of this range from negligible, through parenchymal scarring, to dense and coarse calcification at the site of removal (Fig. 8.21).

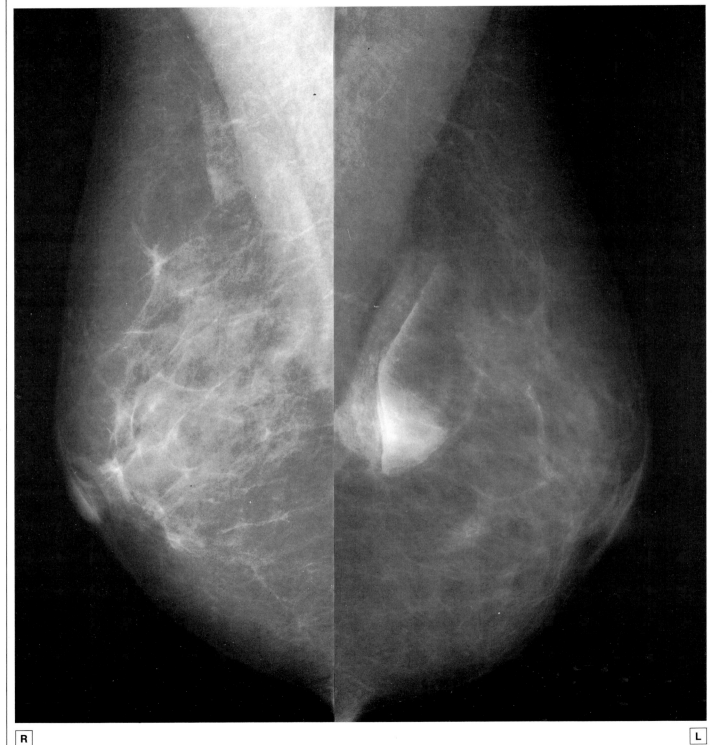

R   L

Fig. 8.21   Several years previously this woman had removal of bilateral failed prostheses. Residual coarse implant bed calcification is seen on the left side. The right side appears normal.

Reduction mammoplasty. Reduction mammoplasty is usually indicated to improve the appearance of patients with macromastia, or to produce a more symmetrical appearance after mastectomy and contralateral reconstruction. Several techniques are used, all of which require relative elevation of the nipple and resection of some of the glandular tissue, with contouring and removal of redundant skin. Some procedures involve resection of the nipple and areola as a full-thickness graft which is then transposed.

Some women who have undergone reduction mammoplasty will show either no significant, or very subtle evidence on mammography. Characteristic mammographic findings have been described (Miller et al 1987), in addition to the standard range of post-surgical changes. Skin thickening either in the periareolar region or inferior to the nipple line is one of the commonest findings, and similarly retraction of the parenchyma inferior to the nipple may be seen. There may be an apparent redistribution of parenchyma from the upper outer quadrant to inferior to the nipple (Fig. 8.22). An abnormal nipple position (usually high in relation to the breast contour) and visible disruption of continuity between the nipple and subareolar ducts are other findings according to the technique used (Fig. 8.23). Retroareolar band-like thickening from fibrosis also occurs.

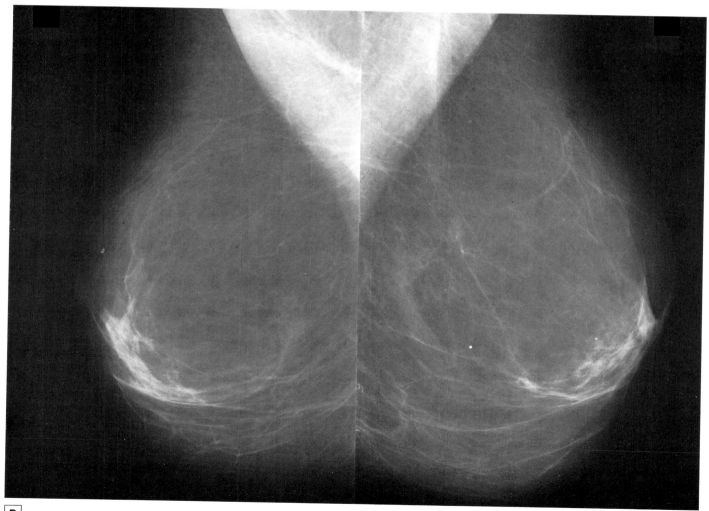

R　　　　　　　　　　　　　　　　　　　　　　　L

Fig. 8.22 Bilateral reduction mammoplasty. There is little to show mammographically; what little residual glandular tissue there is lies inferior to the nipple line.

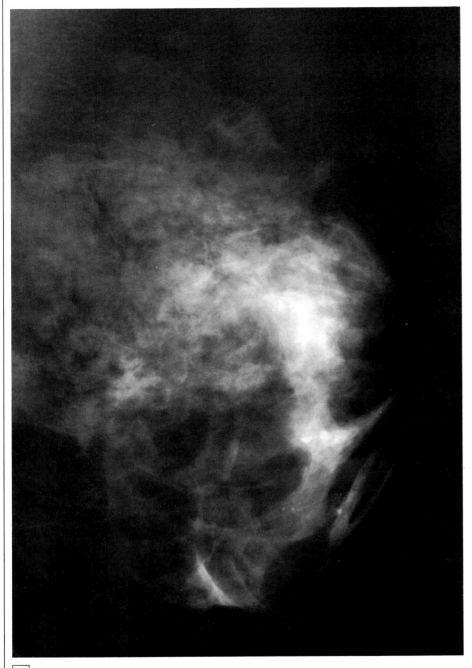

L

Fig. 8.23 Following reduction mammoplasty there is discontinuity of the subareolar duct system.

Changing appearances of scarring, periareolar thickening and inferior contour change have been observed on serial mammography in most patients 2 years following reduction mammoplasty (Brown et al 1987). Asymmetrical densities and benign-appearing calcifications are also identified, with fat necrosis appearing in at least 10%. It should be stressed that many changes seen can be best appreciated following comparison with the preoperative mammograms.

Common causes of palpable lumps after reduction mammoplasty include fat necrosis (Baber & Libshitz 1977), formation of haematomata, benign breast change and, occasionally, newly developed carcinoma (Isaacs et al 1985). It is reasonable to perform a preoperative mammogram in order to detect occult carcinoma before surgery and aid interpretation of subsequent mammograms.

RADIOTHERAPY

Most patients receiving radiotherapy to the breast have had a breast biopsy, but radiotherapy may be used alone to treat large inoperable tumours or Paget's disease of the nipple (Stockdale et al 1989). Many of the mammographic appearances attributable to radiotherapy are similar to those caused by residual tumour, recurrent tumour or surgery, and it can be difficult or impossible to differentiate them.

The mammographic features following radiotherapy are independent of the histology and site of the primary breast tumour (Dershaw et al 1987). They include skin thickening, alteration of the appearance of the subcutaneous tissue, trabeculae and parenchyma, change in the appearance of any residual mass, and the development of calcifications. The post-surgical appearances of parenchymal deformity and scar formation do not appear to be affected by the type of radiotherapy (Buckley and Roebuck 1986, Dershaw et al 1987).

Skin thickening

The relationship between skin thickness and underlying breast disease was recognized long ago (Leitch 1909). The normal range with modern mammographic technique is 0.8–3.0 mm, being greater medially than laterally, inferiorly than superiorly and in small rather than larger breasts (Willson et al 1982). There are many causes of abnormal skin thickening including breast cancer, breast surgery, lymphatic obstruction, radiotherapy, obesity, congestive cardiac failure, dermatological disorders and other causes of inflammation (Morrish 1966). The mammographic appearance of thickened skin is identical whatever the cause (Gold et al 1971), that due to radiotherapy being distinguished only by the way it develops over time. The histological process underlying skin thickening due to radiotherapy is intracellular and extracellular oedema, inflammatory infiltration and collagen bundle oedema (Lever 1967, Libshitz et al 1978). Skin atrophy is a late feature.

External beam radiotherapy, typically 40–50 Gy over 4–6 weeks followed by local tumour-bed boost of another 10–20 Gy, produces less skin thickening than ^{192}Ir implants (Dershaw et al 1987). Skin thickening is reduced by the use of compensators during external beam radiotherapy (Bloomer et al 1976) and by the use of fractionation. Axillary dissection and chemotherapy are likely to increase skin thickening due to radiotherapy.

Almost all patients, except those with peau d'orange, show increase in skin thickness during the first 6 months after radiotherapy, corresponding to the increasing skin oedema seen histologically. Subsequently skin thickness reduces, to be almost normal by 18–24 months in the majority of patients. Dershaw et al (1987) found skin thickening to be present in 96% of patients within 1 year. Libshitz et al (1978) found that 60% of patients with skin thickening due to radiotherapy had normal skin thickness at 2 years, 77% being normal at 4 years.

Hohenberg & Wolf (1983) reported 54% normal at 4 years with another 34% showing partial resolution (Fig. 8.24). Any skin thickening which persists 3 years after radiotherapy is unlikely to resolve further. The time course of these changes in skin thickness does not appear to be influenced by whether external beam or radioactive implant is used (Dershaw et al 1987).

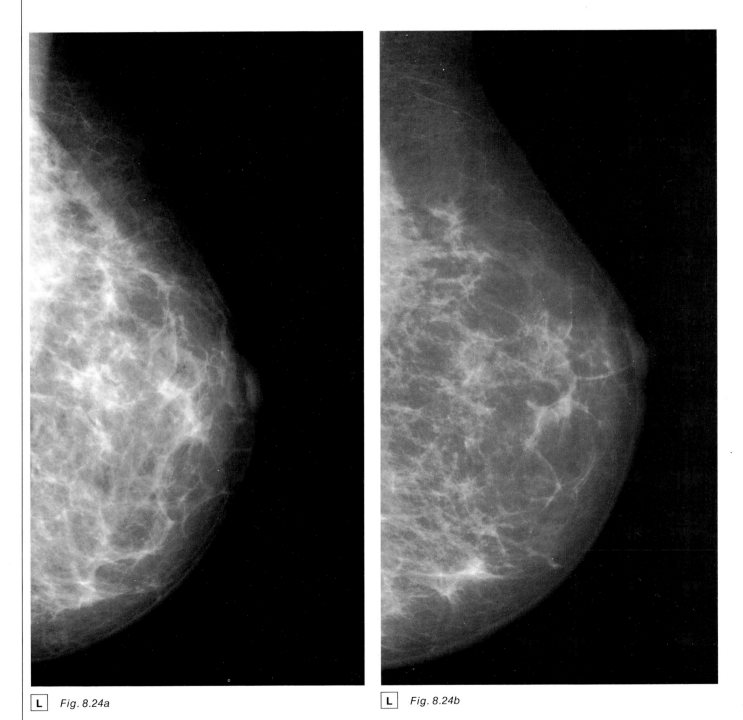

L   *Fig. 8.24a*

L   *Fig. 8.24b*

Fig. 8.24 *a* 15 months following excision biopsy and radiotherapy there is a coarse trabecular parenchymal pattern with skin thickening and residual subcutaneous reaction. *b* 1 year later there is partial resolution of these features. *c* 3½ years following radiotherapy there has been minor further resolution but the changes are now static.

Patients with peau d'orange at the
time of treatment may show reduction
in skin thickness following
radiotherapy (Bloomer et al 1976).

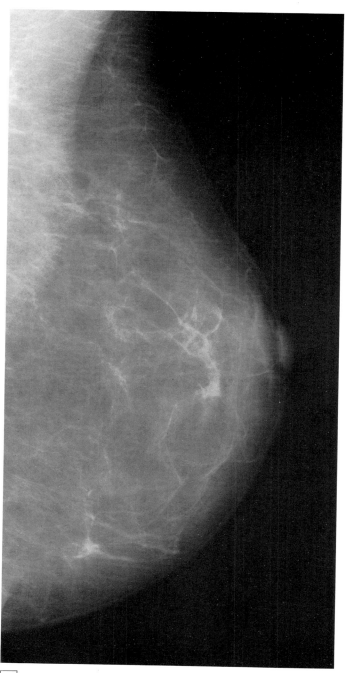

L   *Fig. 8.24c*

Subcutaneous reaction

A subcutaneous reaction is seen in the majority of patients, is most marked at about 6 months after therapy and is largely resolved in most patients by 24 months (Fig. 8.25). The earliest mammographic signs are fine linear subcutaneous opacities, subsequently increasing in number and size. The deep surface of the skin becomes irregular with thorn-like projections.

This reaction is thought to be due to increased blood and lymphatic vessel flow in the subcutaneous fat (Roebuck 1984). Subcutaneous vessels will appear more tortuous but if there is an inoperable tumour being treated by radiotherapy alone, the draining vessels should be reduced in size.

Breast retraction

Breast retraction with loss of volume and increased density is seen in all patients and appears to be dose-dependent (Bloomer et al 1976). It develops over several months and remains stable after about 2 years. Generalized increased fibrosis with loss of fat will contribute to these appearances.

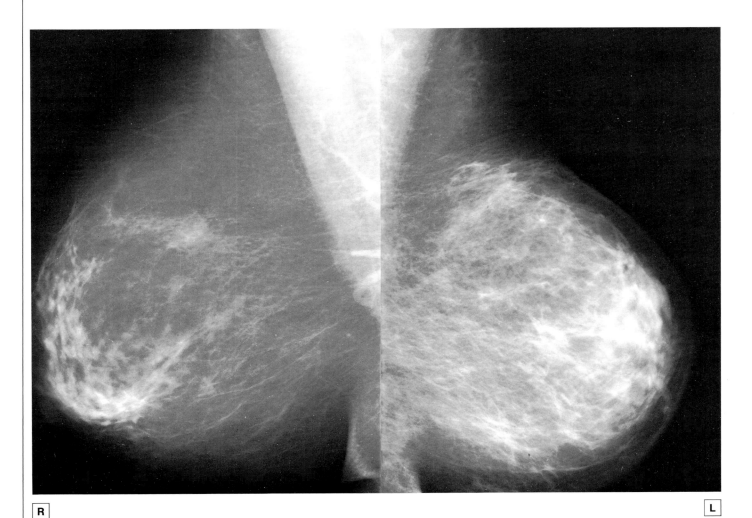

R   L

Fig. 8.25a

Fig. 8.25 *a* 6 months following excision biopsy and radiotherapy on the left side there are typical radiotherapy changes of trabecular thickening, increased density, skin thickening and a subcutaneous reaction. *b* 6 months later there has been partial resolution of these changes. *c* 2 years following radiotherapy these changes have largely but not completely resolved. Localized skin thickening is seen at the site of incision and a calcified area of fat necrosis is present high in the breast.

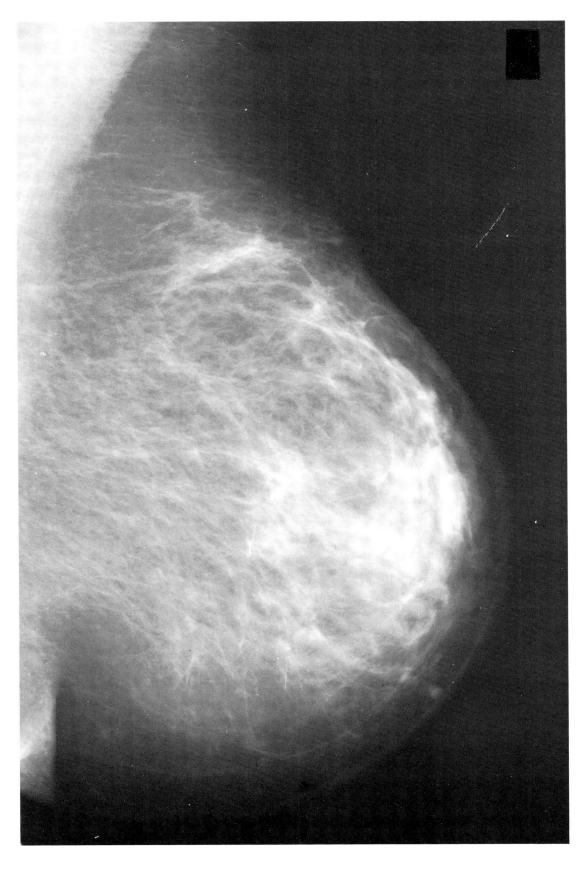

L

Fig. 8.25b

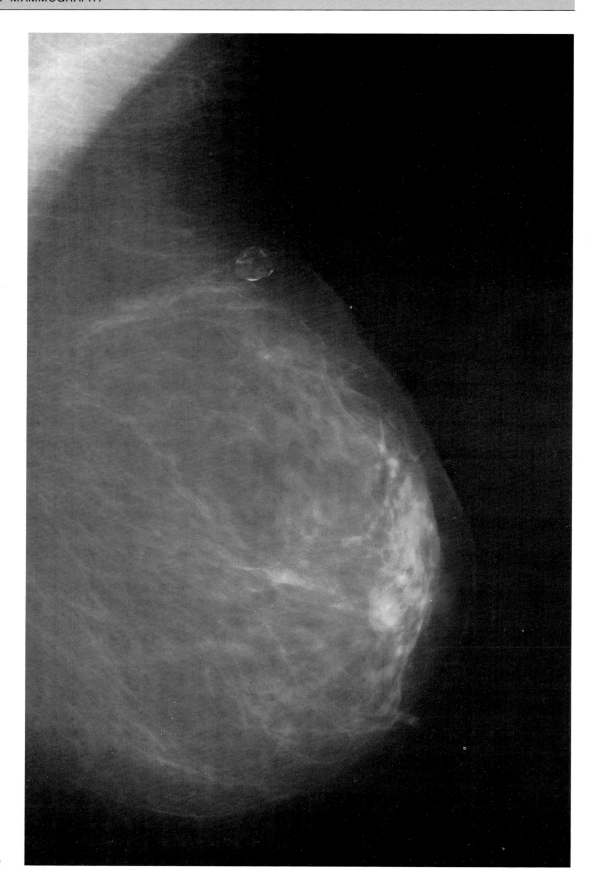

L

Fig. 8.25c

Oedema

Oedema and increased lymphatic drainage result in increased density with trabecular thickening and straightening. These appearances are best seen about 6 months after radiotherapy. The diffuse increase in density tends to resolve over the next 3–6 months, but the coarsening of the trabecular pattern clears more slowly and after 2–3 years any residual trabecular thickening is unlikely to resolve further (Fig. 8.26). It is more likely to return to normal in those patients receiving external beam radiotherapy rather than in those who have had radioactive implants (Dershaw et al 1987). Persistence of these changes is thought to be due to the development of fibrous strands (Paulus et al 1980).

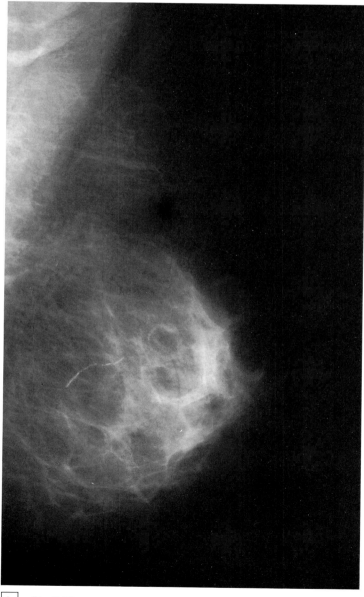

L *Fig. 8.26a*

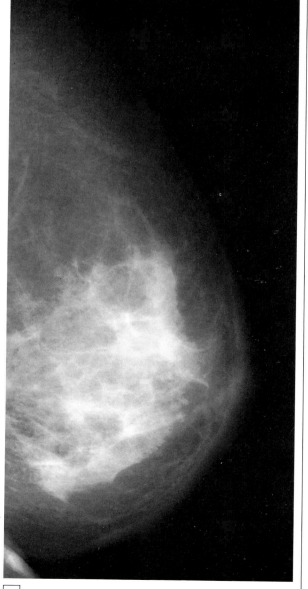

L *Fig. 8.26b*

Fig. 8.26 *a* 9 months after treatment there are typical radiotherapy changes. *b* After 3 years these changes are largely resolved. Calcification has occurred along the line of a Redivac drain.

Alteration of tumour mass

In the management of inoperable breast cancer treated with radiotherapy, mammography has been reported to be more accurate than clinical examination in identifying residual disease, in differentiating fibrosis from disease and in recognizing recurrent disease (Nisce et al 1974). Paulus et al (1980) reported patients treated by radiotherapy alone following diagnostic biopsy, all stage T3 or T4. Most patients had no clinically palpable residual mass immediately following therapy but demonstrated a residual dense area on the mammogram even after the maximum response, (mean time 19 months). Masses which remain apparent on mammography tend to become smaller and less well demarcated, but persistence of a mass after 6 months suggests the presence of residual viable tumour (Bloomer et al 1976). Mid-treatment mammography usually shows minimal change in the appearance of a mass (Nisce et al 1974).

Calcification

Radiotherapy may alter the appearance of calcifications present in the breast at the time of therapy, or may induce new calcifications, the latter not necessarily signifying recurrent malignancy (Libshitz et al 1977). Calcifications may disappear completely, become coarsened in appearance, decrease in size or persist unchanged over a period of months after therapy. Relatively few patients have been studied in whom malignant-type calcifications were present in the breast subjected to radiotherapy (Libshitz et al 1977, Dershaw et al 1987, Buckley & Roebuck 1986). Benign-appearing calcifications have been reported in up to 38% (Libshitz et al 1977, Berenberg et al 1983,

Hohenborg & Wolf 1983, Dershaw et al 1987).

Rebner et al (1989) followed 152 patients who had lumpectomy and radiotherapy, of whom 7% developed suspicious microcalcification as opposed to 11% developing coarse benign-looking calcification. The malignant-looking microcalcification tended to occur earlier than benign-looking calcification, the commonest causes of which are fibrosis, intraductal hyperplasia, fat necrosis or dystrophic change. New calcification occurring after radiotherapy should be treated as suspicious unless demonstrating obvious benign features. Solin et al (1989) biopsied 19 new calcifications following biopsy and radiotherapy, 11 of which were positive for malignancy, this figure bearing no relation to the presence of original tumour calcification.

Bizarre calcification seen at the site of a tumour treated with radiotherapy is probably due to tissue necrosis in the tumour or surrounding tissue. Dystrophic calcification in axillary lymph nodes has also been reported after radiotherapy to the axillary region (Buckley & Roebuck 1986). Suture calcification is more commonly seen after excision biopsy followed by radiotherapy than after biopsy alone. It may not be present at 6 months but frequently increases over the next 2–3 years.

Others

An incidentally reported effect of radiotherapy is the failure of normal lactation hypertrophy in the treated breast. The untreated breast lactated normally (Buckley and Roebuck 1986). Radiotherapy in the augmented breast carries a higher risk of implant encapsulation (Ryu et al 1990).

Recurrent tumour following biopsy and radiotherapy

Several features on mammography raise the possibility of tumour recurrence:

a. Development of a mass
b. Increase in size of a mass
c. Inappropriate increase in skin thickening
d. Increase in subcutaneous reaction, trabecular thickening or parenchymal density
e. Development of malignant-type calcification
f. Increased spacing of calcifications
g. The appearance of dense, rounded axillary lymph nodes.

Some masses which appear after radiotherapy will be benign, but any increase in size of a residual mass or any mass with malignant features is suggestive of recurrence. Skin thickening, subcutaneous reaction, trabecular thickening and parenchymal density may all be affected by processes other than tumour such as infection, but recurrent tumour must be considered if these occur unexpectedly or appear to worsen after they would normally have been expected to resolve, from about 6 months after radiotherapy. The development of malignant-type calcification, or any increase in the amount of suspicious calcification present, is indicative of tumour recurrence; however, failure of calcification to resolve is not necessarily an indication of residual tumour. Increased spacing of calcifications may imply an increase in localized soft tissue due to recurrent tumour. It is possible for tumour to recur even when the malignant-type calcification appears to be diminishing or has completely disappeared (Libshitz et al 1977).

In summary the development of mass or suspicious microcalcification are the two features most likely to indicate recurrent malignancy (Stomper et al 1987, Chaudary et al 1988, Locker et al 1990). New punctate microcalcification occurring is likely to be benign in nature (Dershaw et al 1990). Inflammatory change is also suggestive of recurrent tumour. The mean time of recurrence is between 3 and $3\frac{1}{2}$ years post-treatment and these mostly occur at the primary site (Stomper et al 1987). Another sign described in recurrent malignancy is increased nodularity at the treated site (Paulus et al 1980).

The risk of developing a second breast malignancy after radiotherapy to the breast is unknown. Irradiation therapy for postpartum mastitis, childhood malignancy, benign breast change and breast cancer have all been associated with excess breast cancer after a long latent period (10–15 years) having a greater risk for development in younger women, where the radiogenic risk is greatest (Lipsztein et al 1985). Fibrosarcoma, osteogenic sarcoma and angiosarcoma have been reported to arise occasionally after radiotherapy (Lipsztein et al 1985, Givens et al 1989).

MISCELLANEOUS

Compression rupture of cyst

There have been case reports of compression during mammography rupturing cysts (Novak 1989, Pennes & Homer 1987, Pennes 1986). Additional views of a lesion have shown that it has disappeared without significant discomfort. It has been suggested that this event might occur more commonly with small breasts or large cysts, although in either event it is a rare occurrence. In the UK, mammography equipment conforms to the recommendation that a compression plate should not be able to apply a force of more than 200 N (Department of Health and Social Security 1987). Usually 100–150 N is sufficient to produce adequate compression.

Residual localization needles

On the rare occasions that a hook-wire becomes transected during surgery it is often impossible to locate within the breast and may well present on later mammography (see Chap. 10).

Chrysotherapy

Treatment with gold for rheumatoid arthritis results in its deposition in a number of tissues. Gold has been reported to be present up to 23 years after chrysotherapy (Vernon-Roberts et al 1976). Cases have been reported of gold deposits within an intramammary lymph node (Carter 1988) and within axillary lymph nodes (Bruwer 1987), causing punctate densities simulating microcalcification.

A previously used localization technique involved platinum-coated gold grains (Millis et al 1976). Theoretically, inadequate excision could result in gold deposits in breast tissue.

Chemotherapy

Chemotherapy may increase the degree of skin thickening, trabecular thickening and increased parenchymal density seen in patients also receiving radiotherapy, and greatly reduce the proportion of patients in whom these changes resolve (Dershaw et al 1987). Chemotherapy alone produces skin thickening in some patients, most marked about 6 months after commencement of therapy and subsequently tending to resolve.

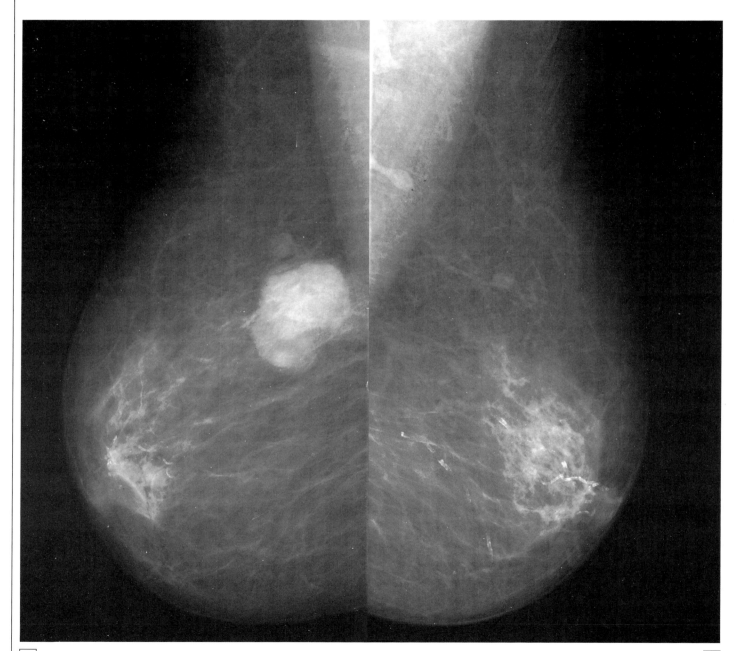

R   L

Fig. 8.27a

Fig. 8.27   Breast cancer treated by tamoxifen alone. *a* The original tumour seen high in the right breast. *b* 10 months later there has been reduction in size and density of the tumour. *c* After 2 years' therapy there has been very significant radiological resolution of the tumour.

Tamoxifen therapy can cause complete or partial regression of all the features of malignancy seen on mammography (Fig. 8.27). Tumour regression to the point of being radiologically occult has been observed, although biopsy of the original site may still show histological evidence of tumour, and if tamoxifen therapy is ceased the tumour may once more become radiologically apparent (Hendriks 1990).

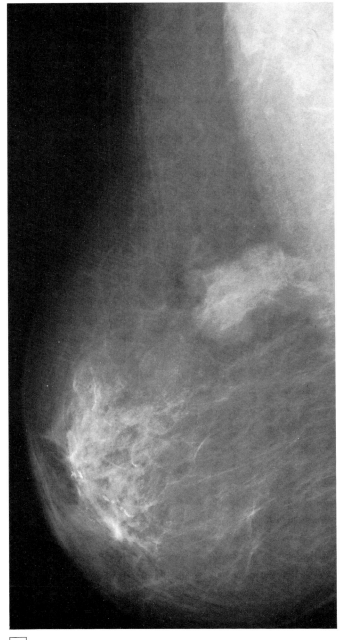

Fig. 8.27b

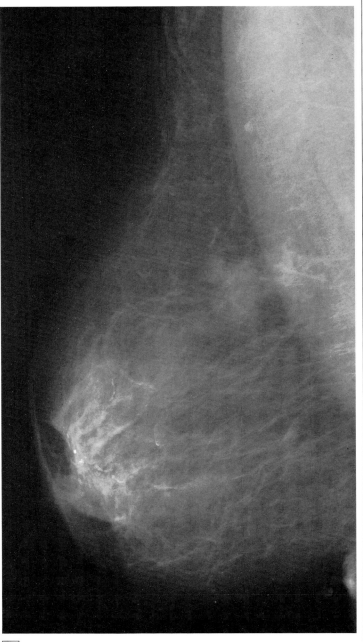

Fig. 8.27c

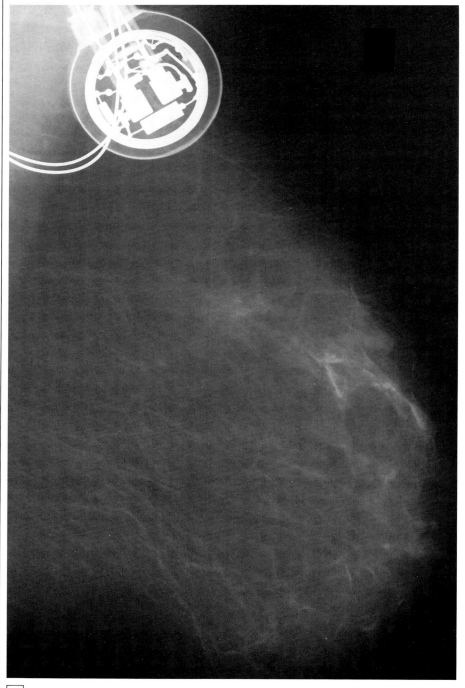

L

Pacemaker insertions

Pacemaker mechanisms placed subcutaneously on the chest wall may obscure breast tissue or make positioning the breast for mammography difficult (Fig. 8.28). The removal of a pacemaker from the subcutaneous tissue over the breast may result in a scar with attendant problems of interpretation.

Post-traumatic fat necrosis

External cardiac massage during resuscitation procedures may result in areas of fat necrosis within the breast tissue (Fig. 8.29).

Fig. 8.28   A pacemaker mechanism has been inserted subcutaneously on the chest wall. Pacemakers may interfere in positioning for mammography and if placed lower down may obscure underlying breast tissue.

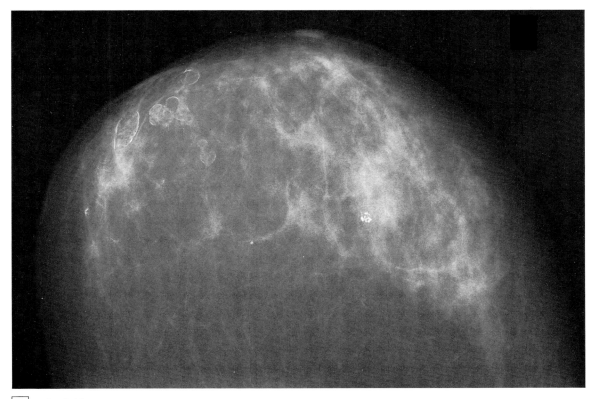

R   *Fig. 8.29a*

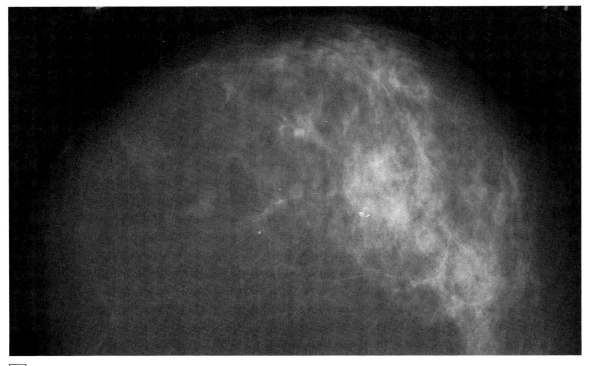

R   *Fig. 8.29b*

Fig. 8.29   *a* Typical areas of calcified fat necrosis are present medially in the breast. *b* 1 year previously these were not present. In the intervening year the patient had required resuscitation with external cardiac massage.

REFERENCES

Andersson I, Fex F, Pettersson H 1977 Oil cyst of the breast following fat necrosis. British Journal of Radiology 50: 143–146

Baber C E, Libshitz H I 1977 Bilateral fat necrosis of the breast following reduction mammoplasties. American Journal of Roentgenology 128: 508–509

Berenberg A L, Levene M B, Tonnesen G L 1983 Mammographic evaluation of the postirradiated breast. In: Harris J R, Hellman S, Silen W (eds) Conservative management of breast cancer: new surgical and radiotherapeutic techniques. Lippincott, pp 265–272

Bassett L W, Gold R H, Cove H C 1978 Mammographic spectrum of traumatic fat necrosis: The fallibility of "pathognomonic" signs of carcinoma. American Journal of Roentgenology 130: 119–122

Bassett L W, Gold R H, Mirra J M 1982 Nonneoplastic breast calcifications in lipid cysts: Development after excision and primary irradiation. American Journal of Roentgenology 138: 335–338

Ben-Hur N, Neuman Z 1965 Siliconoma—another cutaneous response to demethylpolysiloxane. Experimental study in mice. Plastic and Reconstructive Surgery 36: 629–631

Biggs T M, Cukier J, Worthing L F 1982 Augmentation mammoplasty: a review of 18 years. Plastic and Reconstructive Surgery 69(3): 445–450

Bloomer W D, Berenberg A L, Weissman B N 1976 Mammography of the definitively irradiated breast. Radiology 118: 425–428

Boo-Chai K 1969 The complications of augmentation mammoplasty by silicone injection. British Journal of Plastic Surgery 22: 281–285

Brown F E, Sargent S K, Cohen S R, Morain W D 1987 Mammographic changes following reduction mammoplasty. Plastic and Reconstructive Surgery 80(5): 691–698

Bruwer A, Nelson G W, Spark R P 1987 Punctate intranodal gold deposits simulating microcalcifications on mammograms. Radiology 163: 87–88

Buckley J H, Roebuck E J 1986 Mammographic changes following radiotherapy. British Journal of Radiology 59: 337–344

Carter T R 1988 Intramammary lymph node gold deposits simulating microcalcification on mammogram. Human Pathology 19(8): 992–994

Chaudary M M, Girling A, Girling S, Habib F, Millis R R, Hayard J L 1988 New lumps in the breast following conservation treatment for early breast cancer. Breast Cancer Research and Treatment 11: 51–58

Coren G S, Libshitz H I 1974 Fat necrosis of the breast: mammographic and thermographic findings. British Journal of Radiology 47: 758–762

Davis S P, Stomper P C, Weidner N, Meyer J E 1989 Suture calcification mimicking recurrence in the irradiated breast: a potential pitfall in mammographic evaluation. Radiology 172: 247–248

Delage C, Shane J J, Johnson F B 1973 Mammary silicone granuloma. Archives of Dermatology 108: 104–107

Department of Health and Social Security 1987 Guidance notes for Health Authorities on mammographic equipment requirements for breast screening.

Dershaw D D, Shank B, Reisinger S 1987 Mammographic findings after breast cancer treatment with local excision and definitive irradiation. Radiology 164: 445–461

Dershaw D D, Chaglassian T A 1989 Mammography after prosthesis placement for augmentation or reconstructive mammoplasty. Radiology 170: 69–74

Dershaw D D, McCormick B, Cox L, Osborne M P 1990 differentiation of benign and malignant local tumor recurrence after lumpectomy. American Journal of Roentgenology 155: 35–38

Ecklund G W, Busby R C, Miller S H, Job J S 1988 Improved imaging of the augmented breast. American Journal of Roentgenology 151: 469–473

Givens S S, Ellerbroek N A, Butler J J, Libshitz H I, Hortobagyi G N, McNeese M D 1989 Angiosarcoma arising in an irradiated breast. Cancer 64: 2214–2216

Gold R H, Montgomery C K, Minagi H, Annes G P 1971 The significance of mammary skin thickening in disorders other than primary carcinoma: a roentgenologic–pathologic correlation. American Journal of Roentgenology, Radiotherapy and Nuclear Medicine 112(3): 613–621

Hadfield G 1930 Fat necrosis of the breast. British Journal of Surgery 17: 673–682

Hayes H, Vandergrift J, Diner W C 1988 Mammography and breast implants. Plastic and Reconstructive Surgery 82(1): 1–6

Hendricks J 1990 Personal communication

Ho W C 1987 Radiographic evidence of breast implant rupture. Plastic and Reconstructive surgery 79(6): 1009–1010

Hohenberg G, Wolf G 1983 Mammographischfassbare veranberungen bei der teiloperierten und nachbestrahlten brust. Strahlentherapie 159: 622–625

Isaacs G, Rozner L, Tudball C 1985 Breast lumps after reduction mammoplasty. Annals of Plastic Surgery (15)5: 394–399

Jensen S R, Mackey J K 1985 Xeromammography after augmentation mammoplasty. American Journal of Roentgenology 144: 629–633

Klein D L, Sickles E A 1982 Effects of needle aspiration on the mammographic appearance of the breast: a guide to the proper timing of the mammography examination. Radiology 145: 44

Koide T, Katayama H 1979 Calcification in augmentation mammoplasty. Radiology 130: 337–340

Lanyi M 1988 Diagnosis and differential diagnosis of breast calcification. Springer, New York, p 180

Leborgne R 1967 Easteatoneccrosis quistica calcificada de la mamma. El torax 16: 172–175

Lee B J, Adair F E 1920 Traumatic fat necrosis of the female breast and its differentiation from carcinoma. Annals of Surgery 72: 188–195

Leibman S J, Kruse B 1990 Breast cancer: mammographic and sonographic findings after augmentation mammoplasty. Radiology 174: 195–198

Leitch A 1909 Peau d'orange in acute mammary carcinoma: its cause and diagnostic value. Lancet: 861–863

Lever W F 1967 Histopathology of the skin. Lippincott, Philadelphia

Lipshitz H I, Montague E D, Paulus D D 1977 Calcifications and the therapeutically irradiated breast.

American Journal of Roentgenology 128: 1021–1025

Lipshitz H I, Montague E D, Paulus D D 1978 Skin thickness in the therapeutically irradiated breast. American Journal of Roentgenology 130: 345–347

Lipsztein R, Dalton J F, Bloomer W D 1985 Sequelae of breast irradiation. Journal of the American Medical Association 253(24): 3582–3584

Locker A P, Hanley P, Wilson A R et al 1990 Mammography in the preoperative assessment and post operative surveillance of patients treated by excision and radiotherapy for primary breast cancer. Clinical Radiology 41: 388–391

McKinney P, Tresley G 1983 Long-term comparison of patients with gel and saline mammary implants. Plastic and Reconstructive Surgery 72(1): 27–29

Meyer F, Silverman P, Gandbhir L 1978 Fat necrosis of the breast. Archives of Surgery 113: 801–805

Miller C L, Feig S A, Fox J W 1987 Mammographic changes after reduction mammoplasty. American Journal of Roentgenology 149: 35–38

Millis R R, McKinna J A, Hamlin I M E, Greening W P 1976 Biopsy of the impalpable breast lesion detected by mammography. British Journal of Surgery 63: 346–348

Minagi H, Youker J E 1968 Roentgen appearance of fat necrosis in the breast. Radiology 90: 62–65

Minagi H, Youker J E, Knudson H W 1968 The roentgen appearance of injected silicone in the breast. Radiology 90: 57–61

Mitnick J, Roses D F, Harris M N 1988 Differentiation of postsurgical changes from carcinoma of the breast. Surgery, Gynecology and Obstetrics 166: 549–550

Morrish H F 1966 The significance and limitations of skin thickening as a diagnostic sign in mammography. American Journal of Roentgenology, Radiotherapy and Nuclear Medicine 96(4): 1041–1045

Nisce L Z, Synder R E, Chu F C H 1974 The role of mammography in evaluating radiation response of inoperable primary breast cancer. Radiology 110: 85–88

Novak R 1989 Rupture of a cyst during compression at mammography. Acta Radiologica 30(3): 257–258

Ortiz-Monasterio F, Trigos I 1972 Management of patients with complications from injections of foreign materials into the breasts. Plastic and Reconstructive Surgery 50(1): 42–47

Paulus D D, Libshitz H I, Montague E D 1980 Malignant masses in the therapeutically irradiated breast. American Journal of Roentgenology 135: 789–795

Pennes D R 1986 Mammogram as therapy. American Journal of Roentgenology 146: 1100

Pennes D R, Homer M J 1987 Disappearing breast masses caused by compression during mammography. Radiology 165: 327–328

Peters M E, Fagerholm M I, Scanlan K A, Voegeli D R, Kelczi F 1988 Mammographic evaluation of the postsurgical and irradiated breast. Radiographics 8(5): 873–899

Rebner M, Pennes D R, Adler D D, Helvie M A, Lichter A S 1989 Breast microcalcifications after lumpectomy and radiation therapy. Radiology 170: 691–693

Roebuck E J 1984 The subcutaneous reaction: a useful mammographic sign. Clinical Radiology 35: 311–315

Russell F E, Simmers M H, Hirst A E, Pudenz R H 959 Tumors associated with embedded polymers. Journal of the National Cancer Institute 23: 305–315

Ryu J, Yahalom J, Shank B, Chaglassian T A, McCormick B 1990 Radiation therapy after breast augmentation or reconstruction in early or recurrent breast cancer. Cancer 66: 844–847

Sickles E A, Herzog K A 1980 Intramammary scar tissue: a mimic of the mammographic appearance of carcinoma. American Journal of Roentgenology 135: 349–352

Sickles E A, Herzog K A 1981 Mammography of the postsurgical breast. American Journal of Roentgenology 136: 585–588

Sickles E A, Klein D L, Goodson W H, Hunt T K 1983 Mammography after needle aspiration of palpable breast masses. American Journal of Surgery 145: 395–397

Smith D S 1985 False-positive radiographic diagnosis of breast implant rupture: report of two cases. Annals of Plastic Surgery 14(2): 166–167

Solin L J, Fowble B L, Troupin R H, Goodman R L 1989 Biopsy results of new calcifications in the postirradiated breast. Cancer 63: 1956–1961

Stewart F W 1950 Tumors of the breast: atlas of tumor pathology. Armed Forces Institute of Pathology Section 9: 99–104

Stockdale A D, Brierley J D, White W F, Folkes A, Rostom A Y 1989 Radiotherapy for Paget's disease of the nipple: a conservative alternative. Lancet ii: 664–666

Stomper P C, Recht A, Berenberg A L, Jochelson M S, Harris J R 1987 Mammographic detection of recurrent cancer in the irradiated breast. American Journal of Roentgenology 148: 39–43

Symmers W St C 1968 Silicone mastitis in topless waitresses and some other varieties of foreign-body mastitis. British Medical Journal 3: 19–22

Tabar L, Dean P 1985 Teaching atlas of mammography. Thieme-Stratton, New York

Theophelis L G, Stevenson T R 1986 Radiographic evidence of breast implant rupture. Plastic and Reconstructive Surgery 78(5): 673–675

Vernon-Roberts B, Dore J L, Jessop J D, Henderson W J 1976 Selective concentration and localization of gold in macrophages of synovial and other tissues during and after chrysotherapy in rheumatoid patients. Annals of Rheumatic Diseases 35: 477–486

von Hoeffken W, Lanyi M 1973 Rontgenuntersuchung der brust. Georg Thieme, Stuttgart

Willson S A, Adam E J, Tucker A K 1982 Patterns of breast skin thickness in normal mammograms. Clinical Radiology 33: 691–693

Wolfe J N 1979 Problems in the diagnosis of breast disease with special emphasis on "traps". In: Margulis A R, Gooding C A (eds) Diagnostic radiology. Masson, New York, pp 825–846

Wren M W F, Crosbie R B 1968 The radiological features of paraffinomata. British Journal of Radiology 41: 797–798

CHAPTER 9

Breast ultrasound (sonomammography)

P. B. Guyer

HISTORICAL INTRODUCTION

Wild & Neal (1951) were the first to describe breast ultrasound. They used an A-scan method and showed it was possible to differentiate cystic from solid masses. Howry et al (1954) also contributed to the early investigation of the technique, but thereafter interest in the Western hemisphere faded, probably due to the developments in X-ray mammography. However, Japanese workers continued to investigate breast ultrasound (Wagai et al 1967, Kobayashi 1975, 1983), and in the late 1960s there was a revival in interest in the United States (Kelly-Fry et al 1971, Kelly-Fry & Gallagher 1978), in Australia (Jellins et al 1971), and in Europe (Gross & Jacob 1971, Pluygers 1975). Together with continuing studies in Japan (Wagai et al 1977, Kobayashi 1979), a large literature on breast ultrasound developed, and the examination is now widely accepted as a valuable adjunct to X-ray mammography. In Japan, sonomammography is also being assessed as a technique for breast screening (Wagai 1983, Kaneko 1989).

Over the years, techniques of breast ultrasound have changed considerably. Wild and Neal's A-scan method was followed by coupling the breast to the transducer by means of a water bath with the patient supine (De Land 1969) or prone (Wells & Evans 1968, Jellins & Kossoff 1973). There were arguments for and against the use of breast compression (Baum 1977, Maturo et al 1980, Kopans et al 1981). The Japanese developed focused transducers, and linear array transducers were later produced (Rosner et al 1980). Dedicated breast ultrasound apparatus became available commercially from a number of manufacturers towards the end of the 1970s, the patient lying prone with the breast in a water bath. Transducer frequencies of 7.5 MHz were introduced, and were ideally suited to a hand-held realtime technique with or without a stand-off water bath attachment. In our unit we have mainly used a direct-contact B-scan technique. In a review, Lees (1982) concluded that a combination of automated water bath and realtime techniques gave optimum results.

CURRENT APPROACHES

Most manufacturers have ceased the production of static B-scan apparatus, although our technique using a 7.5 MHz transducer with a stepped movement is simple, quick, and thorough, and results in very detailed images. There is little difficulty in imaging subcentimetre solid masses, and there is better definition of the more diffuse benign changes.

The dedicated water bath technique is expensive, takes a minimum of 30 min per patient, and produces a large number of images. It is difficult to relate ultrasound abnormalities to clinically palpable lesions, but it is useful for comparing the two breasts; there may be difficulty in defining subcentimetre masses. However, it continues to be used in a number of centres (Kopans 1984, Richardson et al 1984, Walsh et al 1985, Jackson et al 1986a, Kimme-Smith et al 1986, 1988, Bassett et al 1987).

The favoured technique has become a hand-held, realtime examination using a transducer of 7.5 MHz (Fleischer et al 1985, Hayashi et al 1985, Gold et al 1986, Vilaro et al 1989), usually as part of a general-purpose ultrasound machine. Because it is hand-held, it is possible to miss areas in the breast, and resolution may not be quite that of the static B-scan. However, it does allow focal compression, assessment of the mobility and compressibility of a solid mass, angled views, and the examination of a seated patient. There is some evidence that increasing the transducer frequency to 10 MHz offers additional detail of some features such as the highly-reflective halo around a cancer nidus (Hayashi et al 1985, Hilton et al 1986, Kelly-Fry et al 1988, Funk et al 1989). However, the identification of microcalcifications, apart from a tumour mass, remains a problem for all ultrasound techniques. In the immediate future, Doppler ultrasound offers considerable potential in helping to differentiate benign from malignant lesions by examining the blood supply. Ultrasound computed tomography (UCT), which can measure attenuation and speed of transmission, is not likely to be used clinically in its present form (Scherzinger et al 1989).

NORMAL APPEARANCES, AND VARIANTS

The ultrasound appearances of the breast vary with age (Guyer & Dewbury 1987). The components which can be identified are the highly-reflective glandular and fibrous stromal structures, and the poorly-reflective fatty tissue (Fig. 9.1a–c). The gland elements occupy the central portion of the breast, lying between the subcutaneous and retromammary fat layers; rounded fatty lobules are distributed throughout the glandular tissue in varying amounts. In the young breast there is an overall highly reflective appearance (Fig. 9.1b), with thin or absent subcutaneous and retromammary fat layers, and little or no intramammary fat. Normal ducts,

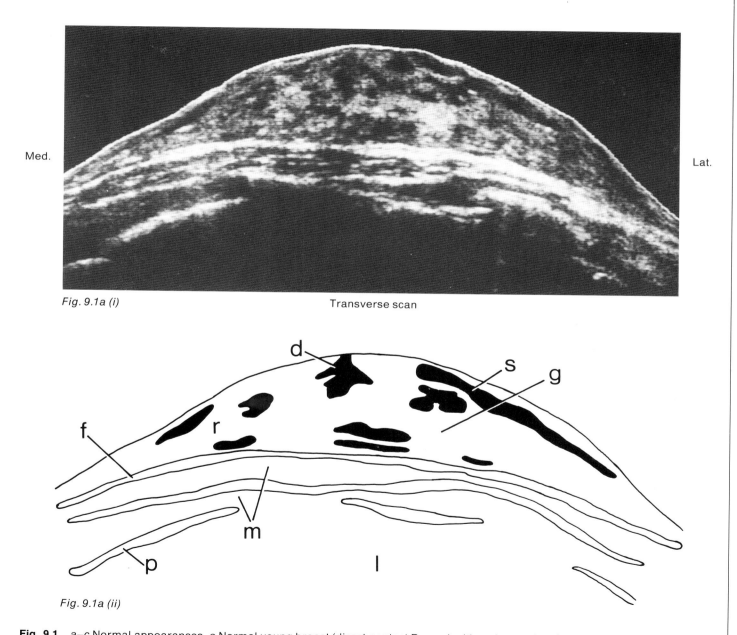

Med.

Lat.

Fig. 9.1a (i)

Transverse scan

Fig. 9.1a (ii)

Fig. 9.1 *a–c* Normal appearances. *a* Normal young breast (direct-contact B-scan) with an incomplete layer of subcutaneous fat (s), a predominantly highly reflective central glandular zone (g), within which ducts (d) are visible, and an incomplete retromammary fat layer (r). The pectoral muscles (m) are separated from the breast by the thin highly reflective layer of prepectoral fascia (f), and another highly reflective layer (p) represents the pleura separating these structures from lung (l).

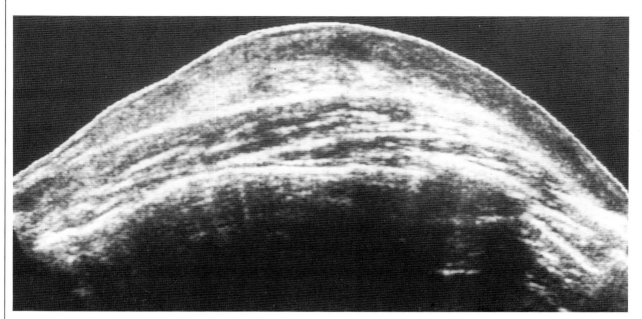

Fig. 9.1b   A variant of normal, showing virtually no fat (direct contact B-scan).

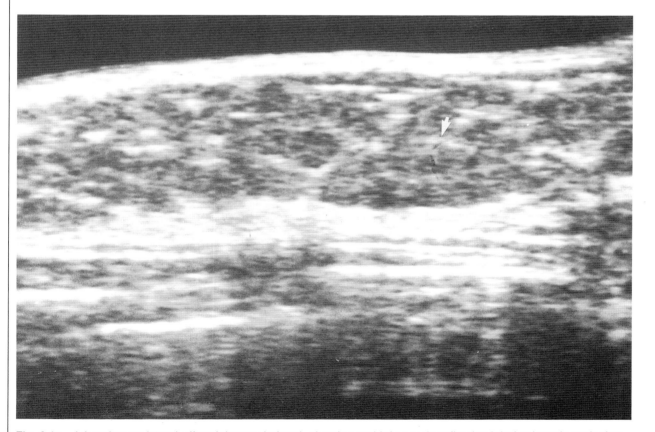

Fig. 9.1c   A fatty breast (stand-off real time technique), showing multiple poorly reflective lobules largely replacing the breast with only a small glandular area (arrow indicates an example of Cooper's ligaments). The pre-pectoral fascia, pectoral muscles, and pleura are visible as in *a*.

when visible, are seen as poorly reflective tubular structures deep to the nipple with a maximum calibre of 3 mm (Fig. 9.1a). In the postmenopausal breast the fatty layers become dominant, and there may be little or no gland tissue visible, although Cooper's ligaments remain as highly-reflective curved or curvilinear structures around the fat lobules (Fig. 9.1c). Ducts may be difficult to identify in this age group. Between these two extremes can be found various combinations, as Kaizer et al (1988) describe, which parallel the range of normal radiological appearances seen in X-ray mammography.

The nipple and areola occasionally give rise to attenuating shadow, which may interfere with identification both of normal structures and pathological features deep to the nipple. This attenuating shadow is attributed to the connective tissue which surrounds the lactiferous ducts; in the non-lactating state the latter are generally invisible, but, during lactation, may reach a diameter of 7–8 mm (Fig. 9.3b). The appearances of the skin vary with technique; with direct-contact B-scans the skin is a single highly-reflective layer, but with stand-off techniques the skin can be seen to consist of two highly reflective zones separated by a thin poorly-reflective layer (Kopans et al 1981) (Fig. 9.1c).

Deep to the retromammary layer of fat, both the pectoralis major and pectoralis minor muscles may be identified, separated from breast tissue by a thin highly reflective zone representing the pre-pectoral fascia. Deep to the pectoral muscles the ribs and costal cartilages may be seen, and, still deeper, the pleura is shown by another thin highly-reflective layer, separating all these structures from the poorly-reflective lung.

The axilla contains mixed echogenic tissue, representing fibro-fatty contents, within which lie the axillary vessels (Fig. 9.2). The pectoral muscles and humeral head may be identified, but normal lymph nodes are invisible.

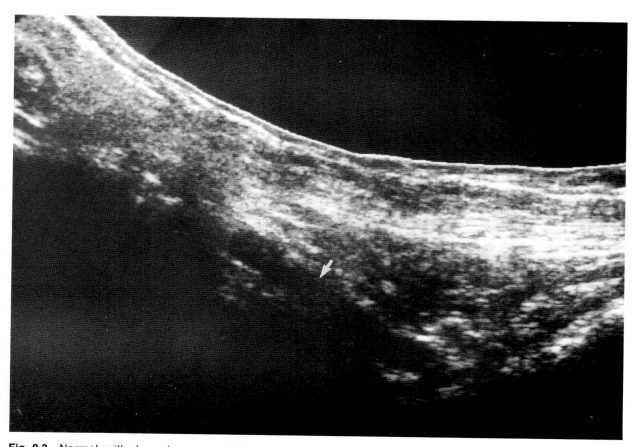

Fig. 9.2 Normal axilla. Largely composed of mixed reflective fibro-fatty tissue within which the axillary artery (arrow) can be seen on this scan.

In pregnancy and lactation the glandular component is dominant, giving a tightly packed highly-reflective appearance to the breast (Fig. 9.3*a*). Ducts may be seen, but are often difficult to identify separately, being filled with the same reflective material. Occasionally galactoceles can be seen as more circumscribed echogenic or mixed-echoic lesions (Fig. 9.3*b*).

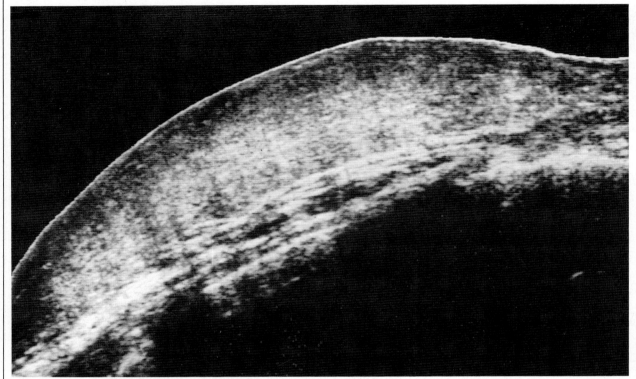

Fig. 9.3a

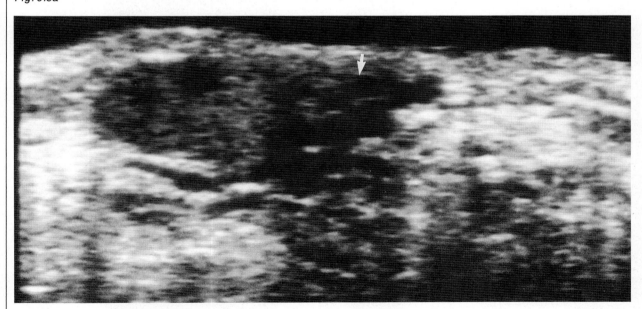

Fig. 9.3b

Fig. 9.3a & b   *a* Lactation. The breast is replaced by tightly packed bright echoes (note good visibility of normal muscles and fascial planes deep to the breast—B-scan). *b* Galactocele. A circumscribed echo-containing mass adjacent to dilated subareolar ducts (arrow) (realtime technique with stand-off water bag).

'Benign breast change' is a term which is now replacing such clinical terms as 'fibroadenosis' and 'fibrocystic disease'. The symptoms of pain and nodularity, often with a cyclical variation, which give rise to these diagnoses, are so common that they can hardly be considered to represent a pathological situation, and they may now be regarded as variants of normal (Hughes et al 1987). The symptoms most commonly affect younger patients and are accompanied by nodular or patchy densities on the X-ray mammograms (Breast Group of the Royal College of Radiologists 1989). Ultrasound reflects these X-ray changes, with a mixed echogenic pattern, replacing the normal uniform architecture, either focally or diffusely (Guyer & Dewbury 1988). Small cysts may be identifiable (Fig. 9.4a–d); the prominent ductal pattern sometimes seen on X-ray mammograms is seldom shown on sonomammography, lending weight to the concept that the X-ray pattern is due mainly to periductal shadowing (Rees et al 1977, Breast Group 1989) rather than duct dilatation. In our experience, benign changes are better appreciated on direct-contact B-scans than on realtime images, largely due to the ability to compare portions of the breast on a single scan of the breast. This decreased definition with realtime techniques may account for the varying reports in the literature on the ease with which changes can be seen (Cole-Beuglet et al 1980, Harper & Kelly-Fry 1980, Maturo et al 1980, Teixidor 1980, Lambie 1983, McSweeney & Murphy 1985). Some authors maintain it is impossible to differentiate benign changes from normal; others describe highly-reflective glandular elements with attenuating shadow due to poor acoustic penetration resulting from

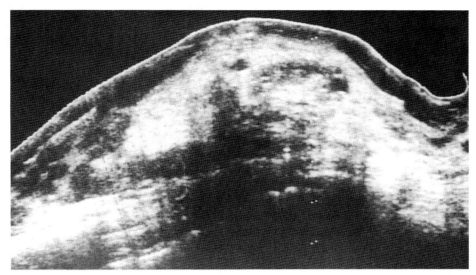

Fig. 9.4a

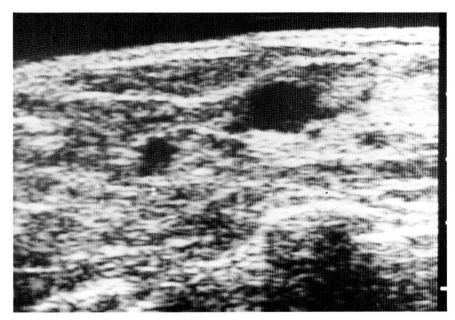

Fig. 9.4b

Fig. 9.4a & b Benign breast change. *a* Glandular components predominate, but are interspersed by small poorly reflective areas and two small, round poorly reflective shadows which are small cysts. *b* Hand-held realtime examination for comparison with *a*. *c* Extensive attenuation obscuring the deeper structures—a variant of benign change attributed to fibrosis of the more superficial layers of the breast. *d* Realtime examination for comparison with *c*—the changes are less marked in this patient.

increased fibrous content of the glandular layer (Fig. 9.4*b*). When widespread attenuating shadow is produced, it may obscure the deeper layers of the breast, making the exclusion of a carcinoma difficult or impossible. The general term 'benign breast change' is preferred because biopsy in patients showing these ultrasound appearances has revealed a very wide range of histological features, and poor correlation with mammograms and sonomammograms (Guyer & Dewbury 1988, Breast Group 1989). Sometimes the ultrasound changes are very focal, raising the possibility of a mass lesion; rarely, diffuse infiltrating carcinoma may mimic these changes (see below).

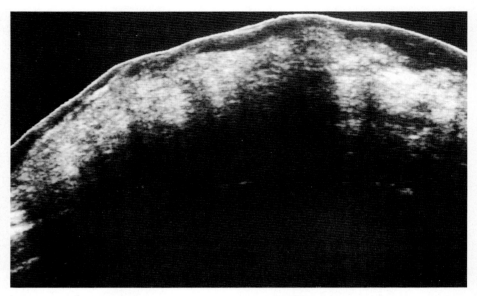

Fig. 9.4c   Benign breast change less marked in this patient (B-scan).

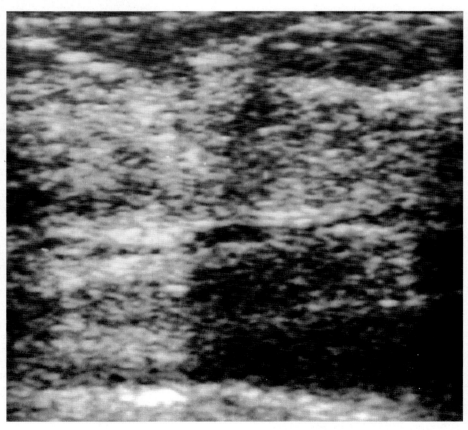

Fig. 9.4d   Realtime.

BREAST CARCINOMA

The principal ultrasound features of a breast carcinoma are a mass, i.e. nidus, a surrounding highly-reflective zone, i.e. halo and retrotumorous attenuating shadow (Kobayashi 1981) (Fig. 9.5a–f). There may be additional features of trabecular distortion (Fig. 9.5b), tissue plane disruption, skin thickening and microcalcification (Fig. 9.5f). These features are seen in varying combinations (Cole-Beuglet et al 1983c). The commonest combination

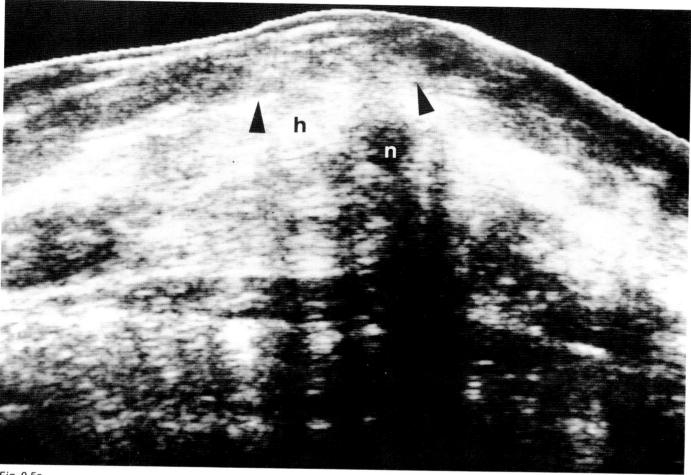

Fig. 9.5a

Fig. 9.5 Carcinoma. *a* Characteristic appearances with an ill-defined tumour nidus (n), a surrounding highly reflective zone ['halo' (h)] and with attenuating shadow deep to the tumour. Because the tumour is fairly superficial, the subcutaneous fat layer has been interrupted by the 'halo' (arrows). This is a B-scan.

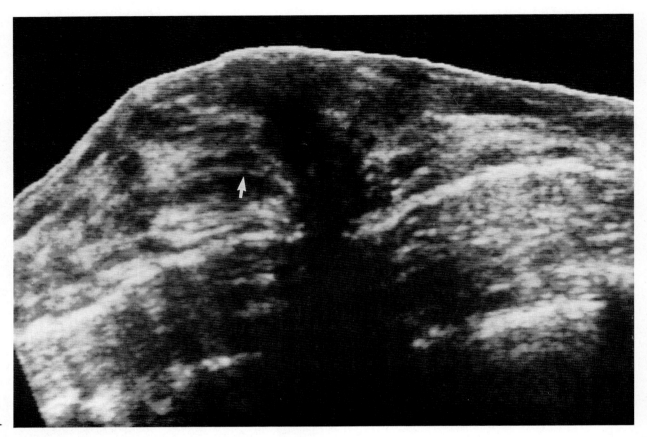

Fig. 9.5b ▷

Fig. 9.5c ▽

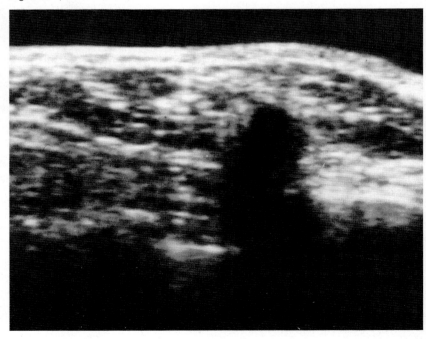

is nidus, halo and shadow, which can be seen in 40% of cancers (Kopans et al 1981, Guyer & Dewbury 1987) (Fig. 9.5a); shadow alone occurs in 20%, and the remaining 40% are approximately equally divided between nidus alone, nidus with halo and nidus with shadow (Harper et al 1983, Egan et al 1984) (Fig. 9.5c). The tumour nidus, when small, is poorly-reflective (Harper et al 1983) with ill-defined margins; the internal echo

Fig. 9.5b & c   *b* An irregular poorly reflective mass with trabeculae being drawn into the deeper portions of the tumour in a curvilinear manner (arrow). This is a B-scan. *c* A common variant of carcinoma: nidus with attenuating shadow, but no halo. (Note normal appearance of double layer to skin with stand-off technique.)

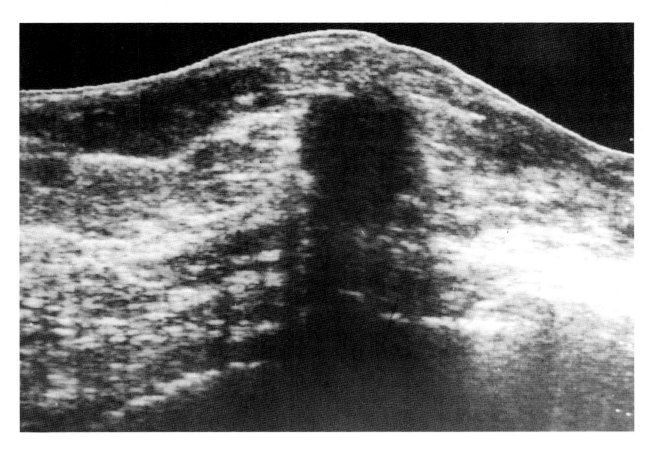

Fig. 9.5d (i) △

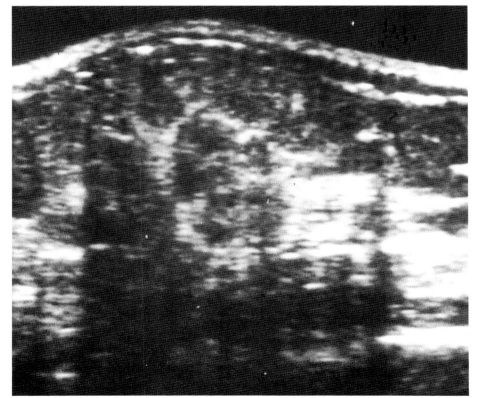

pattern may be even when the nidus is under 1 cm, but tends to become inhomogeneous as the tumour increases in size (Fig. 9.5*d*). With tumours larger than 2 cm the pattern is generally heterogeneous, occasionally with areas of necrosis. From time to time the echo pattern remains homogeneous, even when the nidus

Fig. 9.5d(i) & (ii)   *(i)* A larger, heterogeneous carcinoma with poor border definition and subcutaneous fat interruption (B-scan). *(ii)* Realtime technique: the mass is more deeply placed so there is no fat infiltration.

◁ *Fig. 9.5d (ii)*

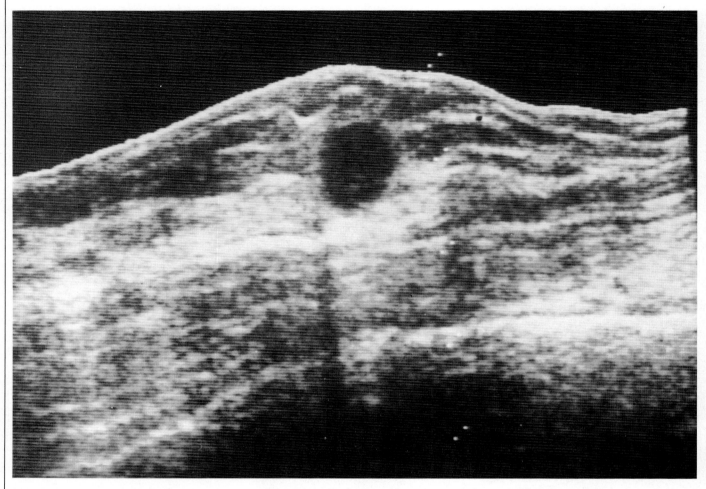

Fig. 9.5e   A more circumscribed tumour with a poorly reflective nidus, a poorly visible halo, and trabecular disturbance laterally. There is no attenuating shadow (B-scan).

exceeds 2 cm. The margins occasionally remain well-defined, although not as sharp as in a typical fibroadenoma—the 'circumscribed cancer' of Kasumi et al (1981, 1982) (Fig. 9.5e). A medullary carcinoma (Fig. 9.5f) typically produces these appearances, but they can also occur in colloid and ductal cancers (Meyer et al 1989). These latter tumour appearances cause problems in differentiating a fibroadenoma from malignant solid masses (Cole-Beuglet 1982a, b, Maturo et al 1982, Rosner & Blaird 1985, with a misdiagnosis rate of 7–10% in either direction, necessitating a cellular fine-needle aspiration, or even biopsy, for diagnosis.

In all, attenuating shadow is a feature of approximately 75% of cancers (Guyer & Dewbury 1987), although Harper et al (1983) quoted a figure of 97%, and Kobayashi (1979) 83%, with tumours over 2 cm in diameter. The attenuating shadow is central, but may not be visible on all scans (Harper et al 1983); many breast masses give rise to edge-refractive shadowing, which is therefore non-specific. The cause of the central attenuating shadow is debated. Kossoff (1988) attributes it to reflection of the ultrasound energy from areas of high impedance within the tumour, absorption, and scatter, but it may be related to the connective tissue content of the carcinoma. Very occasionally accentuation is identified deep to the tumour.

The pathogenesis of the area of high reflectivity (halo) which surrounds some tumours is also debated. Teubner (1989) considers it to be due to the combination of irregular tumour margin, tumour/fat interfaces, and oedema, but it is also possible that neovascularity at tumour margins may be contributory. This feature of halo

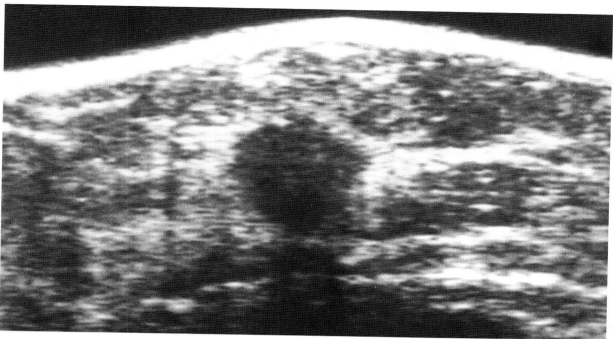

Fig. 9.5f (i) △

Fig. 9.5f (ii) ▽

Fig. 9.5f(i) & (ii) *(i)* A circumscribed tumour with poor border definition, deeply placed in a fatty breast; a medullary carcinoma. *(ii)* Similar mass but with a pronounced 'halo' (realtime technique).

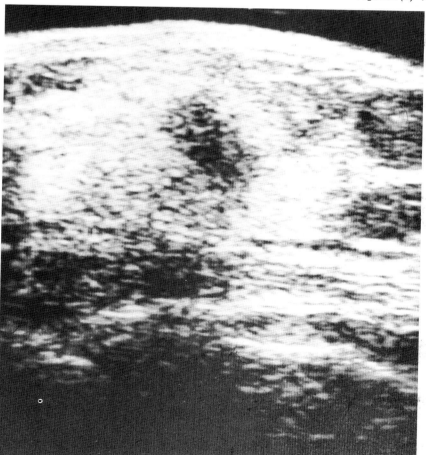

may be identified with varying ease in 70% of carcinomas, and it is claimed it can be more easily identified with a 10 MHz transducer (Kelly-Fry et al 1988).

Tissue plane disruption and trabecular distortion are inconstant features; although the former occurs due to the presence of the mass itself, it is more obvious when the highly-reflective halo is visible, and particularly so with superficial tumours that interrupt the subcutaneous fat layer (Fig. 9.5a–d).

Microcalcifications are unreliably shown as small bright echoes with variable deep attenuating shadow.

Individual microcalcifications of between 100 and 500 µm may be identified within a tumour mass (Fig. 9.5g), but will not be seen when free in the surrounding tissues (Kasumi 1988). X-ray microcalcifications accompanied by ultrasound evidence of a soft tissue abnormality carry a high likelihood of malignancy (Lambie 1983, Guyer & Dewbury 1987). Currently the unreliable demonstration of microcalcifications by ultrasound is an indication that it should not be used as a primary technique for breast cancer detection in a screening programme.

Sometimes carcinoma is diffuse, in

which case it can give rise to two appearances. The first of these is when the breast plate is largely replaced by poorly reflective tissue which does not produce any attenuating shadow; this may be impossible to distinguish from diffuse benign breast change (Kubota et al 1983, Egan & Egan 1984b, Guyer & Dewbury 1987) (Fig. 9.5h), and fine-needle aspiration or biopsy may be needed to establish the diagnosis. This problem arose in four of 481 ultrasonic diagnoses of diffuse benign change in our department (Guyer & Dewbury 1988). The other diffuse change is when there is either widespread involvement of lymphatics by cancer, or following axillary dissection, in which case there is

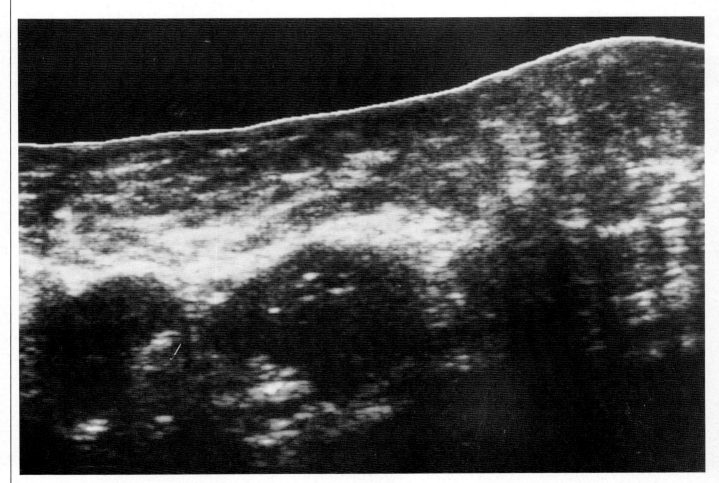

Fig. 9.5g   Axillary ultrasound in a patient with breast carcinoma showing two enlarged poorly reflective nodes, one of which contains multiple small highly reflective areas representing microcalcifications.

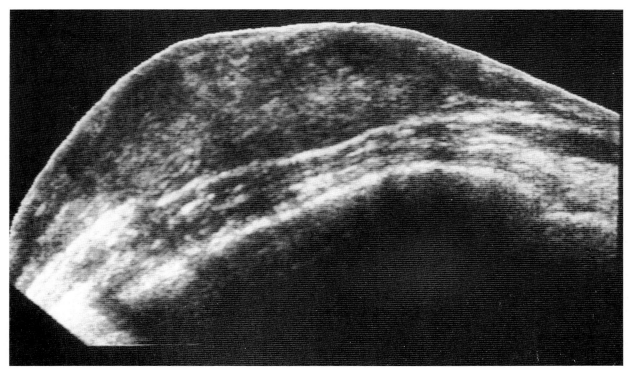

Fig. 9.5h Diffuse carcinoma showing total involvement of the breast by mixed-reflective tissue. The posterior aspect of the breast plate is protruding down towards the pectoral muscles. This appearance needs to be differentiated from diffuse benign change (Fig. 4). (Note the good definition of the pectoral muscles and fascial planes in this B-scan examination.) Reproduced with permission of the publishers from *Sonomammography—An Atlas of Comparative Breast Ultrasound* by P. B. Guyer and K. C. Dewbury; Wiley, Chichester, 1987.

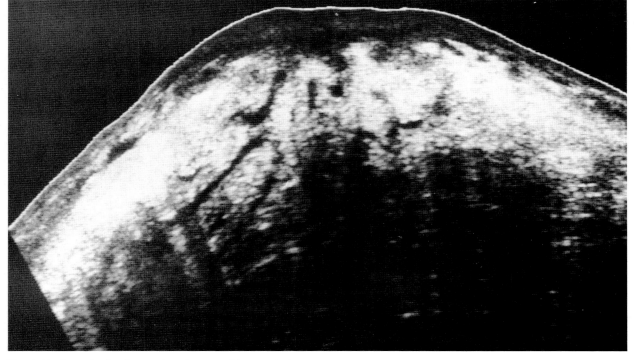

Fig. 9.5i Lymphatic obstruction due to axillary node involvement.

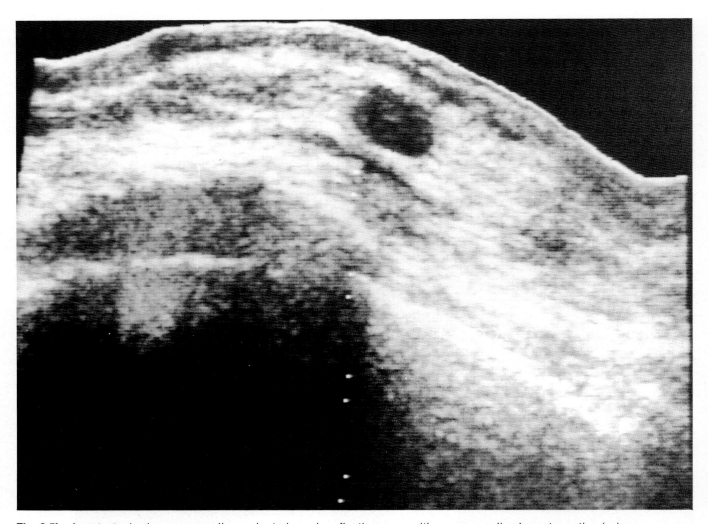

Fig. 9.5j   A metastasis shown as a well-marginated poorly reflective mass with no surrounding breast reaction (primary melanoma). (This needs to be differentiated from a fibroadenoma, which at this depth in the breast tissue, is likely to be relatively highly reflective—see Fig. 9.6a.)

oedema of the breast. The skin will be thickened, and dilated lymphatics may be detected (Fig. 9.5i).

Ultrasound examination of the axilla for nodal involvement in breast cancer is of limited value (Tate et al 1989). Malignant nodes (Fig. 9.5g) may be identified more frequently than by clinical examination, but cannot be readily differentiated from inflammatory enlargement, resulting in false-positive reports. Bruneton et al (1986) recommend a search for axillary nodes to monitor treatment after incomplete dissection, and

following radiotherapy. Huber et al (1989) and Konishi et al (1989) report on the detection of internal mammary node enlargement, the latter noting only a 50% sensitivity.

Metastases to the breast are infrequently seen. Clues to the diagnosis are multiplicity of lesions, their development at a quicker rate than might be expected of a primary lesion, and their failure generally to excite any tissue response, so that they remain circumscribed (Derchi 1985). Those that the author has seen have

generally been poorly reflective (Fig. 9.5j), but one metastasis from a presumed bronchial or thyroid primary was highly reflective.

Lymphoma of the breast is rare. Pope et al (1985) state that it represents 0.5% of all breast malignancy. Our experience suggests that the frequency is even less than this, and Pope himself noted less than 200 cases in the world literature. Two appearances are described—nodal involvement, which is similar to lymphomatous involvement of nodes elsewhere, with a diffuse poorly reflective mass; and diffuse poorly reflective replacement of breast tissue.

BENIGN MASSES

Fibroadenoma, characteristically, is revealed as a solid, well-defined round or lobulated mass (Fig. 9.6a–c) with an even internal echo pattern which, with direct-contact techniques, may be poorly reflective when situated in the near field. However, with stand-off techniques, it is usually shown to be more evenly echogenic. Using water-bath techniques, some authors suggest that it may be difficult to differentiate a fibroadenoma from a fat lobule (Cole-Beuglet et al 1983d, Jackson et al 1986b); mobility of the mass with realtime examination may help here. Border definition is typically good, particularly on the deep aspect, and it may even appear encapsulated due to compression of adjacent tissue (Fig. 9.6a). There is normally no retrotumorous effect, but occasionally either central attenuating shadow (Cole-Beuglet et al 1983d, Harper et al 1983, Egan & Egan 1984b) or accentuation may occur; attenuation is attributable to hyalinization. Fornage et al (1989) recorded 92% fibroadenomas to be poorly reflective, 72% to be homogeneous and 27% with irregular margins. Calcifications may be detected within the mass (Fig. 9.6d), again resulting in retrotumorous attenuation. Any variation of internal echo pattern, or a loss of border definition, should raise a possibility of malignancy, and cytological or histological examination is mandatory (Jackson et al 1986b). The overlap of fibroadenoma and carcinoma is well recognized (Warwick et al 1988) and is reflected in the surgical attitude of excising these masses in patients over the age of 30, only leaving them in situ in younger patients if there is firm cytological proof of their nature.

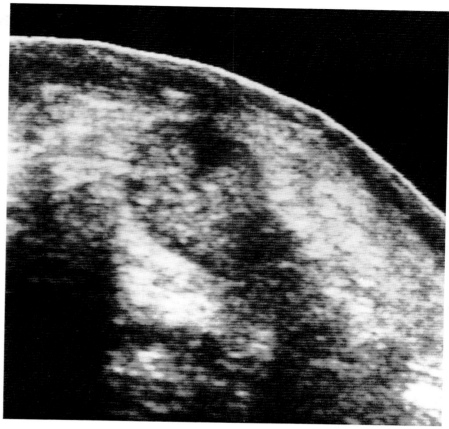

Fig. 9.6a

Fig. 9.6   Fibroadenoma and benign solid masses. *a* Typical appearances, with a well-defined margin except where it is obscured by edge-refractive shadow. The internal echo pattern is even. A little loss of definition superficially due to placement in the near-field.

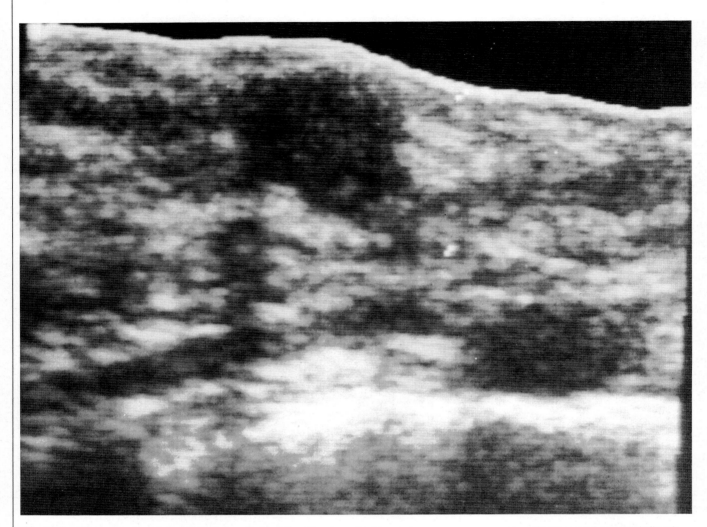

Fig. 9.6b   Fibroadenoma lying in the near-field of the direct-contact transducer: appears poorly reflective and poorly defined; there is no halo or attenuation.

Other features which aid the diagnosis of a fibroadenoma as against a carcinoma are mobility of the mass, its compressibility, and the tendency of the long axis of a fibroadenoma to lie in the line of the tissue planes of the breast (Fornage et al 1989).

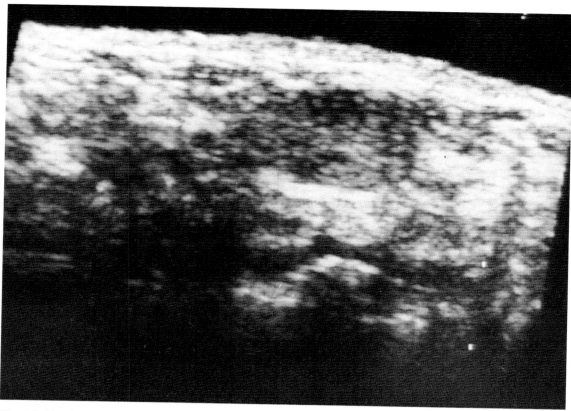

Fig. 9.6c(i) Same as *b*, but using stand-off realtime technique. The fibroadenoma is well-defined and has an even internal echo pattern.

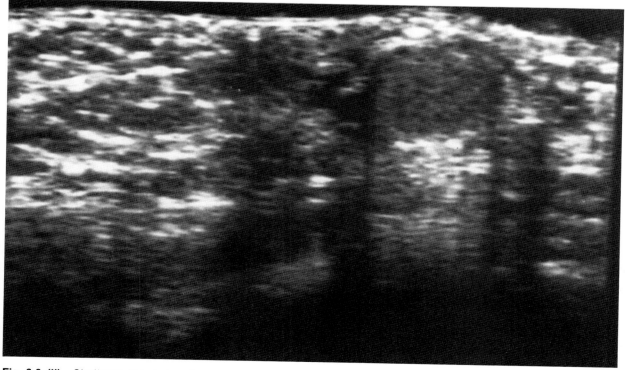

Fig. 9.6c(ii) Similar to (i) but also shows edge refractive shadow.

Other benign solid masses may be indistinguishable from fibroadenoma. These include adenomata and papillomata (Fig. 9.6e); a clue to the latter is the tendency for them to develop adjacent to the nipple, and occasionally a surrounding rim of fluid is seen, indicating an intraductal situation. Haematomata show a rather uneven internal echo pattern in a mass with well-defined margins. From time to time what are diagnosed as benign masses clinically and sonomammographically turn out histologically to be no more than focal collections of fibrous and glandular tissue, variously labelled as fibroadenomatoid change or focal lobular hyperplasia. An adenolipoma (fibroadenolipoma) appears as a well-defined mass but with greater internal echo variation due to the presence of fatty and glandular elements. In these lesions, the X-ray appearance is generally characteristic with ultrasound, i.e. a lipoma is generally well defined with an even internal echo pattern.

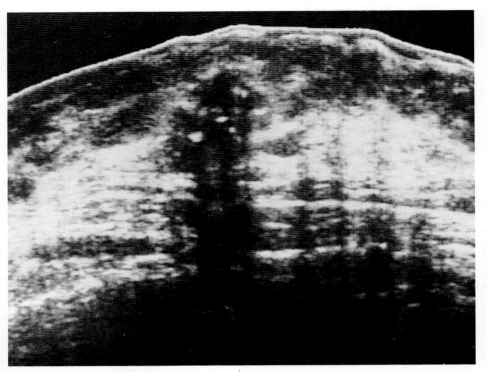

Fig. 9.6d △   ▽ Fig. 9.6e

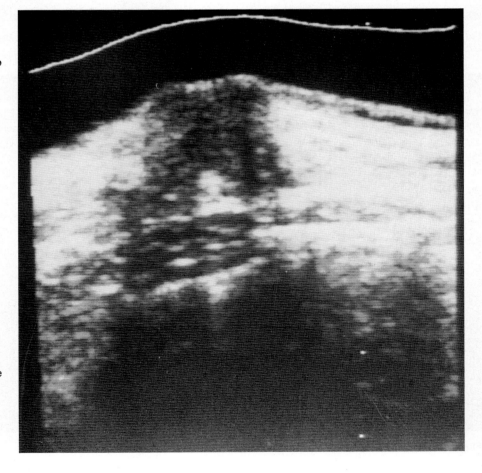

Fig. 9.6d & e   *d* Fibroadenoma with multiple calcifications: resembles a carcinoma but there is no halo (B-scan technique). X-ray showed typical benign calcifications. Reproduced with permission of the publishers from *Sonomammography* (as Fig. 9.5h). *e* Intraductal papilloma. The only suggestive feature is the presence of a solid mass adjacent to the nipple. The presence of fluid around the mass (cf. Fig. 9.7c, intracystic papilloma) would indicate an intraductal situation. Stand-off with B-scan.

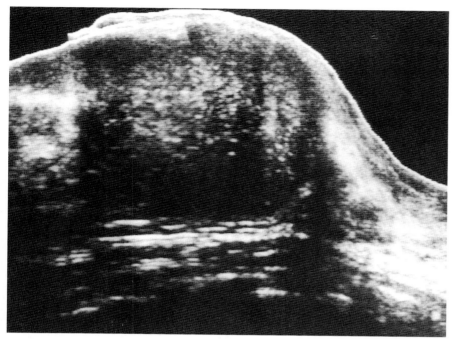

Fig. 9.6f

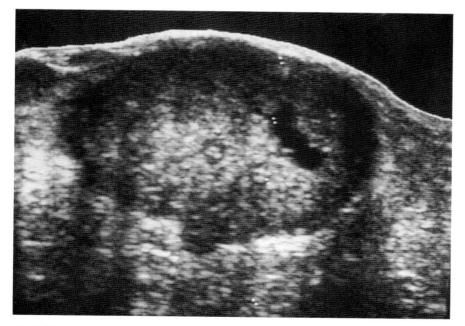

Fig. 9.6g

Fig. 9.6f & g *f* Huge mass with a mainly even internal reflective pattern: giant fibroadenoma. B-scan technique. *g* Phylloides tumour: very similar to *f*, but containing a characteristic fluid cleft.

Large benign solid masses are seen in younger patients as giant fibroadenomata (Steinbeck et al 1983), and, in older patients, as phylloides tumours (Fig. 9.6*f*, *g*). The giant fibroadenoma is well-defined with a very even internal echo pattern; the phylloides tumour is similar, but may show the additional feature of fluid clefts (Cole-Beuglet et al 1983a, Egan & Egan 1984a, Umpleby et al 1989).

Vascular abnormalities may appear as either a solid mass (haemangioma), or as a mainly cystic abnormality (venous malformation). As in the liver, a haemangioma may show a more reflective echo pattern than might be expected for other benign masses, and rather poor border definition. Venous malformation shows characteristic tubular poorly-reflective structures of varying calibre.

Cysts are very common, being detectable in approximately one-quarter of patients aged 35–50 years. They are uncommon under the age of 35, but are becoming more common over the age of 50, due to the increasing use of hormone replacement therapy. When present, they are almost invariably multiple and bilateral. The ultrasound appearances are of a well-defined echo-free mass, round when tense, but flattened when not under tension with retrotumorous enhancement (Fig. 9.7*a*). The ultrasound sensitivity for cysts is almost 100% (Jellins et al 1977), the commonest difficulty being cysts containing turbid fluid which may produce echoes (Fig. 9.7*b*). Under these circumstances, aspiration under ultrasound guidance should clarify the diagnosis. If this fails, excision should be contemplated to ensure the lesion is not a poorly reflective solid tumour, such as a medullary carcinoma, with which there is some ultrasonic overlap. Ultrasound guidance can also be used if attempted cyst aspiration of outpatients is unsuccessful.

Intracystic carcinoma is rare (Reuter et al 1984, Rosner & Baird 1985), but we have seen on a number of occasions synchronous occurrence of cysts and carcinoma. The presence of adjacent malignancy may make an adjacent cyst reappear quickly, and the aspirate from such a cyst may be blood-stained. Unlike intracystic carcinoma, intracystic papilloma is relatively common, and readily diagnosed by ultrasound, when the polypoid mass within the cyst can easily be visualized (Fig. 9.7*c*).

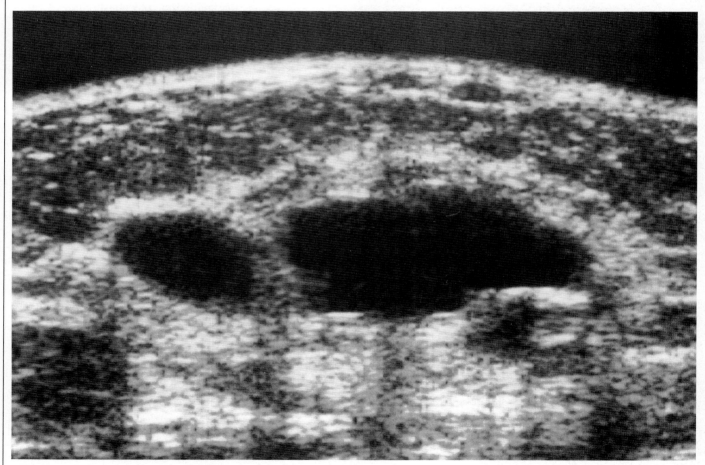

Fig. 9.7a

Fig. 9.7 Cysts. *a* Typical cysts shown by hand-held realtime transducer with a stand-off technique. The cysts are well-defined and echo-free, with accentuation ('bright-up') on the deep aspect. (Note typical double layer to skin with this technique.) *b* Echo-containing cyst: aspiration revealed very turbid contents. (Note thin retromammary fat layer and refractive edge shadowing at cyst edges – B-scan.) Reproduced with permission of the publishers from *Sonomammography* (as Fig. 9.5h). *c* Intracystic papilloma: the papilloma is evenly echo-containing suspended from the anterior wall of the cyst. *d* on p. 234.

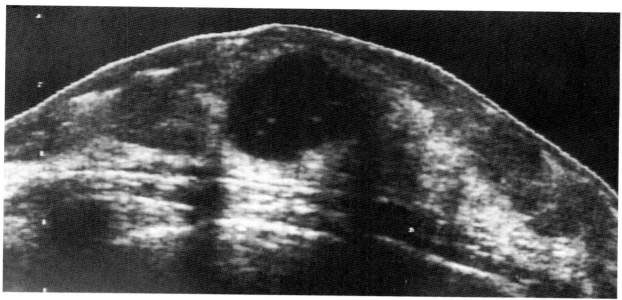

Fig. 9.7b

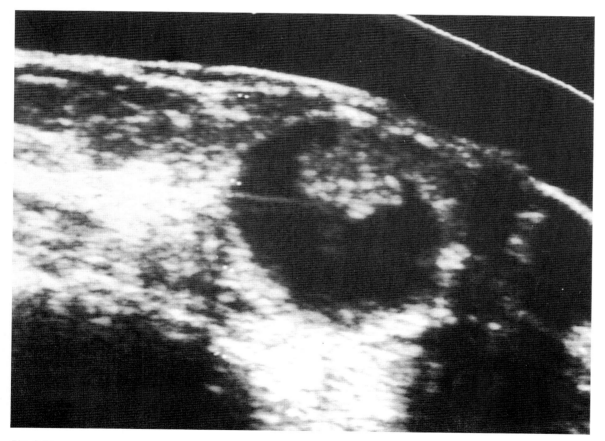

Fig. 9.7c

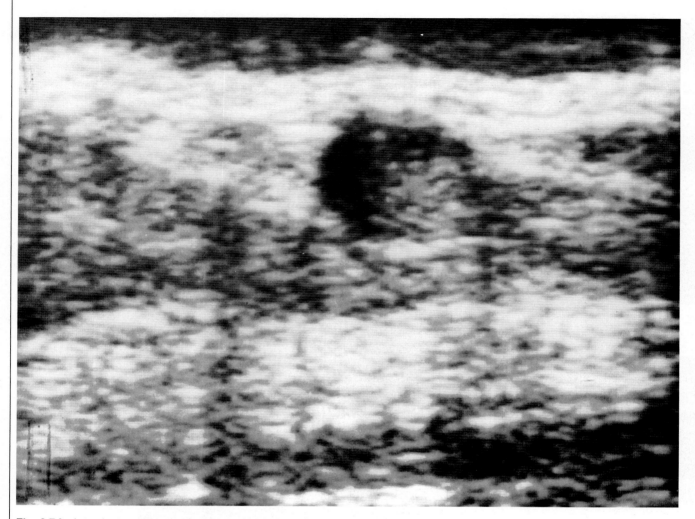

Fig. 9.7d   Intraduct papilloma: similar to *c* but adjacent to the nipple.

MISCELLANEOUS CONDITIONS

Fat necrosis may cause difficulties in diagnosis (McSweeney & Murphy 1985). There are two main features: attenuating shadow, which may be very marked and widespread (Fig. 9.8); and focal, rather poorly defined, poorly reflective masses, which may show areas of fluid within them. The main problem with the attenuating shadow is that it makes it very difficult to exclude a carcinoma. Since fibrosis may be a major feature of these lesions, fine-needle aspiration may prove inadequate, and it may be necessary to proceed to open biopsy.

The focal mass lesions, with partial fluid contents, are very similar to the appearances of a haematoma (Fig. 9.9) (which may in any case proceed to an area of fat necrosis). The aspiration of altered blood from one of the fluid-filled spaces in such a lesion would establish the diagnosis.

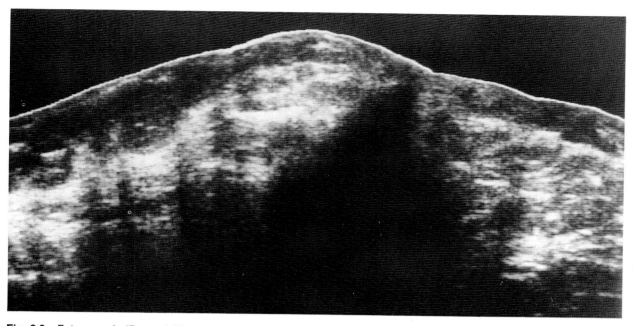

Fig. 9.8 Fat necrosis (B-scan). There is focal attenuating shadow originating from the subcutaneous area and broadening as it goes deeper into the breast. The origin from near the skin is very suggestive of fat necrosis. Reproduced with permission of the publishers from *Sonomammography* (as Fig. 9.5h).

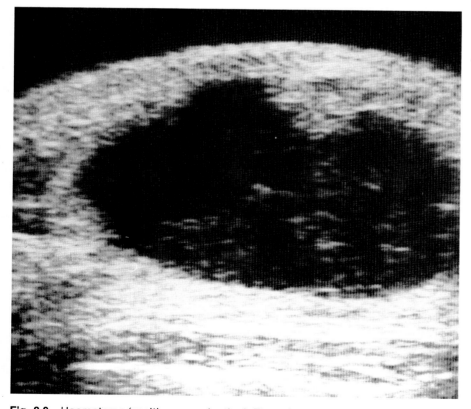

Fig. 9.9 Haematoma (realtime examination). There is an oval cystic space with echoes in the more dependent portions. Aspiration showed altered blood; these changes followed wide local excision.

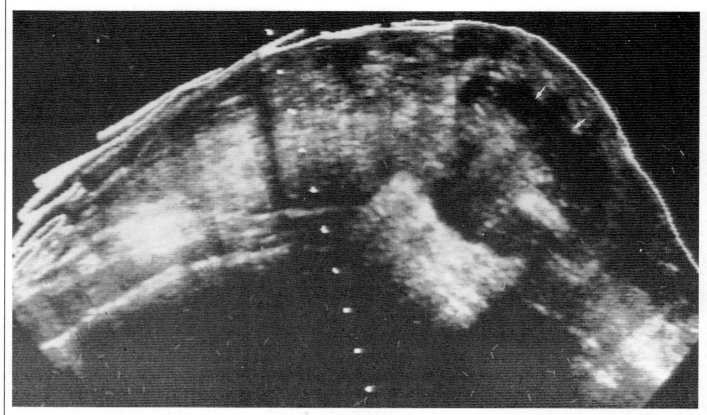

Fig. 9.10a

Fig. 9.10   Abscess. *a* The central portion of the breast is replaced by an echo-containing mass at the margins of which are small echo-free zones, particularly on the right side (arrowed). Aspiration produced pus. B-scan technique. *b* Another abscess, with realtime technique. In this patient the appearances are similar to haematoma—the clinical situation makes the differentiation. Reproduced with permission of the publishers from *Sonomammography* (as Fig. 9.5h).

There is a third focal condition which may mimic these two, and this is an abscess, which may produce a number of poorly reflective areas in a larger area of deranged breast tissue (Fig. 9.10). One feature of an abscess is variable attenuating shadow from portions of the inflamed breast; with these lesions pus may be aspirated from the focal areas of liquifaction. With such overlap of clinical conditions giving a similar ultrasound appearance, the diagnosis will be indicated both by the clinical situation, and the results of aspiration.

Plasma cell mastitis results in focal or more generalized attenuating shadow, with disruption of the tissue planes in the breast; in this situation, the detection of typical tubular calcifications on X-ray mammography will aid the diagnosis.

Duct ectasia can readily be diagnosed by ultrasound when the duct calibre exceeds 3 mm (Fig. 9.3b). However, the frequency of duct dilatation does not, in our view, reach the 23% claimed by Matellana & Orenberg (1983). A solitary dilated duct proximal to a papilloma is well seen, but the papilloma itself may not be identified.

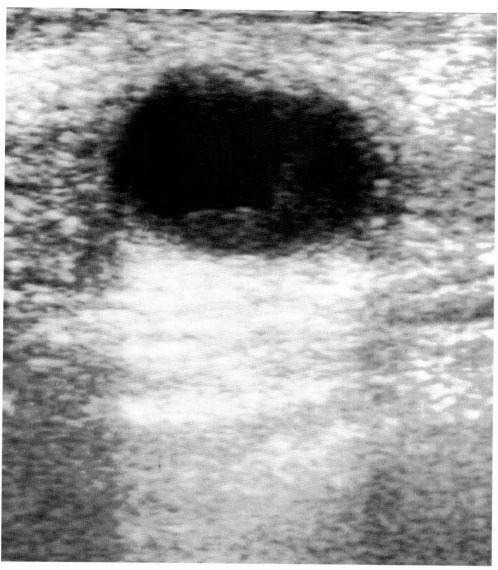

Fig. 9.10b

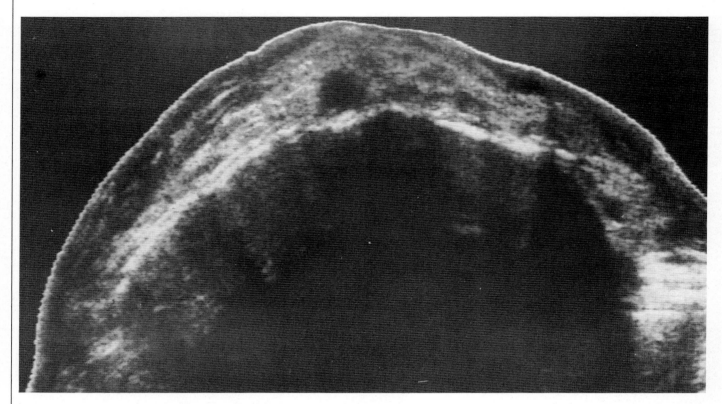

Fig. 9.11   Prosthesis. The augmentation prosthesis is represented by the poorly reflective mass deeply placed in the breast, convex anteriorly. Anterior to prosthesis is a rounded echo-free mass which is a cyst (proved by aspiration).

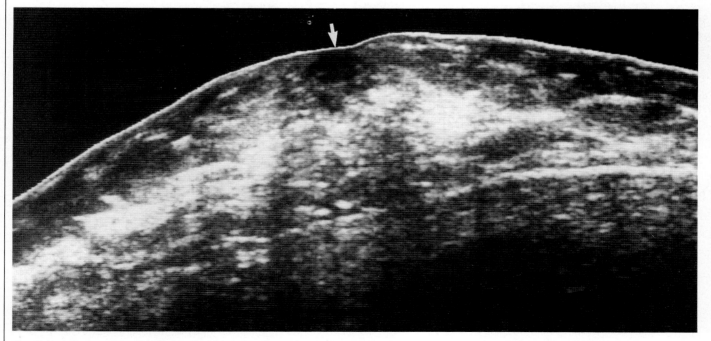

Fig. 9.12   Gynaecomastia. There is generalized swelling of the breast, with rudimentary duct formation (arrowed).

Breast augmentation poses difficulties for X-ray mammography, and ultrasound is the investigation of choice in patients who have undergone this procedure, and who now have symptoms (Cole-Beuglet et al 1983b). With ultrasound, the prosthesis is a poorly reflective structure which is convex superficially, and within which there may be reverberation artefacts. Lesions lying alongside the prosthesis are generally well identified, particularly cysts (Fig. 9.11); however, in the early stages, a carcinoma will need careful differentiation from the results of any surgical scarring that may lie at the margins of the prosthesis.

In the male breast the commonest abnormality is gynaecomastia, which is represented on ultrasound by a general increase in the subcutaneous tissues with a central, poorly defined, poorly reflective area within which rudimentary duct formation may occur (Fig. 9.12). Carcinoma has the same features as in females; cysts have typical appearances but are rare.

LOCALIZATION OF LESIONS

Localization of breast lumps can usefully be achieved employing ulrasound. The simplest method is to identify the lesion within the breast, and mark the skin superficial to this, noting the depth from the skin down to the lesion. It should be ensured that this measurement is made with the patient lying in the operative position. When a breast abnormality which requires localization can be identified both on X-ray and ultrasound, the latter should be used for preoperative localization because it is simpler, quicker, non-invasive, and equally accurate. Ultrasound may also be used to guide a hooked wire to the suspect

lesion (Kopans et al 1984a). A refinement of sonographic localization is for intraoperative localization of impalpable lesions with a small portable ultrasound set in theatre (Schwarz et al 1988).

EFFECTS OF TREATMENT

Treatment to the breast by surgery or radiotherapy produces a number of changes. Following surgery, a common abnormality is a haematoma producing a rounded shadow which, in the early stages, is ill-defined, but later becomes better-defined. Initially, there may be ragged, poorly reflective areas due to altered blood collections, but later these coalesce to produce a fluid space containing echoes, either scattered throughout the fluid collection, or gravitating to its most dependent part. Left without interference, these spaces may persist for several weeks or months, but resolution can be accelerated by repeated aspiration. Associated with this there may be changes of skin thickening, focally increased echogenicity, and trabecular distortion (Calkins et al 1988), resulting in quite marked focal attenuating shadow. Similar, but more widespread features may also follow radiotherapy, when they may persist for several months with decreasing visibility; they may never resolve completely. Eventually a scar results, which is shown sonographically by a narrow band of attenuating shadow extending down from the skin, perhaps associated with persisting trabecular distortion and some residual skin thickening (Cole-Beuglet et al 1980). In the presence of these residual changes, ultrasound is at least as effective as X-ray mammography in identifying any tumour recurrence, which will be shown as a developing poorly-

reflective area within, or adjacent to, the scar.

Attempts at fine-needle aspiration cytology may produce detectable changes in the breast, consisting of poorly-marginated, poorly-reflective areas in the subcutaneous region. However, this procedure is frequently performed on patients in the outpatient clinic prior to imaging, and we have not found that this is a major detriment to the sonographic diagnosis of breast abnormalities. As with localization of occult lesions, ultrasound has been shown to be valuable in guiding fine-needle aspiration, either by marking the skin over the suspect area within the breast (Patel et al 1988), or by guiding a needle into the lesion. For the latter, the tips of most needles can be identified during the procedure as a small reflective focus. The tips of small needles may be difficult to identify, and rough-coated or electronically guided needles have been developed which can be seen more easily sonographically. Up to 92% of carcinomas may yield malignant cells (Fornage et al 1989).

RESULTS OF, AND INDICATIONS FOR, SONOMAMMOGRAPHY

A high ultrasound sensitivity for carcinoma has been recorded, several authors worldwide noting sensitivities of 92–95% (Cole-Beuglet 1982a, Jellins et al 1982, Harper et al 1982, Kelly-Fry 1983, Pluygers et al 1983, Walsh et al 1985, Smallwood et al 1986). Although some authors have commented on the difficulty of identifying subcentimetre malignant lesions (Cole-Beuglet 1982a, Fleischer et al 1983, Kopans et al 1984b, Rosner & Blair 1985, Smallwood et al 1986), we identified 54 cancers in which the nidus was under 1 cm in size, out of the first 287 cancers we recorded (Kelly-Fry (1983) has had similar experience). Of these 287 cancers, 34 were partially or completely obscured by surrounding gland density; in all we found that we were able to be more certain about the diagnosis of malignancy using ultrasound compared with X-ray mammography in just over one-quarter of the cancers, due mainly to tumour identification in X-ray density (Harper & Kelly-Fry 1980, Maturo et al 1982, Kelly-Fry 1983, Pluygers et al 1983, Walsh et al 1985) in symptomatic patients. If ultrasound is used in conjunction with X-ray mammography, the sensitivity for the preoperative identification of cancer rises to 97% (Croll et al 1982, Harper et al 1982, Kelly-Fry 1983, Warwick et al 1988). The significant overlap between circumscribed carcinoma and fibroadenomas (McSweeney & Murphy 1985), 7% of cancers being diagnosed as a fibroadenoma, and a similar proportion of fibroadenomas being regarded as malignant, is an indication for care with such lesions. The insensitivity of ultrasound for microcalcification indicates that, at the moment, it should not be used as a screening technique for breast cancer; Kanecho (1989) found that 34 of 83 proven cancers were not identified with a 7.5 MHz water-bath technique. A major use of ultrasound is to differentiate between cysts and solid lesions, and it can be used effectively in the investigation of the clinically lumpy breast, in which there is X-ray density, by diagnosing unsuspected carcinoma, excluding focal mass lesions, and monitoring or aspirating cysts. The biopsy rate in such instances can be reduced by over 30%, providing aspiration cytology is also undertaken for solid lesions (Fleischer et al 1983, McSweeney & Egan 1983, Rubin et al 1985, Kossoff 1988). The sensitivity of ultrasound for cysts is such that there should rarely be any difficulty over this diagnosis. In patients under the age of 35 years, where X-ray mammographic density may be a restrictive factor, ultrasound can be used as the first investigation in symptomatic patients. It is the initial investigation of choice in the augmented breast. The occurrence of attenuating shadow in association with fibroadenomas or benign breast change may lead to a false-positive diagnosis, and unnecessary biopsy in up to 3% of patients examined. Ultrasound mammography may be done in preference to X-ray mammography in the presence of severe mastalgia, a morbid fear of X-ray mammography, pregnancy, massive breast lesions, failure of previous attempts at cyst aspiration, and severe physical disability.

Although sonomammography is presently unacceptable as a primary breast-screening technique, it does have a valuable role in the assessment of screen-detected abnormalities. It can be used in the exclusion of a mass, in cyst/solid differentiation, in the identification of a mass associated with microcalcifications, in the evaluation of possible trabecular disturbance, and to guide fine-needle aspiration cytology on impalpable lesions.

REFERENCES

Bassett L W, Kimme-Smith C, Sutherland L K, Gold R H, Santi D, King W 1987 Automated and handheld breast ultrasound—effect on patient management. Radiology 165: 103–108

Baum G 1977 Ultrasound mammography. Radiology 122: 199–205

Breast Group of the Royal College of Radiologists 1989 Radiological nomenclature in benign breast change. Clinical Radiology 40: 374–379

Bruneton J N, Caramella E, Hery M, Aubanel D, Manzino J J, Picard J L 1986 Axillary lymph node metastases in breast cancer: preoperative detection with ultrasound. Radiology 158(2): 325–326

Calkins A R, Jackson V P, Morris J G, Stehman F B 1988 The sonographic appearances of the irradiated breast. Journal of Clinical Ultrasound 16(6): 409–415

Cole-Beuglet C 1982a Sonographic manifestations of malignant breast disease. Seminars in Ultrasound 3: 51–57

Cole-Beuglet C, Kurtz A B, Rubin C S, Goldberg B B 1980 Ultrasound mammography. Radiol Clinics of North America 18: 133–143

Cole-Beuglet C, Soriano R Z, Kurtz A B 1983a Ultrasound, X-ray mammography and histopathology of cystosarcoma phylloides. Radiology 146: 481–486

Cole-Beuglet C, Schwartz G, Kurtz A B 1983b Ultrasound mammography for the augmented breast. Radiology 146: 737–742

Cole-Beuglet C, Soriano R Z, Kurtz A B, Goldberg B B 1983c Ultrasound analysis of 104 primary breast carcinomas classified according to histologic type. Radiology 147: 191–196

Cole-Beuglet C, Soriano R Z, Kurtz A B, Goldberg B B 1983d Fibroadenoma of the breast—sonography correlated with pathology in 122 patients. American Journal of Roentgenology 140: 369–375

Croll J, Kotevich J, Tabrett M 1982 The diagnosis of benign disease and the exclusion of malignancy in patients with breast symptoms. Seminars in Ultrasound 3: 38–50

De Land H 1969 A modified technique of ultrasonagraphy for the detection and differential diagnosis of breast lesions. American Journal of Roentgenology 105: 446–452

Derchi L E, Rizzatto G, Giuseppetti G M, Dini G, Garaventi A 1985 Metastatic tumours of the breast. Journal of Ultrasound in Medicine 4: 69–74

Egan R L, Egan K L 1984a Detection of breast cancer. American Journal of Roentgenology 143: 493–497

Egan R L, Egan K L 1984b Automated water bath full breast sonography: correlation with histology in 176 solid lesions. American Journal of Roentgenology 143: 499–507

Egan R L, McSweeney M B, Murphy F B 1984 Breast sonography and the detection of cancer. Recent results in cancer research. Springer, Berlin vol 90, pp 90–100

Fleischer A C, Muhletar C A, Reynolds V H et al 1983 Palpable breast masses: evaluation by high-frequency hand-held realtime sonography and xero-mammography. Radiology 148:813–817

Fleischer A C, Thieme G A, Winfield A C et al 1985 Breast sonography and high frequency handheld realtime sonography. Journal of Ultrasound in Medicine 4: 577–581

Fornage B D, Lorigan J G, Andry E 1989 Fibroadenoma of the breast: sonographic appearances. Radiology 172: 671–675

Funk A, Marque K L, Fendel H 1989 Differential diagnosis of mammary tumours with a 10 MHz probe. Sixth International Congress on the Ultrasonic Examination of the Breast, Paris, 29–30 June, 1989

Gold R H, Bassett L W, Kimme-Smith C 1986 Breast imaging: state of the art. Investigative Radiology 21(4): 298–304

Gross C M, Jacob M 1971 Echographie mammaire et thyroidienne. Journal de Radiologie Médicale 52: 222–228

Guyer P B, Dewbury K C 1987 Sonomammography: an atlas of comparative breast ultrasound. Wiley, Chichester

Guyer P B, Dewbury K C 1988 Sonomammography in benign breast disease. British Journal of Radiology 61: 374–378

Harper P, Kelly-Fry E 1980 Ultrasound visualisation of the breast in symptomatic patients. Radiology 137: 465–469

Harper P, Jackson V P, Bies J, Ransburg R, Kelly-Fry E, Noe J S 1982 A preliminary analysis of the ultrasound imaging characteristics of malignant breast masses compared with X-ray mammographic appearances and the gross and microscopic pathology. Ultrasound in Medicine and Biology 8: 365–368

Harper A P, Kelly-Fry E, Noe J S, Bies J, Jackson V P 1983 Ultrsound in the evaluation of solid breast masses. Radiology 146: 731–736

Hayashi N, Tamaki N, Yonekura Y, Senda M, Yamamoto I, Torizuka K 1985 Real-time sonography of palpable breast masses. British Journal of Radiology 58: 611–615

Hilton S V, Leopold G R, Olson L K, Willson S A 1986 Real-time breast sonography. American Journal of Roentgenology 147(3): 479–486

Howry D H, Stott D A, Bliss W R 1954 Ultrasonic visualisation of cancer of the breast, and other soft tissue structures. Cancer 7: 354–358

Huber C, Renody N, Glunet F, Reynier F 1989 Internal mammary area examination by ultrasound for malignant breast pathology. Presentation at the Sixth International Congress on the Ultrasonic Examination of the Breast, Paris, 29–30 June, 1989

Hughes L E, Mansell R E, Webster D J T 1987 Aberrations of normal development and involution (ANDI). Lancet 2: 1316–1319

Jackson V P, Kelly-Fry E, Rothschild P A, Holden R W, Clark S A 1986a Automated breast sonography using a 7.5 MHz PVDF transducer. Radiology 159(3): 679–684

Jackson V P, Rothschild P A, Kreipke D L, Mail J T, Holden R W 1986b The spectrum of sonographic findings of fibroadenoma of the breast. Investigative Radiology 21(1): 34–40

Jellins J, Kossoff G 1973 Velocity compensation in water-coupled breast echography. Ultrasonics 11: 223–226

Jellins J, Kossoff G, Buddee F N, Reeve T S 1971 Ultrasonic visualisation of the breast. Medical Journal of Australia 6: 305–307

Jellins J, Kossoff G, Reeve T S Detection and classification of liquid-filled masses of the breast by grey-scale echography. Radiology 125: 205–212

Jellins J, Reeve T S, Croll J, Kossoff G 1982 Results of breast echographic examinations in Sidney 1972–9. Seminars in Ultrasound 3: 58–62

Kaizer L, Fishell E K, Hunt J W, Foster F S, Boyd N F 1988 Ultrasonographically defined parenchymal patterns of the breast. British Journal of Radiology 166: 435–439

Kaneko Y 1989 Mass screening for breast cancer by ultrasonic examination. Presentation at the Sixth International Congress on the Ultrasonic Examination of the Breast, Paris, 29–30 June, 1989

Kasumi F, Masshuru H, Fukami A, Kuno K, Kajitami K 1981 Characteristic features of circumscribed cancer. Second International Congress on the Ultrasonic Examination of the Breast, London, p 44

Kasumi F, Fakumi A, Kuno K, Kagitani T 1982 Characteristic echographic features of circumscribed cancer. Ultrasound in Medicine and Biology 8: 369–375

Kasumi F 1988 Can microcalcifications located within breast carcinomas be detected by ultrasound imaging? Ultrasound in Medicine and Biology 14 (suppl 1): 175–182

Kelly-Fry E 1980 Breast imaging. In: Sabagna R E (ed) Diagnostic ultrasound in obstetrics and gynaecology. Harper & Row, Hagerston MD, pp 327–350

Kelly-Fry E 1983 Breast cancer screening for younger United States women. In: Jellins J, Kobayashi T (eds) Ultrasonic examination of the breast. Wiley, Chichester, pp 265–273

Kelly-Fry E, Gallagher H S 1978 A research approach to visualisation of breast tumours by ultrasound methods. In: Ultrasound: its application in medicine and biology. Elsevier, Amsterdam, pp 637–672

Kelly-Fry E, Franklin T D, Gallagher H S 1971 Ultrasound visualisation of excised breast tissue. Proceedings of the Acoustical Society of America, Washington DC, 1971

Kelly-Fry E, Morris S T, Jackson V P, Holden R W, Sanghvi N T 1988 Variation of transducer frequency output for improved detection and characterisation of solid breast masses. Ultrasound in Medicine and Biology 14(1): 143–161

Kimme-Smith C, Bassett L W, King W 1986 Calibration of automated water bath breast ultrasound scanners. Journal of Ultrasound in Medicine 5(12): 271–275

Kimme-Smith C, Bassett L W, Gold R H 1988 Whole breast ultrasound imaging: four year follow-up. Investigative Radiology 21(9): 752–754

Kobayashi T 1975 Ultrasonic diagnosis of breast cancer. Ultrasound in Medicine and Biology 1: 383–391

Kobayashi T 1979 Diagnostic ultrasound in breast cancer: analysis of the retrotumourous echo pattern correlated with sonic attenuation by cancerous connective tissue. Journal of Clinical Ultrasound 7: 471–479

Kobayashi T 1981 current status of sonography for the early diagnosis of breast cancer. Abstract: Second International Congress on the Ultrasonic Examination of the Breast, London, 1981. p 45. British Lending Library, Boston Spa

Kobayashi T 1983 Current status of interpretative criteria for breast tumour. In: Jellins J, Kobayashi T (eds) Ultrasonic examination of the breast. Wiley, Chichester, pp 57–64

Konishi Y, Hashimoto T, Ogata M 1989 Preoperative ultrasound detection of the parasternal lymph node metastases of breast cancer. Presentation at the Sixth International Congress on the Ultrasonic Examination of the Breast, Paris, 29–30 June, 1989

Kopans D B 1984 Early breast cancer detection using techniques other than mammography. American Journal of Roentgenology 143: 465–468

Kopans D B, Meyer J E, Poppe K H The double line of skin thickening on sonograms of the breast. Radiology 141(2): 485–487

Kopans D B, Meyer J E, Lindfors K K, Buchianeri S S 1984a Breast sonography to guide cyst aspiration and wire localisation of occult solid lesions. American Journal of Roentgenology 143: 489–492

Kopans D B, Meyer J E, Sadowsky N 1984b Breast imaging. New England Journal of Medicine 310: 960–976

Kossoff G 1988 Causes of shadowing in breast sonography. Ultrasound in Medicine and Biology 14 (suppl 1): 211–215

Kubota M, Tagima T, Mitomi T, Nanrik, Sakurai I, Kobayashi H 1983 Ultrasonogram of intraductal-spreading breast carcinoma. In: Jellins J, Kobayashi T (eds) Ultrasonic examination of the breast. Wiley, Chichester, pp 103–104

Lambie R W 1983 Sonomammographic manifestations of mammographically detected microcalcifications. Journal of Ultrasound in Medicine 2: 509–514

Lees W R 1982 Breast ultrasonography. In: Sanders R C (ed) Ultrasound annual. Rana Press, New York, pp 301–320

McSweeney M B, Egan R L 1983 Automated breast sonography: comparison with other modalities. In: Jellins J, Kobayashi T (eds) Ultrasonic examination of the breast. Wiley, Chichester, 325–333

McSweeney M B, Murphy C H 1985 Whole breast sonography. Radiologic Clinics of North America 23(1): 157–167

Matellana R, Orenberg C 1983 Ultrasound diagnosis of mammary duct ectasia. In: Jellins J, Kobayashi T (eds) Ultrasonic examination of the breast. Wiley, Chichester, p 319

Maturo V G, Zusmer N R, Gilson A J et al 1980 Ultrasound of the whole breast using a dedicated automated breast scanner. Radiology 137: 457–463

Maturo V G, Zusmer N R, Gilson A J, Bear B E 1982 Ultrasonic appearances of mammary carcinoma with a dedicated whole-breast scanner. Radiology 142: 713–718

Meyer J E, Amin E, Lindfors L K, Lipman J C, Stomper P C, Genest D 1989 Medullary carcinoma of the breast. Radiology 170: 79–82

Patel J J, Gartell P C, Guyer P B, Herbert A 1988 Use of ultrasound localisation to improve results of fine needle aspiration cytology of breast masses. Journal of the Royal Society of Medicine 81(1): 10–12

Pluygers E 1975 Diagnostique ultrasonore par echographie A et B, des affections mammaires. J. Belge Radiol 58: 15–29

Pluygers E, Rombaut M, Dormal C 1983 The accuracy of ultrasonics in the diagnosis of small and subclinical breast cancer. In: Jellins J, Kobayashi T (eds) Ultrasonic examination of the breast. Wiley, Chichester, p 318

Pope T L, Brenbridge A N, Sloop F B,

Morris J R, Carpenter J 1985 Primary histiocytic lymphoma of the breast. Journal of Clinical Ultrasound 13(9): 667–670

Rees B I, Gravelle I H, Hughes L E 1977 Nipple retraction in duct ectasia. British Journal of Surgery 64: 577–580

Reuter K, D'Orsi C J, Reale F 1984 Intracystic carcinoma of the breast: role of ultrasonography. Radiology 153: 233–234

Richardson J E, Olcay S C, Grant E G, Wang P C 1984 Imaging the breast—sonography. Medical Clinics of North America 68(6): 1497–1505

Rosner D, Blaird D 1985 What ultrasound can tell that clinical examination and X-ray cannot. Journal of Surgical Oncology 28(4): 308–313

Rosner D, Weiss L, Norman L 1980 Ultrasonography in the diagnosis of breast disease. Journal of Surgical Oncology 14: 83–96

Rubin E, Miller V E, Berland L L, Han S Y, Koehler R E, Standley R J 1985 Hand-held realtime breast sonography. American Journal of Roentgenology 144: 623–627

Scherzinger A L, Belgam R A, Carson P L et al 1989 Assessment of ultrasound computed tomography in symptomatic patients. Ultrasound in Medicine and Biology 15(1): 21–28

Schwarz G F, Goldberg B B, Rifkin M D, D'Orazio S E 1988 Ultrasonographic localisation of non-palpable breast masses. Ultrasound in Medicine and Biology 14 (suppl 1): 217–229

Smallwood J, Guyer P B, Dewbury K C et al 1986 The accuracy of ultrasound in the diagnosis of breast disease. Annals of the Royal College of Surgeons in England 68: 19–22

Steinbeck R T, Stonaper P C, Meyer J E, Kopans D B 1983 Ultrasound appearances of giant fibroadenoma. Journal of Clinical Ultrasound 11: 451–454

Tate J J, Lewis V, Archer T, Guyer P B, Royle G T, Taylor I 1989 Ultrasound detection of axillary lymph node metastases in breast cancer. European Journal of Surgical Oncology 15: 139–141

Teixidor H S 1980 The use of ultrasound in the management of breast masses. Surgical Gynaecology and Obstetrics 150: 486–490

Teubner J 1989 Diagnostic value of
5 MHz realtime sonography in
preoperative staging of axillary lymph
node metastases. Presentation at the
Sixth International Congress on the
Ultrasonic Examination of the Breast,
Paris, 29–30 June, 1989

Umpleby H, Moore I, Royle G T, Guyer
P B, Taylor I 1989 An evaluation of the
preoperative diagnosis and management
of cystosarcoma phylloides. Annals of
the Royal College of Surgeons in
England 71: 285–288

Vilaro M M, Kurtz A B, Needleman L et
al 1989 Handheld and automated
sonomammography. Journal of
Ultrasound in Medicine 8: 95–100

Wagai T 1983 Results of screening trials in
Japan. In: Jellins J, Kobayashi T (eds)
Ultrasonic examination of the breast.
Wiley, New York, pp 275–281

Wagai T, Takahashi S, Ohashi H,
Ichikawa H 1967 A trial for quantitative
diagnosis of breast tumours by
ultrasonography. Medical Ultrasound 5:
39–40

Wagai T, Tsutsumi M, Takeuchi H 1977
Diagnostic ultrasound in breast disease.
In: Logan W W (ed) Breast carcinoma.
Wiley, New York

Walsh P, Baddesley H, Timms H,
Furnival C M 1985 An assessment of
ultrasound mammography as an
additional investigation for the diagnosis
of breast disease. British Journal of
Radiology 58: 115–119

Warwick D J, Smallwood J A, GuyerP B,
Dewbury K C, Taylor I 1988
Ultrasound mammography in the
management of breast cancer. British
Journal of Surgery 75: 243–245

Wells P N T, Evans K T 1968 An
immersion system for two-dimensional
ultrasonic examination of the human
breast. Ultrasonics 6: 220–228

Wild J N, Neal D 1951 The use of high
frequency ultrasonic waves for detecting
changes of texture in living tissues.
Lancet 1: 655–657

Doppler ultrasound in breast diseases

D. Cosgrove

INTRODUCTION

Since simple diffusion of gases and metabolites is only adequate over short distances, a clone of neoplastic cells that grows larger than a diameter of approximately 1 cm must have the ability to simulate the growth of new blood vessels. At first sight it seems remarkable that tumours should be endowed with this power but it is, in fact, a property of many tissues, being ubiquitous in the embryo and during the normal growth of childhood. It is also activated during healing in most tissues, especially in acute inflammation and in granulation tissue and in the corpus luteum of the ovary.

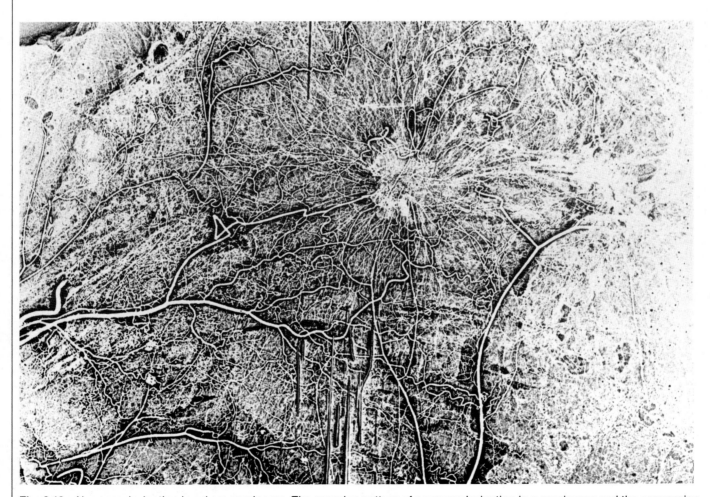

Fig. 9.13 Neovascularization in a 1 cm carcinoma. The complex pattern of neovascularization in a carcinoma and the converging pattern of feeding vessels is demonstrated in this microangiogram of a mastectomy specimen. [Reprinted from *Clinical Ultrasound*, Meire H B, Cosgrove D O and Dewbury K C (eds), Churchill Livingstone, London, 1992. Figure courtesy of Mr J Alan McKinna, Surgeon to the Breast Unit, Royal Marsden Hospital, London.]

The neovascularization is stimulated by angiogenesis factors, compounds secreted by the neoplastic cells (Feldman 1969, Folkman et al 1971, Schor & Schor 1983) that cause new vessels to bud from the adjacent vasculature and grow into the mass from its periphery, forming a tortuous meshwork of small vessels which intertwine and anastomose chaotically (Fig. 9.13). They are also abnormal in structure in that they lack a muscular layer to their walls and therefore do not develop the normal vasomotor tone in response to neural messages or vasoactive hormones and drugs.

These considerations underlie both the potential and the limitations to the uses of Doppler in the investigation of breast disease (and equally in other parts of the body). Obviously, tiny tumours cannot be expected to give Doppler signals, while inflammatory lesions, both infective and non-infective, are likely to produce similar signals to malignancy. In addition, the limits to sensitivity of the equipment available means that the weak signals from small tumours may not be detectable.

On the other hand, in the breast, several favourable factors combine to make this one of the most promising applications of Doppler (Merrit 1987, Nelson & Pretorious 1988). Because the ultrasound beam needs to penetrate for only a few centimeters, high frequencies can be used for Doppler studies—this improves the ability to detect low-velocity flow. Unlike many areas in the body, especially the abdomen, interference from unwanted signals due to cardiac and respiratory movements is minimal.

Because the neovascularization results in a tangle of vessels, there is likely to be some blood flowing towards or away from the transducer regardless of its orientation relative to the mass (Strickland 1959). This means that maximum-intensity Doppler signals can be received from the tumour vessels whatever the direction of the beam, simplifying the problem of locating small vessels. Unlike the usual situation with normal vessels where the Doppler angle is critical, changing the angle when the tortuous vessels of a malignant tumour are being studied simply picks up different portions of the same vessels rather than revealing otherwise undetected vessels. On the negative side, this tortuosity means that only short segments of each vessel are detected at any one time, so that their total number and length are greatly underestimated.

These anatomical considerations apply to the abnormal new vessels within and at the margins of the tumour. The supply vessels that feed the tumour as well as the breast itself, however, retain their normal straight or gently curved configuration so that, for these, the beam-vessel angle is critical. In these vessels an increase in flow velocity in response to the demand of the tumour and the presence of arteriovenous shunts may be expected and is likely to be proportional to the size of the tumour. In addition, alterations in the flow pattern reflecting the lack of vasomotor tone of the tumour vessels may occur. This is depicted on Doppler as a relative increase in diastolic flow compared with the normal resting breast where the arteriolar sphincters have sufficient tone to close more-or-less completely in diastole. Ratios of the peak systolic to lowest diastolic Doppler frequency shift (e.g. the resistance index) are higher in such a normal bed than in an artery supplying a bed with neovascularization (Burns & Jaffe 1985). This change to a 'low impedance' flow pattern is likely also to be apparent only with larger masses.

CLINICAL STUDIES

The earliest studies of breast vasculature employed relatively simple continuous wave (CW) Doppler systems which are very sensitive to flow, even of low velocity, but provide only minimal anatomical information (Fig. 9.14). However, they are well-suited to the study of the supply vessels, both those in the vicinity of a mass and the main lateral thoracic and internal mammary arteries. The largest study (of over 400 cases) (Burns et al 1982, 1984, Minassian & Bamber 1982, Bamber et al 1983) demonstrated high velocity flow in the arteries supplying the breast that contained carcinomas in 73% of cases, and there were parallel alterations in a number of features of the Doppler spectrum, especially the peak velocity, when compared to the unaffected side. A striking change in

the sound output from the CW systems was noted in the form of a higher-pitched and rough sound that was characteristic of arteries supplying carcinomas. There was no asymmetry in patients with benign breast change but some 35% of fibroadenomas did have asymmetrical flow, though the difference was not as marked as with the carcinomas and the characteristic 'tumour sound' was rarely present. Subsequent studies have confirmed that these findings are reproducible and changes through the normal menstrual cycle, as well as in carcinomas treated with chemotherapy, have been demonstrated (Sambrook et al 1987).

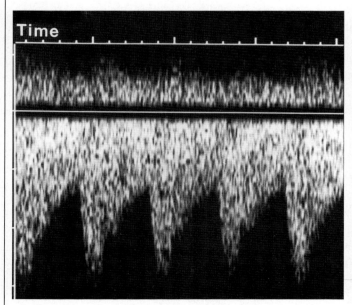

Fig. 9.14a

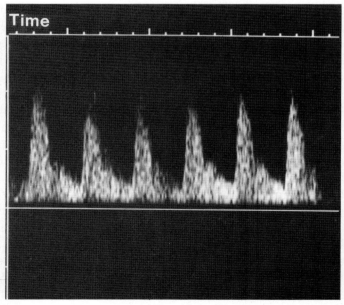

Fig. 9.14b

Fig. 9.14   Continuous-wave Doppler. The spectral tracings show Doppler shift (*x*-axis, in kHz) with time (*y*-axis) from arteries supplying the breast that contains a carcinoma (*a*) and from the normal side (*b*). Note the higher peak shifts (corresponding to higher flow velocities) on the tumour side and the relative increase in diastolic velocity. There is also more signal at low velocities in the tumour-bearing breast, perhaps because of flow disturbances. [Flow towards the probe is conventionally depicted above the line and flow away, below; this depends on the orientation of the transducer and is unimportant in this type of study. In (*a*) an accompanying vein lying in the region of Doppler sensitivity has given signals in the reverse direction.]

The CW study is difficult to perform, involving a tedious slow search through the whole volume of the breast. On the presumption that these difficulties would be eased if more anatomical information were available to guide placement of the Doppler beam, duplex pulsed Doppler was applied enthusiastically to the problem of diagnosis of breast carcinoma (Fig. 9.15). Although good results were reported (Schoenberger 1988) and the addition of Doppler was shown to improve diagnostic accuracy (Jellins 1988), in fact the vessels involved are usually too small to be resolved on the B-scan, so that the added anatomical information proved only to be helpful in locating the tumour mass and the technique remains tedious (Jackson 1988). A new feature of the pulsed Doppler studies is that abnormal signals were found at the margins and even within the tumour masses.

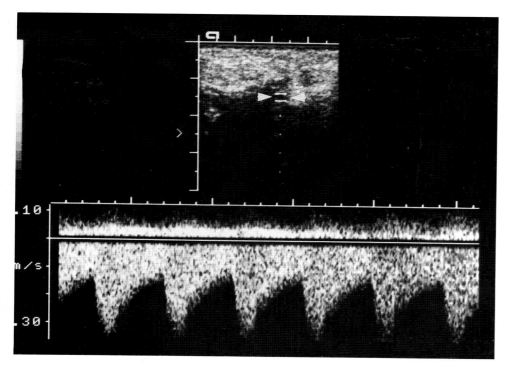

Fig. 9.15 Pulsed-wave Doppler. The facility for simultaneous imaging and Doppler ('duplex scanning') shows that these spectral signals arise from vessels at the margin of this carcinoma. The sensitive Doppler gate is indicated by the parallel bars (arrowheads) on the dotted line that represents the line of the Doppler beam. The spectral tracing is the same as that used for continuous-wave Doppler (Fig. 9.14) and the waveform shows the typical malignant features of high peak systolic velocity and continuous diastolic flow.

Colour Doppler (CD) has proved to be more interesting, partly because of the direct display of vessels it provides but also because of its apparent sensitivity to low-volume and low-velocity flow, so that minute vessels are readily demonstrated both around and within masses (Cosgrove et al 1990) (Fig. 9.16). The technique is simpler than either the CW or the pulsed Doppler duplex methods (Adler et al 1990), though some technical problems remain, notably the motion artefacts produced by bulk movements of the tissue during the scanning action, the low frame rate that precludes a rapid search and the fact that the blood pressure in the tiny vessels is so low that they are easily obliterated by even slight pressure with the transducer.

Vessels can be demonstrated in and around almost all carcinomas (55/56; Cosgrove et al in press) and they usually have the expected tortuous configuration. There is a tendency for larger masses to have more vessels, though vessels can be found in tumours as small as 5 mm in diameter.

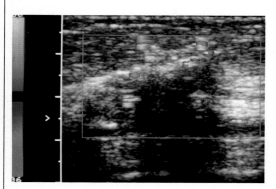

Fig. 9.16a

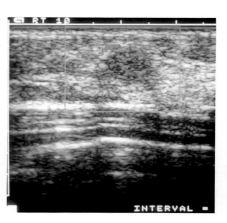

Fig. 9.16b

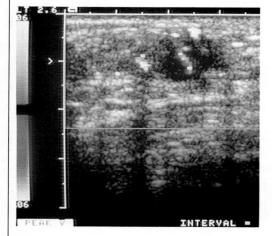

Fig. 9.16c

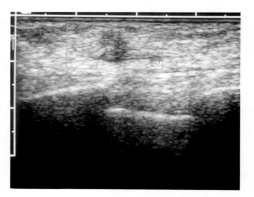

Fig. 9.16d

Fig. 9.16 Colour Doppler in carcinomas. *a* Large carcinoma showing colour signals both at the margin and within the lesion. Note the tortuous vessels. *b* Small (8 mm) carcinoma with a prominent tortuous vessel at the tumour margin as well as a central vessel. *c* 1 cm non-shadowing carcinoma with two vessels shown within the lesion as well as several at its anterior edge. *d* A small (5 mm) carcinoma with a single prominent vessel.

The most striking vascularity is seen in inflammatory carcinomas while scirrous tumours tend to be less vascular, presumably because only the cellular components are vascularized.

Benign lesions generally are poorly vascularized and no colour Doppler signals can be obtained (Fig. 9.17). Cysts, of course, are avascular and are not considered further in this discussion except to note that the finding of vessels in a lesion taken to be a cyst on ultrasound imaging reclassifies it as non-cystic and should lead to further investigation. Benign breast change (BBC or ANDI) is rarely vascular (4/97; Cosgrove et al in press), occasional exceptions being encountered in examples where the histology shows florid changes; presumably here it is the inflammatory component that excites the vascular response. The fact that BBC is usually 'CD-negative' is most helpful in the differential diagnosis of the otherwise confusing focal or localized form in which a region of altered architecture with shadowing may suggest a carcinoma.

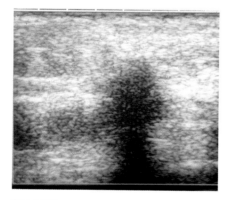

Fig. 9.17a

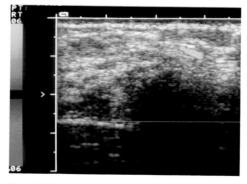

Fig. 9.17b

Fig. 9.17 Benign breast change. *a* Focal benign breast change: the absence of colour signals is reassuring in cases where the grey scale scan is highly suspicious. Histology of this lesion showed fibroadenosis. *b* In occasional cases (0.5%) a single vessel is associated with a worrying region of benign mammary change. Probably this vessel is actually a normal breast vessel that happens to lie close to the suspicious region; criteria to distinguish normal from pathological breast vessels have not yet been established. In other cases, histology reveals an inflammatory component to the benign changes.

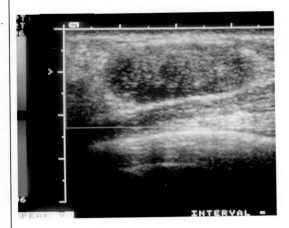

Fig. 9.18a

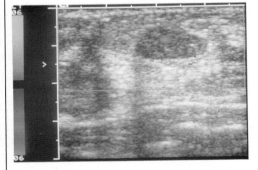

Fig. 9.18b

Fig. 9.18   Fibroadenomas: colour Doppler. *a* Large fibroadenoma with no colour signals. This is the typical pattern, even for large lesions. *b* Vascular fibroadenoma: about 20% of fibroadenomas are associated with one or occasionally two vessels.

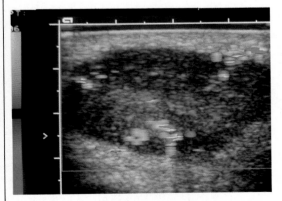

Fig. 9.19   Phylloides tumour. These are often vascular; this example contains several vessels and its margin is also vascularized.

As with the early CW studies, fibroadenomas are sometimes 'CD-positive' (6/33; Cosgrove et al in press): in about one-fifth of cases one or, sometimes two, vessels can be demonstrated within or at the margin of the lesion (Fig. 9.18). In contrast to the convoluted vessels that are typical of malignancy, they are straight or gently curved and many, in fact, are probably normal breast vessels that happen to become involved in the fibroadenoma. Larger fibroadenomas and the fleshy juvenile types are more commonly vascular. While these 'false-positives' undoubtedly weaken the value of CD as a diagnostic tool, the absence of colour signals from a doubtful region is reassuring and, more importantly, any region that does show colour Doppler signals requires a biopsy.

A few rarer pathologies are also vascular: phylloides tumours usually show several vessels (Fig. 9.19), as do metastases to the breast—both of these need the same initial management as breast carcinomas, so the finding of vascularity is diagnostically helpful. Inflammatory processes are a striking exception to the lack of vascularity in benign pathologies in general: the inflammatory capsule around an abscess typically shows a higher vascular density even than an inflammatory carcinoma though there are no vessels in the cavity itself (Fig. 9.20). Among the rarer disorders that are notably avascular are granulomas and fibrosis; in the latter case, the absence of colour signals is helpful in the otherwise difficult problem of differentiating scarring from recurrence. Involved lymph nodes are variably vascular and it is not yet clear whether Doppler will be of help in distinguishing reactive from involved nodes.

The seemingly reasonable suggestion that the vascularity of tumours would correlate with their invasiveness does not seem to be borne out on a histological comparison (Cosgrove et al in press). Prospective studies will be needed to evaluate its potential in defining patients at high risk of recurrence or metastasis. However, in patients treated medically prior to surgery ('primary medical treatment'), the colour Doppler signals reduce or disappear as the tumour responds (Kedar et al in press); sometimes the vascular changes precede shrinkage and this is often easier to document than the change in volume.

Overall therefore Doppler, and especially colour Doppler, is emerging as a useful additional feature in the differential diagnosis of breast masses that can be used alongside the established morphological and dynamic features. It is particularly helpful in highlighting those carcinomas that are inapparent on the grey scale scan (Fig. 9.21)—those that do not shadow are of the same reflectivity as the surrounding tissue or have infiltrated widely (e.g. extensive inflammatory carcinomas). It is also useful in locally recurrent carcinomas which are frequently difficult to differentiate from postoperative scarring. The lack of signals from benign breast change is especially reassuring when focal fibrotic regions are encountered: though they are often suspicious on realtime imaging, the lack of vascular signals indicates that they are benign.

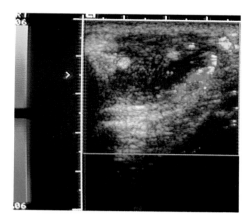

Fig. 9.20 Breast abscess. The margins of an abscess are usually very vascular. This corresponds with the inflammatory capsule demonstrated on histology.

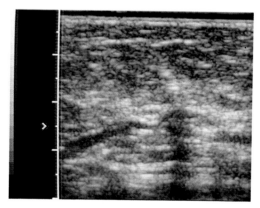

Fig. 9.21a

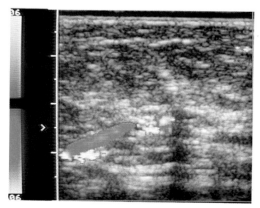

Fig. 9.21b

Fig. 9.21 Inapparent carcinoma. *a* On the greyscale the tumour mass is hard to detect—it was, in fact, missed during the first (realtime) part of the study. *b* Colour Doppler signals highlight the lesion.

REFERENCES

Adler D A, Carson P L, Rubin J M, Quin-Reid D 1990 Doppler ultrasound color flow imaging in the study of breast cancer. Ultrasound in Medicine and Biology 16: 553–559

Bamber J C, Sambrook M, Minassian H, Hill C R 1983 Doppler studies of blood flow in breast cancer. In Jellins J, Kobayashi T (eds) Ultrasonic examination of the breast. Wiley, Chichester, pp 371–378

Burns P N, Jaffe C C 1985 Quantitative flow measurements with Doppler ultrasound. Radiological Clinics of North America 23: 641–657

Burns P N, Halliwell M, Wells P N T, Webb A J 1982 Ultrasonic Doppler studies of the breast. Ultrasound in Medicine and Biology 8: 127–143

Burns P N, Davies J D, Halliwell M, Virjee J, Wells P N T 1984 Doppler ultrasound in the diagnosis of breast cancer. In: Leopold G R (ed) Clinics in diagnostic ultrasound. Churchill Livingstone, New York, vol 12, pp 41–56

Cosgrove D O, Bamber J C, Davey J B, McKinna J A, Sinnett H D 1990 Colour Doppler signals from breast tumours. Radiology 176: 175–180

Cosgrove D O, Kedar R P, Vagios E et al Colour Doppler in the differential diagnosis of breast masses. Radiology, in press

Feldman F 1969 Angiography of cancer of the breast. Cancer 23: 803–809

Folkman J, Merler E, Abernathy C, Williams G 1971 Isolation of a tumour factor responsible for angiogenesis. Journal of Experimental Medicine 33: 275–278

Jackson V P 1988 Duplex sonography of the breast. Ultrasound and Medicine in Biology 14 (suppl 1): 131–137

Jellins J 1988 Combined imaging and vascularity assessment of breast lesions. Ultrasound in Medicine and Biology 14 (suppl 1): 121–130

Kedar R P, Cosgrove D O, Bamber J C, Smith I E, Al Murrani B, Svenssn W E Colour Doppler in breast carcinoma treated with primary medical therapy. Radiology, *in press*

Merritt C R 1987 Doppler color flow imaging. Journal of Clinical Ultrasound 15: 591–597

Minassian H, Bamber J C 1982 A preliminary assessment of an ultrasonic Doppler method for the study of blood flow in human breast cancer. Ultrasound in Medicine and Biology 4: 357–364

Nelson T R, Pretorius D H 1988 The Doppler signal: where does it come from and what does it mean? American Journal of Roentgenology 151: 439–447

Sambrook M, Bamber J C, Minassian H, Hill C R 1987 Ultrasonic Doppler study of the hormonal response of blood flow in the normal human breast. Ultrasound in Medicine and Biology 13: 121–129

Schoenberger S G 1988 Breast neoplasms: duplex sonographic imaging as an adjunct to diagnosis. Radiology 168: 665–668

Schor A M, Schor S L 1983 Tumour angiogenesis. Journal of Pathology 141: 385–413

Strickland B 1959 The value of arteriography in the diagnosis of bone tumours. British Journal of Radiology 32: 705–713

CHAPTER 10

Localization of impalpable breast lesions

N. M. Perry

INTRODUCTION

Accurate localization of impalpable breast lesions for biopsy was first described by Dodd et al 1965. The commonest occult lesion requiring localization will be microcalcification (63%, Yankaskas et al 1988; 60%, Rosenberg et al 1987; 54%, Chetty et al 1983), either with or without an associated mass or area of parenchymal distortion.

The rate of positive malignancy yield from such procedures in published series varies from 10.7% (Proudfoot et al 1986) up to 35% (Hermann et al 1987) and 44% (Barnard et al 1988). Local diagnostic criteria will be the chief determining factor for this figure, but it will also be influenced by whether the population is symptomatic or screened, the age groups of the women concerned and the availability of fine-needle aspiration cytology (FNAC). An experienced screening centre using FNAC on its incident screening rounds might expect a positive malignancy yield from such localization procedures to be in the order of 75%. The variable predictive value of diagnostic biopsies makes paramount factors such as safety and comfort, the need to excise the least possible volume for accurate histological diagnosis and at the same time allow satisfactory postoperative cosmesis (Gallagher et al 1989).

The amount of breast tissue removed in excision of impalpable lesions has varied from quadrantectomies, to unguided estimated excisions averaging 6.4 cm maximum diameter (Roses et al 1980), and guided excision biopsies averaging 4.9 cm (Norton et al 1988) and 4.1 cm (Hoehn et al 1982). Tinnemans et al (1987) report a mean volume excised of 63 cc, as opposed to Gallagher et al (1989) who, using accurate localization methods, achieved a median specimen volume of 6.0 cc and median maximum specimen diameter of 2.5 cm. Minimal excision refers primarily to diagnostic biopsies; surgical guidelines for the UK Breast Screening Programme quote an upper limit of 20 g for the majority of these procedures. Lesions having been shown to be positive for malignancy on FNA require a reasonable margin of excision in order to avoid the necessity for additional clearance later.

TECHNIQUES

Since Dodd's initial description, many different techniques and variations of them have been described and reviewed (Hall & Frank 1979, Hoehn et al 1982, Svane 1982, Feig 1983, Kopans & Swann 1989). Visual assessment from mammography with subsequent unguided generous biopsy has been used, and even recommended—Prorok et al (1983) stating localization to be time-consuming and unnecessary. Quadrantectomy, which also has been advocated, is unjustified for women with benign lesions.

Surface marking with opaque markers (Frankl & Rosenfeld 1975, Malone et al 1975) and either surface diagrams or grid references in relation to the nipple (Berger et al 1966, Curcio 1970, Stevens & Jamplis 1971) attempted to provide a more accurate method. These had some success with lesions situated not far from the skin surface or in a readily identifiable relationship to the nipple. The inherent problem with these methods is the internal spatial alteration between a compressed breast pulled away from the chest wall in the erect or sitting position for mammography and the flattened supine anterior oblique position of the breast on the operating table.

Most other localization methods involve placement of a marker to the lesion as accurately as possible to guide the surgeon. The marker, or at least its method of delivery, should be radio-opaque to allow the radiologist to confirm position, as well as readily visible to the surgeon.

MARKERS

These include dye or other visible materials delivered to the site of the lesion via a needle (the spot method), or variations of a self-retaining hooked wire.

The spot method was first described to localized lung abscesses (Rabin 1941) but was later applied to breast localization (Hollender & Gros 1965, Simon et al 1972, Egan et al 1976, Horns & Arndt 1976). Dyes used include Methylene Blue, Evans Blue, Toluidine Blue, Isosulfan Blue, Indigo Carmine and Indocyanide Green.

Estimates of position of the lesion are made from the control mammograms and a needle inserted as close as possible to the lesion and confirmed on check mammograms. The dye is then injected, and some radiologists advocate either leaving a trail of dye along the track to the skin surface to guide the surgeon or leaving the needle in place. Radio-opaque contrast material can be added for final confirmation of position mammographically although this has caused problems of precipitation, granuloma formation and obscuration of detail on specimen radiography depending upon which contrast is used (Hall & Frank 1979). There is also at least a theoretical risk of contrast reaction.

Toluidine blue causes less patient discomfort and has a smaller diffusion rate than Methylene Blue with no alteration in cell architecture (Czarnecki et al 1989). Hirsch et al (1989a) report interference of Methylene Blue with oestrogen receptor assay—which remains unaffected by Isosulfan Blue (Hirsch et al 1989b). Other marking substances used include platinum-coated gold grains (Millis et al 1976), metal pellets (Barth et al 1977), stainless-steel suture threads (Bolmgren et al 1977) and carbon powder suspension (Svane 1982).

Dyes will diffuse into breast tissue at varying rates and ideally require operation within 4 h in order to maintain accurate localization. Injection into a duct will result in more rapid and widespread diffusion. Carbon, particularly in colloidal form, diffuses little. Svane (1982) quotes one case where 57 days elapsed between spot localization and excision without diffusion of the carbon.

Needle markers (20–25 gauge) may be used and once positioned kept in place by taping to the skin surface (Threatt et al 1974). Muhlow (1974) described placing two needles at right angles to guide the surgeon. The risk of trauma to the breast or of needle dislodgement is a real one; changes in position have been observed even on respiration (Horns & Arndt 1976).

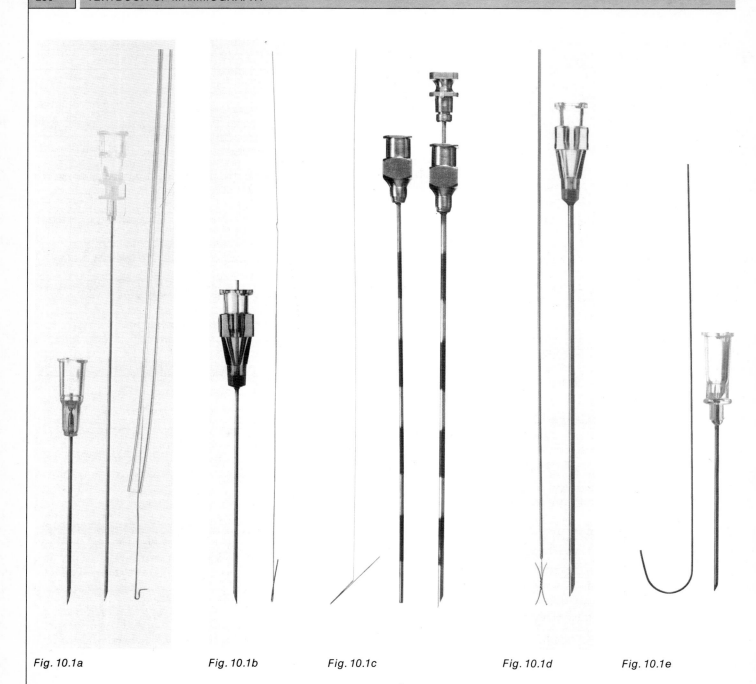

Fig. 10.1a   *Fig. 10.1b*   *Fig. 10.1c*   *Fig. 10.1d*   *Fig. 10.1e*

Fig. 10.1   Some examples of available needle assemblies. *Left to right a* A simple hook wire which may be introduced via a 21 gauge, 5 cm needle or a 22 gauge, 9 cm spinal needle. A plastic sleeve is used to protect the wire from bending during packing and sterilization. For insertion of the assembly the wire should be placed through the lumen of the needle so that the hook sits well down in the bevel of the needle. *b* A spring hook wire able to be contained within the lumen of the introducing needle, or after-loaded. (William Cook Europe Limited, Letchworth, Herts SG6 1JF, UK). *c* The Nottingham wire (Medi Plus, Bourne End, Slough, Bucks SL8 5YS, UK) with introducing trochar and cannula, having 1 cm markings to aid accuracy during adjustment. Despite its configuration the wire may be easily after-loaded. A blunt-ended post-localization surgical stiffening cannula is also shown, able to be fed over the wire during the biopsy procedure. *d* The Reidy Cross Hook wire (Cook). It cannot be after-loaded and the wire remains intraluminally until the introducing needle is accurately placed. *e* The Mammalok (Namic; Henleys, London N8 0DL, UK) curved retractable localization wire assembly.

The commonest marking device now used is a variant of the hook wire (Fig. 10.1) first described by Frank et al (1976). This consisted of a 25 gauge wire with its distal tip bent back to form a hook, using a 9 cm needle for delivery. Once positioned the needle was removed leaving the wire in place, its hook providing some degree of stability. Kopans & De Luca (1980) modified this by fashioning a spring hook able to be contained within the lumen of a 20 gauge needle during placement, withdrawal of the needle then allowing the hook to reform in the breast tissue. Further slight modification (Kopans & Meyer 1982a) allowed a spring hook wire to be after-loaded through a needle which thereby could be used for FNAC once positioned accurately. Homer et al (1981) developed a technique of stiffening the localizing wire during surgery by passing a cannula over it, enabling the surgeon to locate more readily the hook of the wire during surgery in addition to preventing its transection during excision. Homer (1985b) also developed a curved ended lockable sturdy wire able to be contained in a 20 gauge needle (Namic Mammalok). Some wires now have a thickened segment proximal to the spring hook in order to resist surgical transection.

Other recent developments include a cross-hook spring-loaded wire (Reidy), a retractable barb (Hawkins), a coiled wire correctable twist-marker (BIP) and a spring-loaded T-bar (Nottingham), having good self-retaining properties in breast tissue. There may be difficulty in removing the cross-hook wire for pathological sectioning of the excised specimen. It is possible to form hook wires and spring hook wires in the department in conjunction with a standard 20 gauge spinal needle or 21 gauge, 5 cm needle, to save expense. An ordinary hook wire requires a small skin incision and some skill to place incrementally with accuracy as it cannot be pulled back. Both these problems are avoided by the use of a spring hook wire. Without the need for a skin incision, some units do not use local anaesthetic for insertion of their spring hook wires (Landercasper et al 1987).

Placement of marker

Whichever marking device is chosen there are two basic methods of placing it; either an anterior approach—including ultrasound and CT—or a parallel-to-chest-wall approach including stereotaxis. No matter which method is used it is essential to explain the procedure fully and carefully to the woman, gain her confidence and encourage her to relax as far as possible. The procedures described relate primarily to wire markers.

Anterior approach (Fig. 10.2). Control mammograms are taken in the true lateral and craniocaudal projections. These films allow confirmation of the presence of the lesion, adequacy of technical factors and enable accurate measurements to be made of the position of the lesion relative to the nipple, which of course must be in profile. Such measurements can be made on the control mammograms in a linear fashion directly superior or inferior and medial or lateral to the nipple so that there is a clear idea of the exact site of skin entry in relation to the nipple line. It is also possible to estimate the site of skin entry by measuring in a radial fashion round the appropriate skin surfaces as judged from the control films. The radial method sometimes allows a shorter approach and can avoid aiming a needle assembly directly at the chest wall. The angle and depth of entry can also be assessed from the control mammograms (Feig 1983).

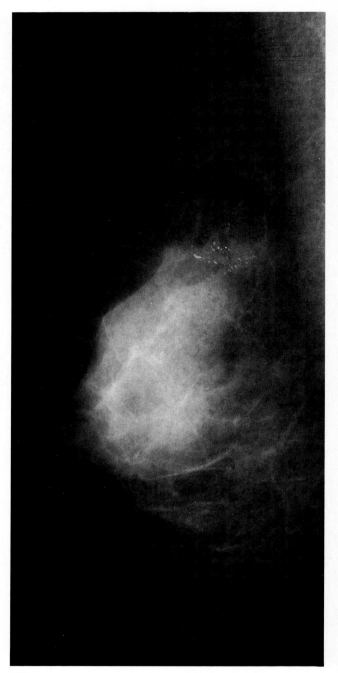

R   *Fig. 10.2a*

Fig. 10.2 Anterior approach hook wire localization. *a and b* A cluster of microcalcification is identified superior and lateral to the nipple line.

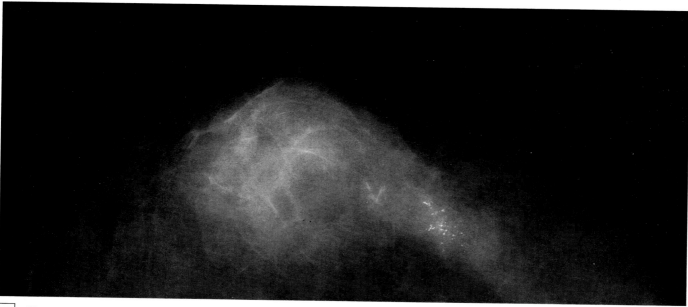

R *Fig. 10.2b*

Before transferring these measurements to the skin of the breast, approximately 10% reduction should be made on the measurements taken from the control mammograms to allow for geometric and compression magnification. With the woman in the sitting or supine position, the measurements are transposed to the skin using a ruler and marking pen. A round or ring-ended object such as a needle holder is then pressed onto the skin at this site in order to indent it temporarily prior to skin cleansing which might otherwise wash off the mark.

Suitable skin cleansing and local anaesthesia is then provided. A 2 mm skin incision with a scalpel blade allows entry of the needle assembly without undue pressure or sudden giving way. The assembly is aimed according to the depth of the lesion and the method of measuring used. Either the radiographer or the free hand of the radiologist supports the breast during this procedure. There is often a degree of error of judgment at this stage, and if a simple hook wire assembly is used it is advisable not to place it to the full estimated depth of the lesion at first pass, but to stop short and to take check views in both projections to gauge the adjustment necessary to obtain satisfactory final position. If a spring hook wire is used, placement to the estimated full depth may be made on the first pass, as the assembly is withdrawable if the needle lies too deep on the check mammogram.

Following any necessary adjustments as determined by check mammograms, the needle is removed, leaving the wire in place, and final films are performed. A second wire should be placed if the first wire is more than 2 cm from the lesion. The final films should be clearly marked, and with a descriptive report should accompany the patient to theatre. The breast is carefully dressed with gauze having tied a loose knot in the end of the wire or coiling it in order to prevent travel of the wire through the skin into the breast. It is inadvisable to fix the protruding wire directly to the skin, as any such fixation tends to dislodge the hook of the wire with any significant movement of the breast. It is better to have 2 or 3 cm of 'slack' in the wire at the skin surface to accommodate such breast movement.

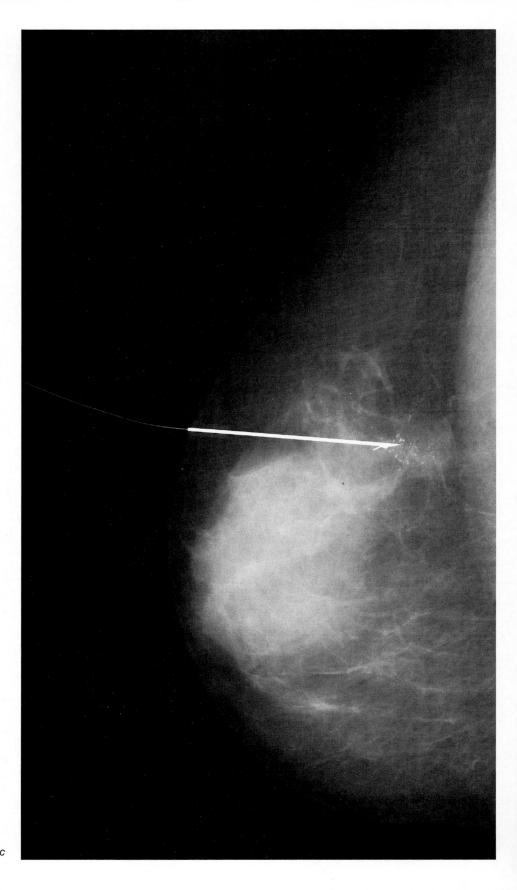

R   Fig. 10.2c

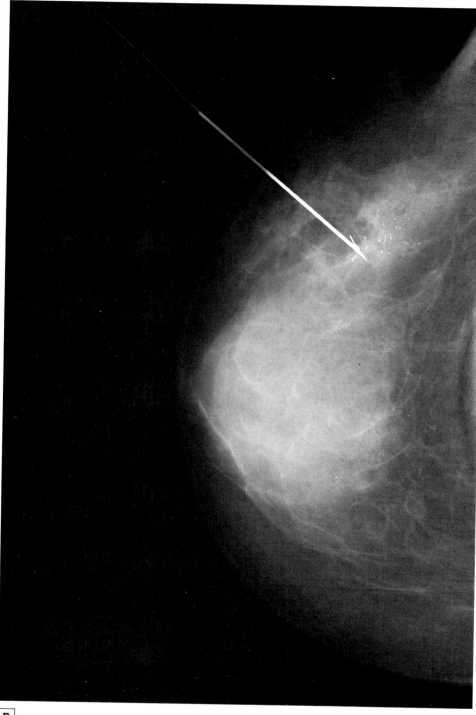

R

Fig. 10.2d

Fig. 10.2c & d   Following radial measurements around the skin surfaces, the hook wire assembly is inserted towards the cluster of calcification. The hook wire is demonstrated to be sitting well down in the bevel of the needle.

Further protection is afforded by the wearing of a loose-fitting bra, and the woman should go back to the ward and later to theatre without any further interference to the dressing. As a general rule excision should be performed within 24 h of placement. Although not ideal, it is possible for the woman to travel to a different hospital for excision of the lesion.

The advantages of this method are that it is simple and requires a minimum of equipment. However, it does require some degree of experience and skill to obtain accuracy and carries a potential risk of puncture of the chest wall due to the anterior nature of the approach, although this risk is considerably diminished with use of a 5 cm needle.

Computed tomography and ultrasound localization. These are both variations of the anterior approach.

Ultrasound provides a quick and efficient method of localization for sonographically identifiable solid lesions or areas of architectural distortion. Needle assemblies may either be placed with triangulation (Kopans et al 1984), with the free hand or with the aid of a fixed angled needle holder attached to the probe, with the line of the needle path demonstrated on the screen. The patient is positioned supine anterior oblique with the ipsilateral arm curled around her head. This position is comfortable, carries less risk of syncope, allows a short skin-to-lesion course and is similar to the surgical position for excision.

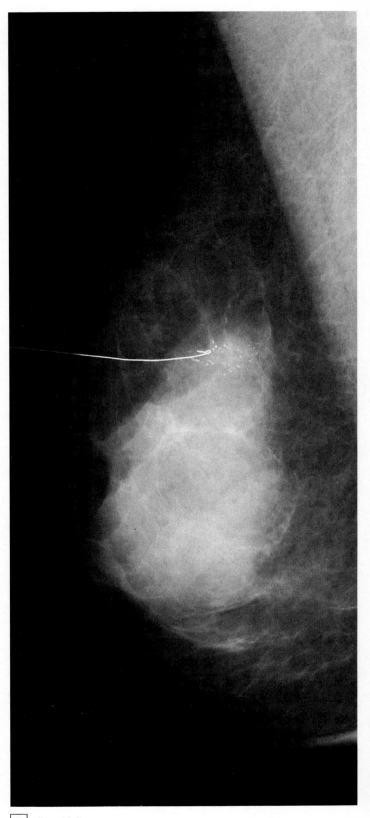

R   *Fig. 10.2e*

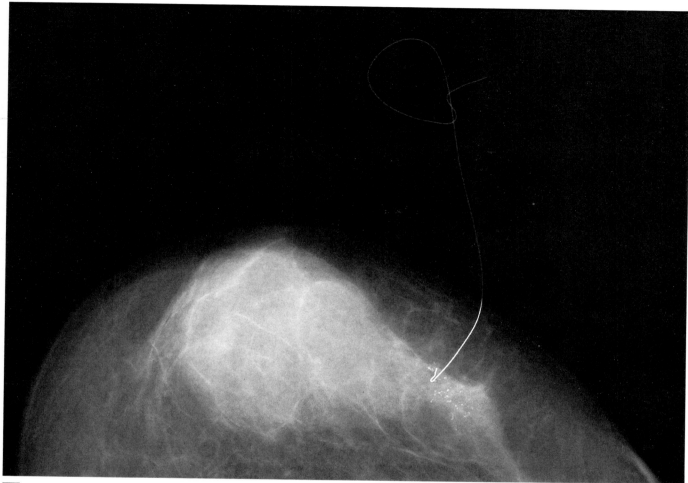

R *Fig. 10.2f*

Fig. 10.2e & f The needle has been removed from the wire. A loose slip knot is tied in the free end of the wire and the final films are then sent to theatre with the patient with accompanying descriptive report.

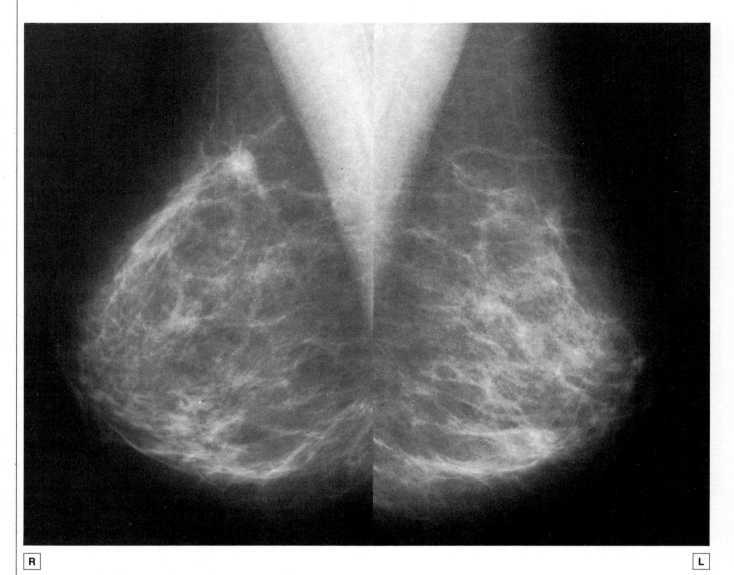

R   L

Fig. 10.3a

Fig. 10.3   Ultrasound localization. *a* A small carcinoma is seen high above the right nipple line. *b* Ultrasound confirms the presence of a small hypoechoic irregular mass with a surrounding irregular echogenic halo. *c* Under ultrasound control a hook wire assembly is inserted adjacent to the lesion. The bright focus of echogenicity is identified adjacent to the tumour nidus.

The usual preliminary procedures of explanation, skin cleansing, local anaesthetic and a small skin incision are performed. A small amount of sterile couplant material may be necessary during needle placement. The technique of using a 5 cm, 21 gauge needle with hook wire is well suited for this method as there should be no need for pull-back. Mammograms are obtained with the wire in situ to confirm position for the surgeon (Fig. 10.3).

An increasingly used method of localization for sonographically identifiable but impalpable FNAC-proven cancers is that of ultrasound-guided skin marking. In the anterior oblique position the skin is marked with a suitable marking pen directly over the lesion. The size of lesion and its depth relative to the skin is clearly stated in the report to the surgeon. This method is quick, comfortable and easily tolerated. Its accuracy is quite sufficient for proven malignant lesions which require a satisfactory margin of excision.

Computed tomography has no routine place in localization procedures but has been described as useful for deep lesions seen only on one view (Kopans & Meyer 1982b). Obvious disadvantages include time, expense, lack of availability, partial voluming and inability to detect small clusters of microcalcification.

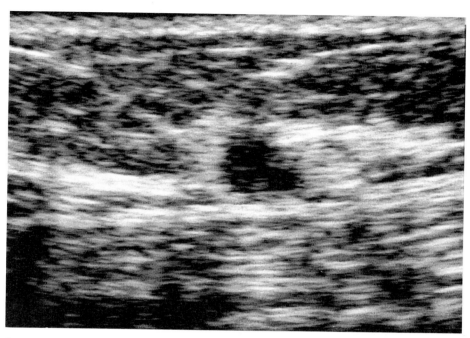

Fig. 10.3b

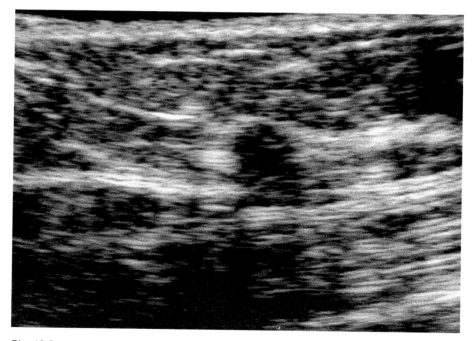

Fig. 10.3c

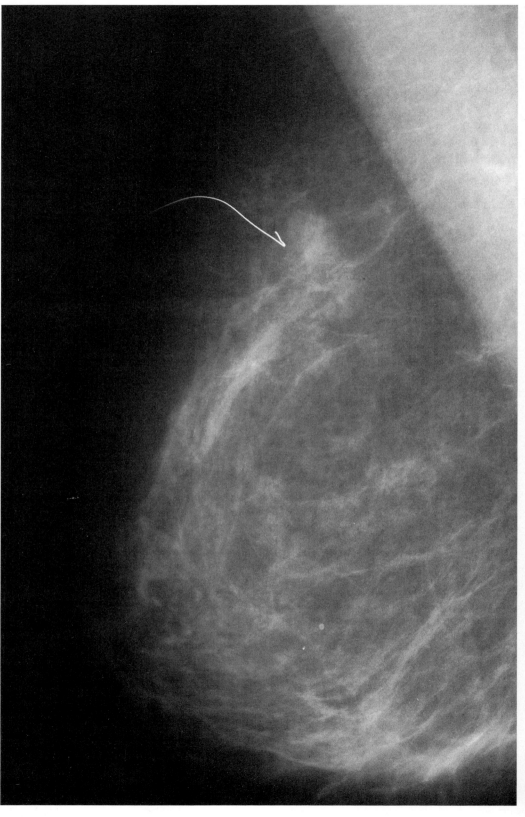

Fig. 10.3d   Final films confirm position for the surgeon.

Approach parallel to chest wall. This method requires use of a perforated or fenestrated plate (Fig. 10.4), or a stereotactic device. A perforated plate for compression was first described by Melander (1972) and further identified as a localization tool by Muhlow (1974) and Oleson & Blichert-Toft (1979). Once the woman has been fully informed of the procedure, her breast is compressed, with the top Perspex compression plate placed on the surface of the breast most likely to allow the shortest skin approach. This is usually superior or lateral because the majority of lesions are in the upper or outer parts of the breast. A mammogram is taken which allows the lesion to be related to one of the numbered holes on the perforated plate or to a grid-marking reference on the fenestrated plate.

Following suitable skin cleansing and local anaesthetic, a spring hook needle assembly is placed accurately to the lesion, or through it according to the reference points on the compression plate. The collimator light beam is helpful at this stage to confirm perpendicularity of the assembly by superimposition of the shadow of the needle hub to the entry site. An assessment of the depth of placement may be made by study of the control mammograms, particularly the orthogonal view. In other words with the breast compressed in the craniocaudal position, a study of the lateral control view will allow depth assessment.

After this initial placement of the needle assembly through the perforated or fenestrated plate, it is largely a matter of experience whether one takes a control view in this position or not. It is vital, however, that when releasing the breast from compression under the localizing plate, great care is taken to avoid catching the needle assembly on the plate because the breast tends to spring back towards the chest wall. This is less likely to occur with the fenestrated plate and can also be avoided by positioning hands under the compression plate before release in order to hold the breast still.

When released, the localizing compression plate can be replaced with a standard Perspex plate for the orthogonal view. Once this view has been processed, assessment can be made of the position of the needle tip in relation to the lesion and any

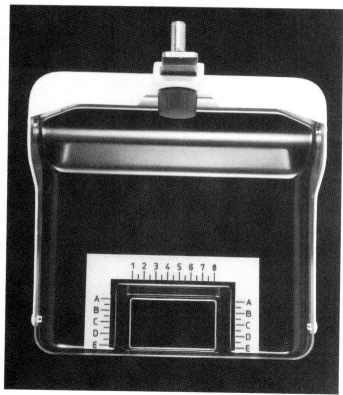

Fig. 10.4a

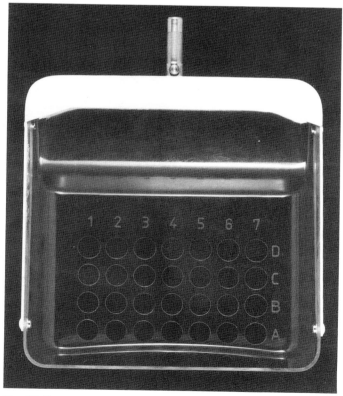

Fig. 10.4b

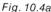

Fig. 10.4 *a* Fenestrated and *b* perforated compression plates for localization.

necessary alteration, e.g. pulling back the assembly by 1–2 cm in relation to the skin surface to obtain depth accuracy, can be performed. For greatest accuracy it is best to keep the breast compressed in the orthogonal projection until this adjustment is made and the wire has been placed through or pushed out of the needle with subsequent needle removal.

Operator experience results in a faster procedure, thereby minimizing compression discomfort for the woman. Most women are able to tolerate compression for up to 5 or 10 min, and it is courteous during such procedures to use a 90 s film cycle as opposed to 3 min. The strength of compression does not necessarily have to be as much as that used for standard diagnostic mammography, but must

be sufficient to provide the radiographic clarity necessary to identify the lesion and to prevent movement of the breast under the plate.

It is generally preferable to place the hook of the wire just deep to the lesion (Figs 10.5 and 10.6) so that any movement of the wire will tend to pull the hook into the lesion rather than

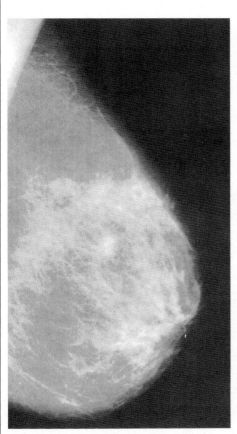

Fig. 10.5a

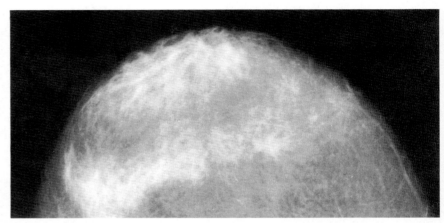

Fig. 10.5b

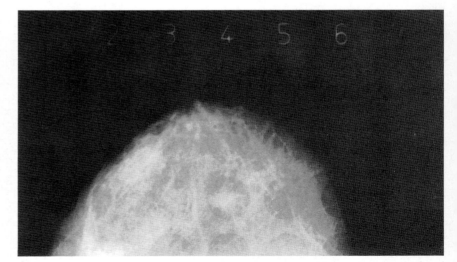

Fig. 10.5c

Fig. 10.5 The Nottingham wire assembly. *a and b* A small stellate opacity is demonstrated just above the nipple line and medial to it. *c* The lesion lies directly below one of the holes in the perforated plate. *d* The needle assembly is placed directly through the lesion. *e* The orthogonal projection confirms position with relation to the lesion and allows estimation of pull-back required. *f and g* Following removal of the trochar, the wire has been after-loaded down the cannula which is then removed leaving the wire accurately in place. *Fig. 10.5g & h appear on p. 270.*

away from it. Final clearly labelled mammograms with the wire in place should be returned to the ward or theatre with an accompanying descriptive report. The use of dressing gauze and a loose-fitting bra is again advised. Tying a knot in a spring hook wire is difficult if not impossible due to the characteristics of the wire. However, it is possible to coil the wire round on itself while still leaving 2 or 3 cm of clear wire at the skin surface.

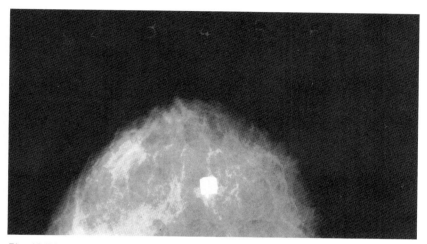

Fig. 10.5d

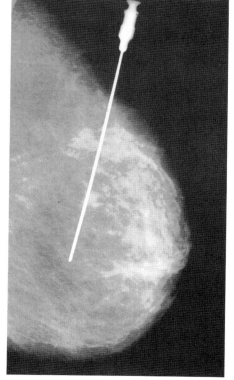

Fig. 10.5e

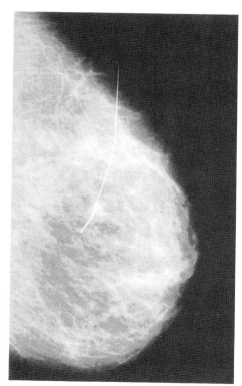

Fig. 10.5f

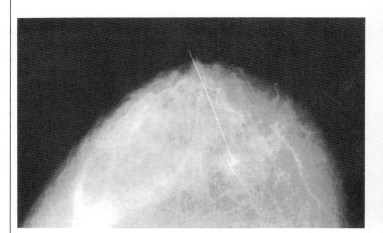

Fig. 10.5g   After removal of cannula.

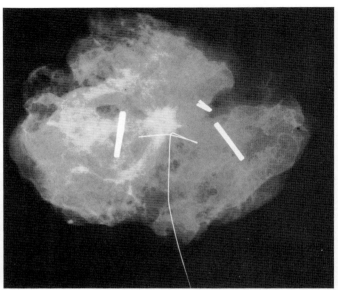

Fig. 10.5h   Specimen radiography confirms accuracy of placement of the wire.

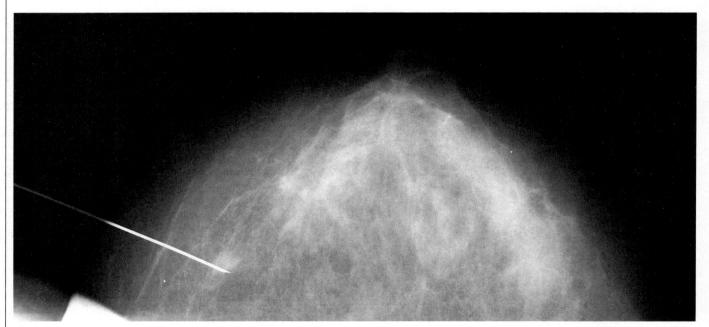

R

Fig. 10.6a

Fig. 10.6   The Mammalok assembly. *a* The needle has been positioned close to a small irregular opacity. *b and c* The curved ended wire has been placed just deep and around the lesion, and the needle withdrawn.

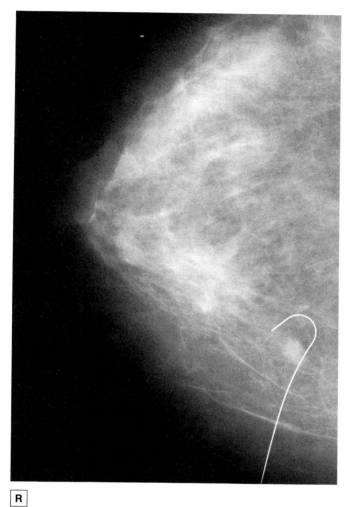

R

Fig. 10.6b

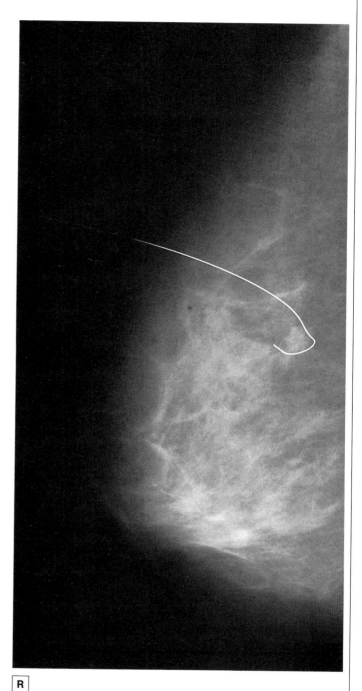

R

Fig. 10.6c

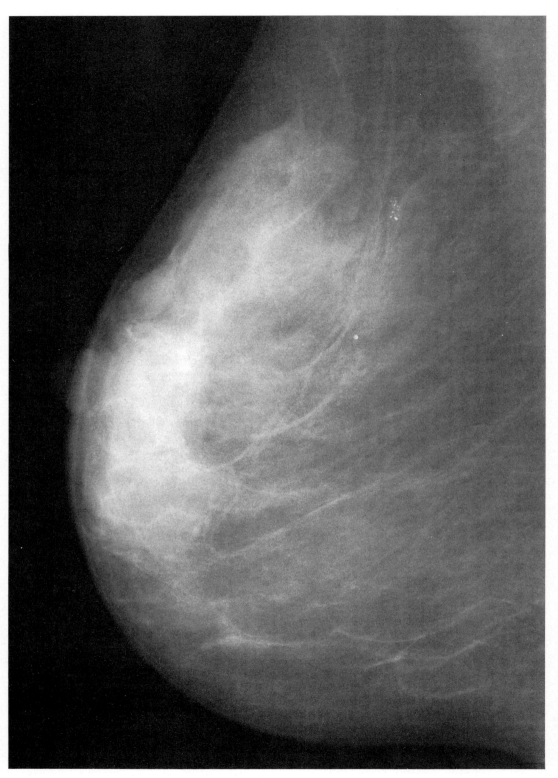

R

Fig. 10.7a

Fig. 10.7   Use of perforated plate. *a* A cluster of microcalcification is seen high above the nipple line. *b* The perforated plate has been applied and the wire assembly inserted through the appropriate hole. Although it is preferable to have the lesion in question directly under one of the holes, as demonstrated it is quite possible to angle the assembly. It is important that the radiologist carefully supervises release of compression with this plate in order not to detach the needle. *c* is on p. 274.

It is quite possible to use a simple hook wire assembly with this approach (Fig. 10.7), but the technique requires greater skill for accuracy. An intermediate siting view for depth will be necessary because it is difficult to pull back the assembly unless the breast tissue is particularly fatty.

A different method of assessing depth of the lesion in the approach plane has been described (Soholm & Conrad 1989). The control mammogram in the orthogonal plane is used to estimate the depth of the lesion as a ratio to the whole breast thickness— the ratio is then assumed to stay constant for the thickness of the compressed breast, e.g. a lesion one-third of the depth of the breast on the control orthogonal view will be 1.5 cm deep if the compressed breast thickness is 4.5 cm.

The advantages of parallel approach are greater accuracy, speed and safety. These outweigh a slightly longer skin-to-lesion approach surgically. It is possible to angle the assembly through the compression plate to attempt a shorter skin distance (see Fig. 10.7). This requires considerable experience in order not to lose accuracy; and special care not to dislodge the needle on compression release. The long skin-to-lesion approach is avoidable if the surgeon approaches the lesion at a different angle through a separately placed incision to the site of wire entry. In this case it is useful to place a simple radio-opaque marker such as a ball-bearing on the skin at the estimated depth of the breast lesion

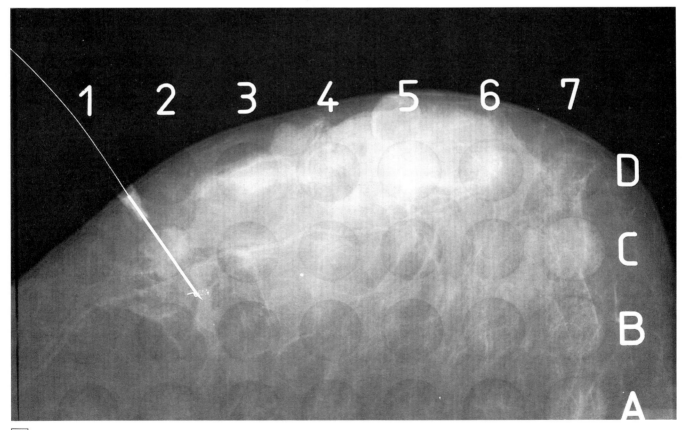

R

Fig. 10.7b

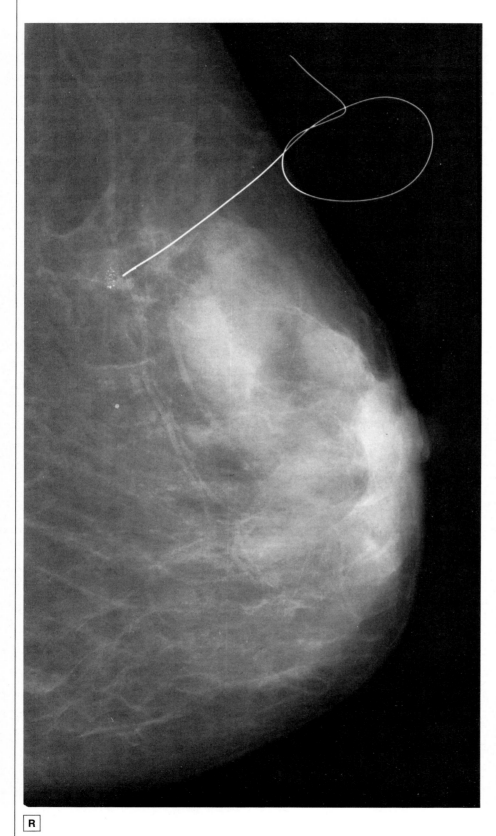

Fig. 10.7c Fixed film confirms position.

just before taking the final orthogonal localization view. The surgeon will then be able to relate the site of the skin marker to the true position of the breast lesion and hook in order to estimate the site of his approach incision.

Stereotaxis. Stereotactic localization is a variant of the parallel approach using computations of stereoscopic measurements first described by Price & Butler (1971) and developed by Bolmgren et al (1977). While the depth of the lesion can be accurately assessed to 1 mm, the assembly should still be placed a little deep to the lesion to allow for the natural resistance and spring-back of breast tissue under compression. A spring hook wire is required as a hook wire will not pass through the needle holders of the device.

A further cause of inaccuracy using stereotaxis is the problem of target mobility (Dowlatshahi et al 1989). The target lesion may deviate away from the localizing needle path with subsequent inaccuracy of placement.

SPECIAL PROBLEMS

Lesions identified on one view only
Such lesions create the problem of depth judgement on the orthogonal view, and of course it is first of all vital to ensure that the lesion is genuine and not artefactual. Ultrasound can be used if the lesion is sonographically identifiable, and stereotactic localization may be suitable if available. However, lesions seen only on one view are often sufficiently awkwardly placed that it is uncomfortable for the woman to hold position in the stereotactic device for an adequate length of time.

A method of depth judgement using parallax in the standard fenestrated plate approach has been described by Kopans et al (1987). Once the needle assembly is placed through the lesion, compression is carefully eased and the breast and needle repositioned elsewhere in the window of the compression plate. This allows a second view to be taken with the beam at an angle to the needle. Comparative measurements are then taken for the apparent length of the needle on the film, and the relationship of tip to lesion is expressed as a ratio with the true measured length of the needle. The needle is then further positioned accordingly.

An additional method (Yagan et al 1985) uses angulation and triangulation. With the breast in the standard approach position, an opaque skin marker is placed directly over the lesion. A tube tilt of 30° is employed to take a further view, and assessment is made of the true depth of the lesion by geometric calculation.

Inferior lesions

10–20% of lesions requiring localization are situated inferiorly in the breast. Standard parallel approach could result in an unnecessarily long course through the breast. Anterior approach methods avoid this problem (Fig. 10.8), as do parallel-to-chest-wall approaches using the medial or lateral positions.

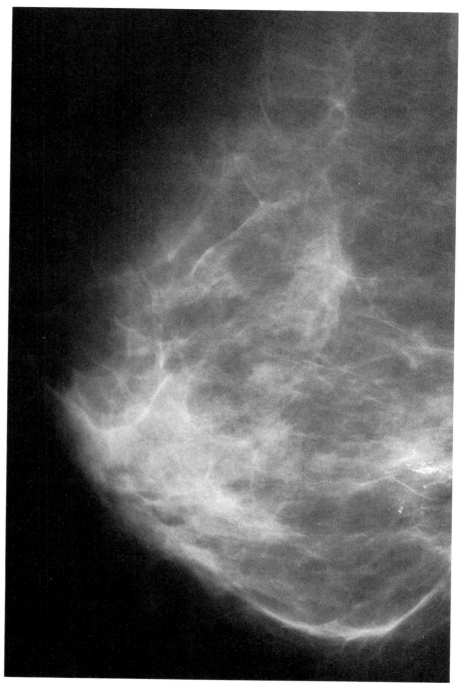

R

Fig. 10.8a

Fig. 10.8 Localization of inferior lesions. *a* Branching malignant microcalcification is identified deep and inferior to the nipple line. *b* is on p. 276, *c* and *d* are on p. 277, *e* is on p. 278.

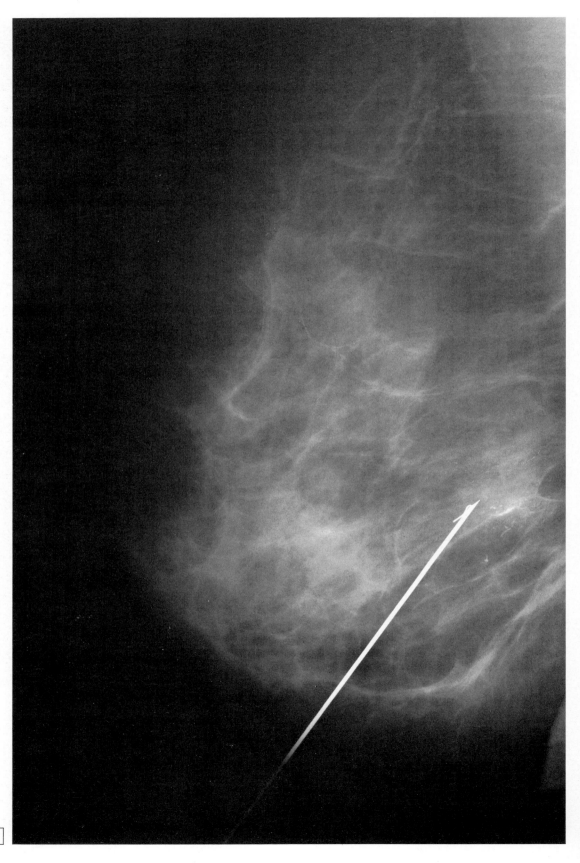

Fig. 10.8b R

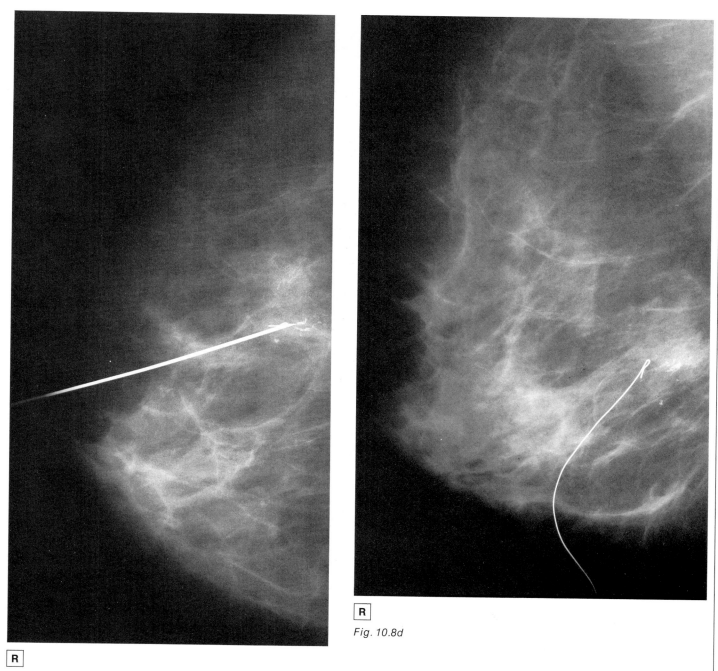

R

Fig. 10.8d

R

Fig. 10.8c

Fig. 10.8b, c & d   *b and c* Using an anterior approach with radial skin markings and with the assistance of the radiographer holding the breast up to enable inferior access, the hook wire assembly has been introduced adjacent to the microcalcification. *d and e* (overleaf) Final films confirm position for the surgeon.

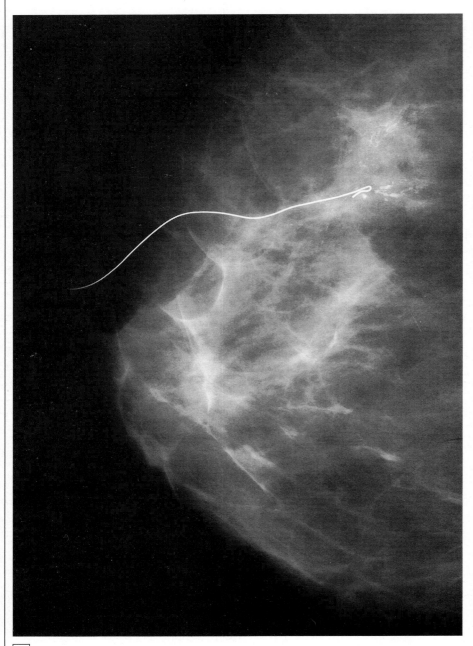

R

Fig. 10.8e   Final film confirms the position for the surgeon.

Pisano & Hall (1989) describe placing the patient in the lateral decubitus position on a couch and employing a standard fenestrated plate method applied to the inferior aspect of the breast, with a horizontal beam. Homer (1987) recommends placing a metallic skin marker directly under the lesion on the craniocaudal projection, then taking the orthogonal projection to allow estimates of depth and angulation from the site of entry so marked. The needle assembly is then positioned with the patient lying supine and the breast supported and compressed by the free hand of the operator.

Cancellation of procedure

The procedure should be abandoned if either the radiologist is not convinced there is a lesion on the control mammograms, or if he is equally convinced that the lesion has been better demonstrated and exhibits benign features. Meyer et al (1988) report 8.8% of localizations cancelled on the day of the procedure. They were all localization referrals from outside hospitals. Listed causes for cancellation include no mass being apparent, sonographic demonstration of simple cysts, skin calcification, superimposition of benign calcification and cyst rupture during control mammography.

COMPLICATIONS

Failure to excise the lesion

Failure rates at biopsy are variable (2.1%, Tinnemans et al 1987; 2.5%, Landercasper et al 1987; 3%, Gisvold & Martin 1984; 3.75%, Chetty et al 1983; 4%, Yankaskas et al 1988; 8.9%, Proudfoot et al 1986). The figure depends upon the expertise of the radiological and surgical team and the communication between them. The commonest cause of failure has been stated to be the lack of radiological and surgical communication (Bigongiari et al 1977), but lack of specimen radiography, inaccurate marker placement and other marker mishaps also account for failure.

Accuracy of placement varies according to the technique and equipment used. Gisvold & Martin (1984) report two or more simple hook wires being required in 20% of cases, and Goldberg et al (1983) report 15%. In most centres a second wire is inserted if the first is 2 cm or more away from the lesion. In the Tinnemans (1987) series (hook wire) 72% of hooks were placed within 1 cm of the lesion. The Goldberg (1983) series (hook wire) placed 83% within 1 cm and 96% within 1.5 cm. Gisvold & Martin (1984), using spring and hook wires, placed 78% within 1 cm. Gallagher et al (1989), using only a spring hook assembly, placed the wire within 2 mm of the lesion in 96% with a second wire being required in 1%. Dowlatshahi et al (1989) report a stereotactic localization series with an accuracy of 96% placed within 2 mm of the lesion.

On published results a spring hook wire assembly placed parallel to the chest wall has been shown to be the most accurate method. It must be remembered that fatty breast tissue may not retain the hook close to the lesion even if it has been placed accurately, as breast fat tends towards liquidity at body temperature. Such movement in fatty breasts may be resisted by the 'T-bar' shape of the Nottingham wire.

Accuracy in spot localization in part depends upon the time of the procedure in relation to the placement of the marker and also to inadvertant entry of the ductal system (Wayne & Darby 1977).

Syncope

True syncope occurs in approximately 2% of localization procedures although exact figures are difficult to obtain. A couch should be available and the patient should not be left unattended while films are being checked (Homer 1985a). Many patients complain of slight dizziness and feeling hot during localization procedures; this can be overcome with encouragement and advice as to regular deep breathing. It is important to ensure that the room used for localization is not small and stuffy or crowded with too many observers. The presence of a nurse or second radiographer, however, is invaluable.

Wire mishaps

It is possible for the entire length of wire to be enveloped by a large breast following deep placement. Once lost the wire is difficult to retrieve and in one case migrated 2 months later to the neck (Davis et al 1988). To avoid this, use of a sufficiently long wire or a simple loose knot in the free end of the wire should suffice. Use of the shortest approach is recommended in such cases. Cutting off excess wire is to be avoided. Taping, suturing and clipping the wire at the skin surface are other possibilities though they carry a definite risk of deep dislodgement from the lesion with breast movement. Such fixation is to be avoided before check mammograms for the surgeon have been performed, because the compression may well dislodge the hook if the wire is fixed at the site of skin entry.

Migration of the hook wire into the pleural space has been reported (Bristol & Jones 1981), possibly encouraged by sudden movement or pectoral muscle contraction. Syncope with the needle assembly in position can result in the patient falling and knocking the end of the needle against either the equipment or floor, forcing the needle tip further into the breast and possibly causing a pneumothorax. This is less likely with a parallel approach but remains a possibility with a long needle assembly whichever method is used. Some radiologists prefer to use a 5 cm needle to minimize this risk.

Transection of the wire occasionally happens during surgery and was reported in three of 100 cases (Homer 1983). Subsequently the hook is very difficult to locate and remove (Fig. 10.9). Use of a post-localization stiffener in theatre should avoid this problem, as should the use of a wire with a thickened segment proximal to the hook. Options for further management would then include second localization or long-term follow-up. Surgical handling of the wire has, in the past, resulted in removal of the wire from the breast before biopsy or dislodgement from the lesion, causing failure of excision. Care should be taken on removing the dressings and also during biopsy not to apply excessive traction to the hook.

Breakage of the wire during placement has been reported (Landercasper et al 1987): this can theoretically occur with pull-back of a hook wire assembly in order to reorientate, which can bring the hook away from the tip of the needle and bend the wire over the bevel. Further pushing may then transect the wire proximal to the hook.

Tumour cell seeding

Seeding along fine-needle tracks has been documented with prostatic, pleural, pulmonary, pancreatic and renal tumours. Such seeding is a theoretical possibility with localization needle assemblies. The size of the needle has been stated to be important with more risk being attached to larger diameter needles (Kline & Neal 1978). The seeding caused by fine needles, however, may be an underestimated risk (Denton et al 1990).

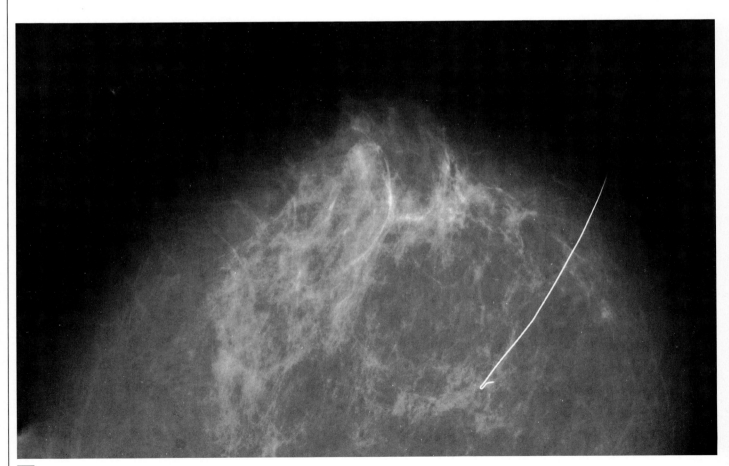

R

Fig. 10.9a

Fig. 10.9   Retained hook. *a* Accurate wire localization of a small faint cluster of microcalcification has been obtained. *b* Transection of the hook occurred during surgery and relocation was not possible. The follow-up film of 6 months later shows the hook to be still present although it has pulled back a small amount.

No known case of breast cancer seeding from aspiration or localization has been reported, although in some techniques the track is excised with the lesion. Kopans et al (1988) found no increase in local recurrence rate following localization but stressed the importance of a parallel approach; an anterior approach having potential to seed deeper into the breast, or into the pectoral or pleural compartments. In conclusion it may be safest to place the assembly as close as possible adjacent to the lesion rather than through it.

Miscellaneous
Haematoma formation, infection, intercostal nerve damage and pneumothorax are occasional complications.

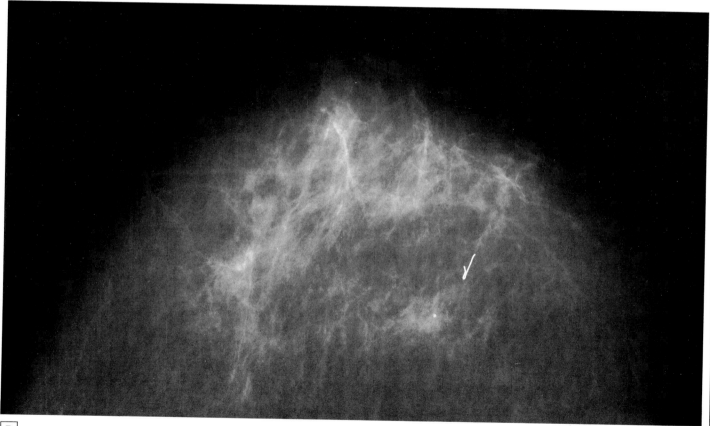

R

Fig. 10.9b

SPECIMEN RADIOGRAPHY

This was first described in 1951 by Leborgne and also described by Patton et al (1966) and Egan (1969). It is an essential part of accurate localization biopsy technique, allowing the surgeon to judge adequacy of excision. A dedicated facility may be used, e.g. Faxitron (Vinten Instruments, Weybridge, Surrey), or if closely situated, departmental mammography will provide excellent imaging. Minimum delay for the surgeon is necessary, however, as he awaits confirmation of excision before skin closure. A clip or suture suitably placed on the excised tissue will aid later orientation of it in relation to the biopsy bed (Fig. 10.10). A second excision may be required if the lesion is not present on the first radiograph (4%, Gallagher et al 1989; 19%, Chetty et al 1983).

If the specimen contains the lesion it is helpful for the radiologist to guide the pathologist by X-raying the specimen on an opaque grid system and marking the lesion with a simple needle, or X-raying slices of the specimen numbered by the pathologist and indicating which slice to study. This helps minimize the number of tissue sections required to be looked at by the pathologist. Coating the specimen surface with Indian Ink aids pathological assessment of excision margins.

The addition of specimen radiography does add some anaesthetic time to the procedure. Depending upon local conditions the additional time required is approximately 6 min (Landercasper et al 1987).

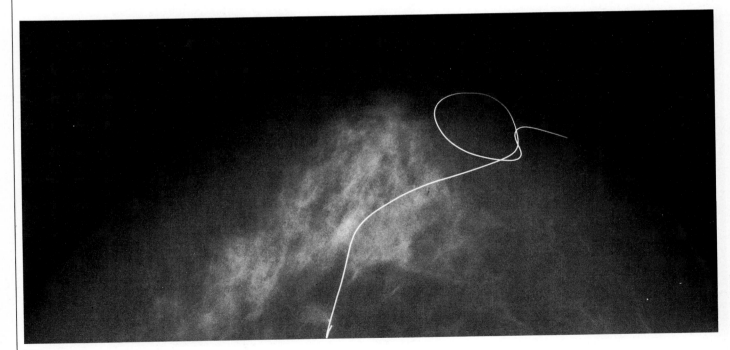

L *Fig. 10.10a*

Fig. 10.10 Specimen radiography. *a* A small irregular soft tissue opacity has been localized deep in the breast. *b* Specimen radiography confirms excision of the lesion. A suture can be seen on the edge of the excised specimen; this acts as a marking device for the surgeon in order to relate anatomically the excised specimen to the remaining biopsy bed if any further excision is required. *c* The specimen has been sectioned and the tumour can be clearly seen in the slice numbered (*H*). This reduces unnecessary section examination by the pathologist.

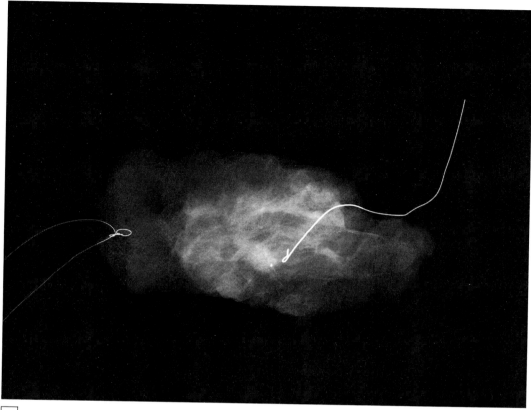

L *Fig. 10.10b*

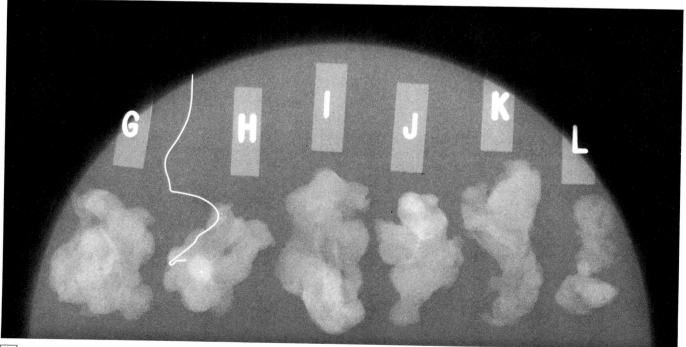

L *Fig. 10.10c*

OUTPATIENT LOCALIZATION BIOPSY

Significant cost savings can be achieved by performing localization as an outpatient procedure followed by biopsy under local anaesthetic on the same day (Landercasper et al 1987). Homer et al (1984) calculated a cost differential of five times for inpatient biopsy with an average 2.6 day stay compared to outpatient biopsy. Deep lesions and anxious or unco-operative patients are not ideally suited for outpatient procedures. Silverstein et al (1987) gave general anaesthetic only to those women with multiple hook wires or with an obvious cancer requiring a clear margin of excision.

Norton et al (1988) report outpatient procedures having a three-times-increased failure rate, a 6% wound infection rate and requiring an additional 10/15 min per case as opposed to those under general anaesthetic. Their mean time for surgical biopsy under local anaesthetic was 48 min compared to 34 min under general anaesthetic. One-third of the women in their series complained of pain under local anaesthetic.

In the main, the current practice in this country is for the localization biopsy procedure to be done under general anaesthetic as an inpatient. Whether this practice alters significantly with regard to a changing economic climate remains to be seen.

REFERENCES

Barnard N J, George B D, Tucker A K, Gilmore O J A 1988 Histopathology of benign non-palpable breast lesions identified by mammography. Journal of Clinical Pathology 41: 26–30

Barth V, Behrends W, Haase W 1977 Methode zur praoperativen Lokalisation nicht palpabler suspekter Mikroverkalkungen im Brustdrusenkorper. Radiologe 17: 219

Berger S M, Curcio B M, Gershoncohen J, Isard H J 1966 Mammographic localization of unsuspected breast cancer. American Journal of Roentgenology 96: 1046–1052

Bigongiari L R, Fidler W, Skerker L G, Comstock C, Threatt B 1977 Percutaneous needle localization of breast lesions prior to biopsy. analysis of failure. Clinical Radiology 28: 419–425

Bolmgren J, Jacobson B, Nordenstrom B 1977 Sterotaxic instrument for needle biopsy of the mamma American Journal of Roentgenology 129: 121–125

Bristol J B, Jones P A 1981 Transgression of localizing wire into the pleural cavity prior to mammography. British Journal of Radiology 54: 139–140

Chetty U, Kirkpatrick A E, Anderson T L et al 1983 Localization and excision of occult breast lesions. British Journal of Surgery 70: 607–610

Curcio B M 1970 Technique for radiographic localization of nonpalpable breast tumours. Radiological Technology 42: 155–160

Czarnecki D J, Feider H K, Splittgerber G F 1989 Toluidine blue dye as a breast localization marker. American Journal of Roentgenology 153: 261–263

Davis P S, Wechsler R J, Feig S A, March D E 1988 Migration of breast biopsy localization wire. American Journal of Roentgenology 150: 787–788

Denton K J, Cotton D W K, Nakielny R A, Goepal J R 1990 Secondary tumour deposits in needle biopsy tracks; an underestimated risk? Journal of Clinical Pathology 43: 83

Dodd G D, Fry K, Delany W 1965 Pre-op localization of occult carcinoma of the breast. In: Nealon T F (ed) Management of the patient with cancer. Saunders, Philadelphia, pp 88–113

Dowlatshahi K, Gent H J, Schmidt R, Jokich P M, Bibbo M, Sprenger E 1989 Nonpalpable breast tumours: diagnosis with stereotaxic localization and fine needle aspiration. Radiology 170: 427–433

Egan R L 1969 Fundamentals of mammographic diagnosis of benign and malignant diseases. Oncology 23: 126–148

Egan J R, Sayler C B, Goodman M J 1976 A technique for localizing occult breast lesions. Cancer 26: 32–37

Feig S A 1983 Localization of clinically occult breast lesions. Radiologic Clinics of North America 21: 155–171

Frank H A, Hall F M, Steer M L 1976 Preoperative localization of nonpalpable breast lesions demonstrated by mammography. New England Journal of Medicine 295: 259–260

Frankl G, Rosenfeld D D 1975 Xeroradiographic detection of occult breast cancer. Cancer 35: 542–548

Gallagher W J, Cardenosa G, Rubens J R, McCarthy K A, Kopans D B 1989 Minimal volume excision of nonpalpable breast lesions. American Journal of Roentgenology 153: 957–961

Gisvold J J, Martin J K 1984 Prebiopsy localization of nonpalpable breast lesions. American Journal of Roentgenology 143: 477–481

Goldberg R, Hall F M, Simon M 1983 Preoperative localization of nonpalpable breast lesions using a wire marker and perforated mammographic grid. Radiology 146: 833–835

Hall F M, Frank H A 1979 Preoperative localization of nonpalpable breast lesions. American Journal of Roentgenology 132: 101–105

Hermann G, Janus C, Schwartz I S, Krivsky B, Bier S, Rabinowitz J G 1987 Nonpalpable breast lesions; accuracy of prebiopsy mammographic diagnosis. Radiology 165: 323–326

Hirsch J I, Banks W L, Sullivan J S, Horsley J S 1989a Effect of Methylene blue on Oestrogen receptor activity. Radiology 171: 105–107

Hirsch J I, Banks W L, Sullivan J S, Horsley J S 1989b Noninterference of Isosulfan blue on oestrogen receptor activity. Radiology 171: 109–110

Hoehn J L, Hardacre J M, Swanson M K, Williams G 1982 Localization of occult breast lesions. Cancer 49: 1142–1144

Hollender L F, Gros C M 1965 Rontgenuntersuchung der klinish nicht tastbaren Mammacarcinome. Langenbecks Archiv fur Klinische Chirurgie 313: 380

Homer M J 1983 Transection of the localization hooked wire during breast biopsy. American Journal of Roentgenology 141: 929–930

Homer M J 1985a Breast imaging: pitfalls, controversies, and some practical thoughts. Radiologic Clinics of North America 23: 459–472

Homer M J 1985b Nonpalpable breast lesion localization using a curved-end retractable wire. Radiology 157: 259–260

Homer M J 1987 Preoperative needle localization of lesions in the lower half of the breast. American Journal of Roentgenology 149: 43–45

Homer M J, Fisher D M, Sugarman H J 1981 Post-localization needle for breast biopsy of nonpalpable lesions. Radiology 140: 241–242

Homer M J, Smith T J, Marchant D J 1984 Outpatient needle localization and biopsy for nonpalpable breast lesions. Journal of the American Medical Association 252: 2452–2454

Horns J W, Arndt R D 1976 Percutaneous spot localization of nonpalpable breast lesions. American Journal of Roentgenology 127: 253–256

Kline T S, Neal H S 1978 Needle aspiration biopsy: a critical appraisal. Journal of the American Medical Association 239: 36–39

Kopans D B, De Luca S 1980 A modified needle-hookwire technique to simplify preoperative localization of occult breast lesions. Radiology 134: 781

Kopans D B, Meyer J E 1982a Versatile spring hookwire breast lesion localizer. American Journal of Roentgenology 138: 586–587

Kopans D B, Meyer J E 1982b Computed tomography guided localization of clinically occult breast carcinoma: the 'N' skin guide. Radiology 145: 211–212

Kopans D B, Swann C A 1989 Preoperative imaging—guided needle placement and localization of clinically occult breast lesions. American Journal of Roentgenology 152: 1–9

Kopans D B, Meyer J E, Lindfors K K, Bucchianeri S S 1984 Breast sonography to guide cyst aspiration and wire localization of occult solid lesions.

American Journal of Roentgenology 143: 489–492

Kopans D B, Waitzkin E D, Linetsky L et al 1987 Localization of breast lesions identified on only one mammographic view. American Journal of Roentgenology 149: 39–41

Kopans D B, Gallagher W J, Swann C A et al 1988 Does preoperative needle localization lead to an increase in local breast cancer recurrence. Radiology 167: 667–668

Landercasper J, Gunderson S B, Gunderson A L, Cogbill T H, Travelli R, Strutt P 1987 Needle localization and biopsy of nonpalpable lesions of the breast. Surgery, Gynaecology and Obstetrics 164: 399–403

Leborgne R 1951 Diagnosis of tumors of the breast by simple roentgenography, calcifications in carcinomas. American Journal of Roentgenology 65: 1–11

Malone L J, Frankl G, Dorazio R A, Winkley J H 1975 Occult breast carcinomas detected by Xeroradiography: clinical considerations. Annals of Surgery 181: 133–136

Melander O 1972 Therapeutiques non multilantes des cancereuses du sein. Symposium International Strasbourg

Meyer J E, Sonnenfeld M R, Greenes R A, Stomper P C 1988 Cancellation of preoperative breast localization procedures: analysis of 53 cases. Radiology 169: 629–630

Millis R R, McKinna J A, Hamlin I M E, Greening W P 1976 Biopsy of the impalpable breast lesion detected by mammography. British Journal of Surgery 63: 346–348

Muhlow A 1974 A device for precision needle biopsy of the breast at mammography. American Journal of Roentgenology 121: 843–845

Norton L W, Zeligman B E, Pearlman N W 1988 Accuracy and cost of needle localization breast biopsy. Archives of Surgery 123: 947–950

Oleson K P, Blichert-Toft M 1979 Preoperative needle marking of nonpalpable breast lesions. Fortschritte Rontgenstrahlen 131: 331

Patton R B, Poznanski A K, Zylak C J 1966 Pathologic examinations of specimens containing nonpalpable breast cancers discovered by radiography. American Journal of

Clinical Pathology 46: 330–334

Pisano E D, Hall F M 1989 Preoperative localization of inferior breast lesions. American Journal of Roentgenology 153: 272

Price J L, Butler P D 1971 Stereoscopic measurement in mammography. British Journal of Radiology 44: 901

Prorok J J, Trostle D R, Scarlato M, Rachman R 1983 Excisional breast biopsy and Roentgenographic examination for mammographically detected microcalcification. American Journal of Surgery 145: 684–686

Proudfoot R W, Mattingly S S, Stalling C B, Fine J G Nonpalpable breast lesions; wire localization and excision biopsy. American Surgeon 52: 117–122

Rabin C B 1941 Precise localization of pulmonary abscesses by the spot method. Journal of Thoracic Surgery 10: 662–664

Rosenberg A L, Schwartz G F, Feig S A, Patchefsky A S 1987 Clinically occult breast lesions: localization and significance. Radiology 162: 167–170

Roses D F, Harris M N, Gortstein F, Gumport S L 1980 Biopsy for microcalcification detected by mammography. Surgery 87: 248–252

Silverstein M J, Gamagami P, Rosser R J et al 1987 Hooked wire directed breast biopsy and overpenetrated mammography. Cancer 59: 715–722

Simon N, Lesnick G J, Lerer W N, Bachman A 1972 Roentgenographic localization of small lesions of the breast by the spot method. Surgery, Gynaecology and Obstetrics 134: 572–574

Soholm S, Conrad C 1989 Preoperative needle marking of non-palpable breast lesions. Acta Radiologica 30: 223–224

Stevens G M, Jamplis R W 1971 Mammographically directed biopsy of nonpalpable breast lesions. Archives of Surgery 102: 292–295

Svane G 1982 A stereotaxic technique for preoperative marking of non-palpable breast lesions. Acta Radiologica Diagnosis 24: 145–151

Threatt B, Appelman H, Dow R, O'Rourke T 1974 Percutaneous needle localization of clustered mammary microcalcifications prior to biopsy. American Journal of Roentgenology 121: 839–842

Tinnemans J G M, Wobbes T, Hendriks J H C L et al 1987 Localization and excision of nonpalpable breast lesions. Archives of Surgery 122: 802–806

Wayne R W, Darby R E 1977 Injection Mammography. Journal of the American Medical Association 237: 2219–2220

Yagan R, Weisen E, Bellon E 1985 Mammographic needle localization of lesions seen in only one view. American Journal of Roentgenology 144: 911–916

Yankaskas B C, Knelson M H, Abernethy M L, Cuttino J T, Clark R L 1988 Needle localization biopsy of occult lesions of the breast. Investigative Radiology 23: 729–733

CHAPTER 11

Fine needle aspiration cytology of breast lesions

Marigold Curling

INTRODUCTION

History

The aspiration of breast cysts is recorded as early as 1835. This was followed in 1853 by Sir James Paget's description of malignant cells in Paget's disease of the breast. These cells he described with great accuracy: "Many of the cells of cancer may be somewhat like gland cells yet can be distinguished singly and much more plainly in their grouping. They are heaped together disorderly and seldom have any lobular or normal arrangement". There were a few other series of fine-needle aspirations (FNAs) in the literature at the end of the nineteenth and early twentieth centuries in spite of 200 FNAs reported by Dugeon with an accuracy of 98% in 1927 and a series from the Memorial Hospital in New York (Martin & Ellis 1930). (This series reduced the number of frozen sections requested as definitive surgery was performed on the positive result of aspiration cytology; Bauermeister 1980).

It was not until 1968 when Franzen reported a series of 3479 consecutive aspirations with an accuracy for carcinoma of 92.1% that FNAs began to be of generally accepted value.

FNA and biopsy

It is usually accepted that aspiration is by fine needle and produces material for cytological smears. This must be distinguished from needle 'biopsy' (trucut biopsy) which produces a core of tissue for histological diagnosis.

It is important to distinguish these two procedures. The accuracy of each, providing sufficient material from the lesion is available, depends on the experience and expertise of the cytopathologist or histopathologist.

Advantages of FNA

The first is the simplicity of the technique and the accuracy in competent hands (Zajicek 1974, Preece 1989). FNA is now the method of choice at most centres (Shabot et al 1982). This technique is acceptable to most patients, the equipment is inexpensive and the procedure takes only a few minutes, and is relatively painless. It is possible for the smears to be stained and reported in outpatient departments (Duguid et al 1979, Frable 1984, Zuk et al 1989). This is becoming essential and is now demanded by many surgeons and radiologists and should be available in all specialist centres. Where possible the cytopathologist should be present in the outpatient department or during radiological assessment by ultrasound, stereotaxis or perforated plate procedures, not only to assess that material aspirated is adequate, but to make a rapid diagnosis (this should be possible in rather more than 80% of cases) (Dent et al 1986, Nicholson et al 1988). This rapid reporting avoids delay and helps to allay the patient's anxiety by reducing waiting time for the result. Inadequate aspirates can be repeated at the same visit. The diagnosis can be discussed with the patient and, if this is cancer, staging investigations and treatment can be planned at this first visit. Hospital facilities are therefore more economically used. It is also possible to reduce unnecessary surgery in some benign conditions (Strawbridge et al 1981, Trott et al 1981). It is becoming accepted practice to leave confirmed fibroadenoma in young women once the diagnosis is established. Adequate aspirates from patients with benign breast lesions may be referred back to a 6 month, 1 year or routine screening follow-up, depending on the radiologist's opinion.

The biopsy compares unfavorably with this; the histological processing and reporting taking at least 24 hours. Other disadvantages of biopsy is that it is a painful procedure even with local anaesthetic and it can cause extensive bruising.

It is important that if the patient is to have a mammogram this should be arranged prior to the FNA or biopsy because the X-ray picture may be distorted by the needle tract or bleeding. In the case of FNAs the breast architecture usually returns to its previous state within 6 weeks but with biopsy there may be scarring and permanent distortion. If the FNA has been performed before mammography it is essential that the radiologist is notified.

Accuracy

There are many reports as to the accuracy and sensitivity of FNAs in breast cancer (Zajicek et al 1967, Hogbin 1977, Strawbridge 1981, Trott 1982, Kwok et al 1988, Naylor 1988, Palombini et al 1988, Falco et al 1989, Rangwala et al 1989, Walloch 1989, Wilkinson et al 1989, Gelabet et al 1990).

The sensitivity reported in the literature varies from just over 50% to 99%. There are many factors which influence the accuracy. Skill in taking the aspirate and experience in interpretation are of the greatest importance. A large enough cell sample is dependent on several factors, the site of the lesion (Kreuzer & Zajicek 1972, Kline 1979), the palpability and the histological type (Anderson et al 1986, Lamb & Anderson 1989). Even more important than the size of the lesion is the aspirator (Dixon et al 1983, Dixon et al 1986, Barrows et al 1986). Anderson showed that when FNAs were performed by multiple aspirators the malignant and suspicious aspirates were only 59%. However, if there was one dedicated aspirator this increased to 99%. There is also an increase in positive aspirates, if these are repeated up to three times in a clinically or mammographically suspicious lesion. Again it was shown that accuracy is significantly improved with increasing experience of the aspirator (Ingram et al 1983).

It is of no importance whether the aspirator is a clinician, radiologist or a pathologist as long as he understands fully the technique, how to obtain sufficient material, spread this on the slides, fix or air dry these slides correctly and to maintain constantly high-quality smears.

The advantage of the pathologist who reports the smears also performing the aspirates is that this usually produces the best results. If there is inadequate material the pathologist quickly improves. Another advantage is to obtain a clinical impression of the lesion while performing the aspirate.

Aspiration by the cytopathologist is the usual practice in Sweden, perhaps the home of FNAs. Elsewhere there are too few cytopathologists to perform as well as interpret the aspirates; although, as has been already stated, this practice is becoming more frequently demanded. Where it is not possible for the pathologist to do the aspirates it must be the pathologist's responsibility to teach the technique and assure quality control both in the technique and in interpretation of the material. Again, accuracy is improved with experience and it is essential that a cytopathologist has considerable

experience before taking up an appointment involving breast aspiration cytology (Royal College of Pathologists Working Group 1990).

Technique

Most aspirators use their own adaptations to a standard technique. The essentials are to use a 21–23 gauge needle and a 10 ml syringe. Sometimes a 20 ml syringe is used and also frequently a syringe holder, which makes fixing the lump and aspirating at the same time considerably easier— but this is not essential and many adequate aspirates are produced just with a 10 ml syringe without the holder. The lump may be fixed with the hand flat between the index and third finger or held between finger and thumb. No local anaesthetic is needed. The needle is passed through the skin and into the lesion. It is possible with little experience to appreciate the texture and consistency of the lesion, the hard gritty feel of a ductal carcinoma, the firm rubbery feel of a fibroadenoma and the softness of a lipoma etc. Once in the lesion, it is possible to move the needle very gently within the lesion, thus breaking up the tissue and by capillary attraction alone, allowing some of the material to pass up the needle. The next manouver is to start aspiration and maintain the pressure while rotating the needle; the cutting edge of the needle will again break up the tissue. Next, the needle must be moved quite vigorously to and fro within the lesion and radially in five or six directions until material just enters the syringe (it is unnecessary to have material actually in the syringe as this is difficult to extract and becomes rapidly air-dried). The pressure is gently released and the needle extracted from the lesion. It is a good idea to give the patient cotton wool to

press on the lesion to prevent bruising; no plaster is needed. This pressure should be continued while the slides are being prepared. Immediately the needle is removed from the lesion the syringe is taken off and filled with air, the needle replaced and the material ejected onto two named glass slides, which should be marked, fixed and air dried. The slide which is to be fixed is spread as for a blood film and fixed immediately with alcohol or a cytospray fixative. The other slide is then spread and should be gently waved in the air for rapid drying. This allows a more satisfactory Diff Quik or May–Grünwald Geimsa staining. It is important that the spreading should be even and neither too thin nor too thick; if too thick the cells will be heaped up in groups and it will not be possible to see the nuclear detail clearly. This can also be made difficult if the material is expressed too rapidly or forcefully onto the slide; there will be many small air bubbles trapped in the fatty material, making it difficult to see the epithelial nuclei. The nuclei will also be difficult to see in heavily blood-stained smears. If there is delay in fixing the smear, and it becomes air-dried, the nuclei fail to take up the Papanicolaou stain and the smear is impossible to interpret. All these are very important features and good technique is essential for accurate results.

Staining

Perhaps even in a textbook of radiology staining of smears should be discussed. If possible air-dried and alcohol-fixed smears should be prepared. Essentially the cytopathologist needs all the help possible and as some carcinomas may show little atypia, the nuclear detail is better demonstrated in the alcohol-fixed smears, while any difference in nuclear size or pleomorphism is better seen in the stained dry smears.

A rapid method of staining dry smears which is now the usual practice in outpatients departments is using Diff Quik stain. This includes a fixative and two stains. The smears are given a few dips in the fixative and a few dips each in staining solutions 1 and 2. They are then washed and are ready to be screened unmounted; the whole process taking a very few minutes with excellent staining very similar to the longer process of May–Grünwald Giemsa staining.

The practice which is sometimes used of rinsing the needle and syringe and filtering through a millipore filter (Coleman et al 1975) cannot be used for rapid results. It is very time-consuming if there are a number of aspirates and it is more satisfactory to make direct smears as already discussed. If there is insufficient material to make direct smears, there is usually too little on the filter to make an unequivocal diagnosis and in these the aspirate should be repeated. However, the millipore filter technique may be used to prepare breast cyst fluids. Again, this is time-consuming and a better method is to centrifuge the fluid, if there is a good deposit, to do a direct smear, while if there appears little cellular material the cytocentrifuge technique can be used.

Complications of FNA

There are no contraindications. Tumour implants in the needle tract, a complication which worries some clinicians, have not been reported in breast lesions. In any case the needle tract in cases of carcinoma will be removed at surgery or included in the field of radiation.

Indications of FNA

These may be divided into aspiration of cysts, aspiration of palpable lumps and aspiration of impalpable lesions. These will be discussed together.

1. Identification of cysts. The diagnosis of cysts can usually be made clinically; occasionally if the cyst is very tense it may feel hard and be mistaken for a solid lesion
2. To investigate any palpable lump, benign or malignant
3. To confirm clinically or mammographically suspected malignancy
4. To confirm inoperable carcinoma prior to radiotherapy (Wallgren et al 1978)
5. To investigate suspected recurrence or lymph node metastases
6. To distinguish between suppurative and neoplastic disease
7. To confirm clinical fibroadenoma in young women so that surgery may be postponed or avoided (Linsk et al 1972)
8. To add negative cytology to the clinical and X-ray impressions that the lesion is benign
9. Receptor studies and immunocytochemistry can now be performed when sufficient material is available (Silfverswärd et al 1980, Curtin et al 1982)
10. The use of FNA in diagnosis of impalpable lesions has now become established. Although the interpretation of these 'screening lesions' appears to be more difficult, even when sufficient material is obtained, it is possible when using stereotaxis (Svane 1983, Svane & Silfverswärd 1983, Gent et al 1986, Bibbo 1988, Azavedo et al 1989, Dowlatshabi et al 1989) ultrasound (Harper 1988, Hogg 1988) or perforated plate localization (Alberhasky 1989, Helvie 1990) to make a diagnosis. It is also possible to obtain material by aspiration before a guidewire insertion, prior to surgical biopsy and to confirm the diagnosis before excision.

REPORTING

Most cytopathologists will report FNAs as inadequate, benign, suspicious or malignant. The National Health Service Breast Screening Programme (NHS BSP; Royal College of Pathologists Working Group 1990) divides the suspicious groups into those which are most likely benign and those probably malignant using a numerical system of 1–5. The system of reporting makes no difference as long as the clinician and radiologist have full understanding.

Cytological findings

It is essential to understand the cytopathologist's problems and it is important to have a general knowledge of the basic patterns and criteria for diagnosis of the various pathological lesions, both benign and malignant.

Benign lesions

1. Cysts
2. Benign breast change (fibrocystic disease)
3. Sclerosing adenosis
4. Radial scar
5. Changes of pregnancy and lactation.

The last four lesions may be present with or without proliferative changes and atypia.

Basic benign pattern (Fig. 11.1)
1. Frequently few epithelial cells are obtained and more than one aspirate may have to be performed to obtain adequate epithelial cells for assessment.
2. Epithelial cells are arranged in small cohesive groups.
3. The presence of bipolar nuclei either singly or in pairs is typical of a benign lesion (Fig. 11.2).
4. Apocrine metaplastic cells may also be present.

Problems in diagnosis of benign lesions
A two-cell-type population (epithelial or myoepithelial cells), the presence of 'bare' nuclei even when there is loss of cohesion in the groups and variation of nuclear size and shape should persuade the cytopathologist that the lesion is benign. Apocrine metaplastic cell nuclei when present without cytoplasm being larger than ductal epithelial cells and having a prominent nucleolus may cause problems for the inexperienced cytopathologist. Misinterpretation of these cells is the commonest cause for a false-positive report.

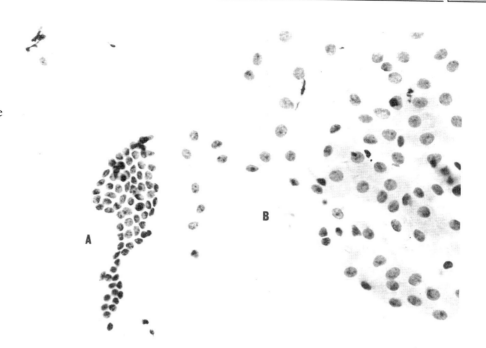

Fig. 11.1 Benign breast change. A, benign ductal epithelial cells; B, apocrine metaplastic cells.

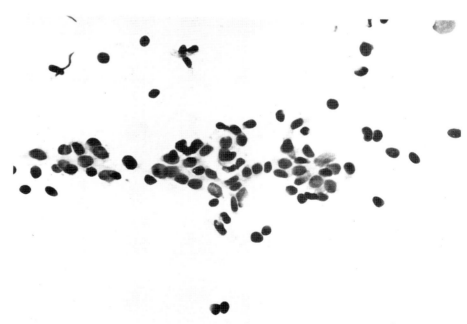

Fig. 11.2 Benign breast change. Ductal epithelial cells, single and pairs of bipolar 'naked' nuclei (sentinel cells).

Simple cysts

These can be included under the heading of benign breast change. They may vary in size and cellular content. The fluid may be clear or cloudy, green or brown and almost cell-free or may contain ductal epithelial cells, apocrine metaplastic cells and 'foamy' macrophages (Figs 11.3–11.5).

So rarely are malignant cells found in cyst fluids that examination is only necessary if the lump has not completely disappeared after aspiration, the cyst is recurrent or it is heavily blood-stained (McSwain et al 1978, Cowen & Benson 1979, Strawbridge et al 1981).

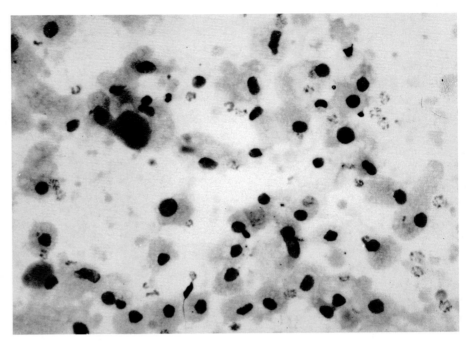

Fig. 11.3 Cyst fluid contents. 'Foamy' macrophages, degenerate cells and cell debris.

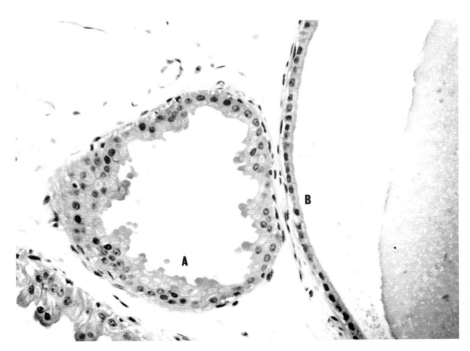

Fig. 11.4 Histological section showing cystic changes. A, cyst lined by apocrine metaplastic cells; B, cyst lined by ductal epithelial cells.

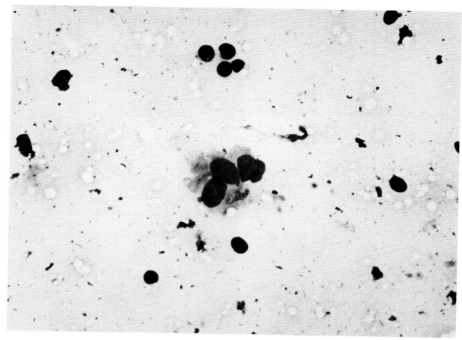

Fig. 11.5 Benign breast change. B; polar cells and larger nuclei. To the inexperienced cytologist these may be mistaken for malignant cells. However, these nuclei show no variation in size or shape.

Two lesions which are included under benign changes are *sclerosing adenosis* and *radial scars*. Both of these may appear clinically and mammographically suspicious of malignancy. Cytology may be of no help; the cells obtained in the aspirate of both these lesions will be benign although they may show some atypia (Figs 11.6, 11.7). It is important that only positive cytology is of value and therefore suspicion clinically or mammographically even in the presence of benign cytology must warrant a biopsy.

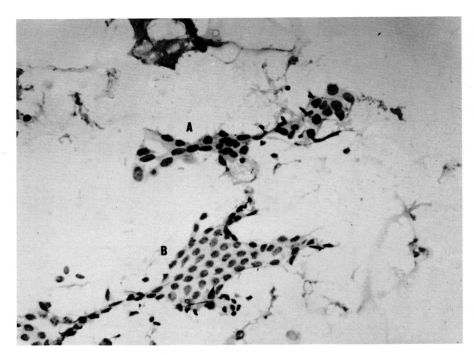

Fig. 11.6   Hyperplasia. A, slightly atypical nuclei with some variation in shape and size; B, a sheet of benign epithelial cells.

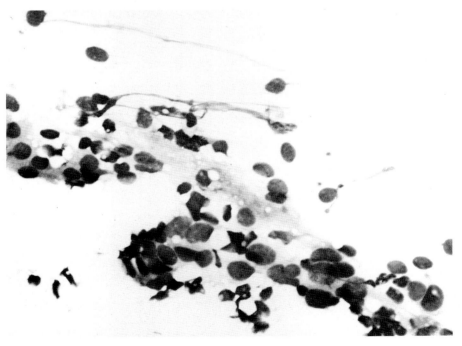

Fig. 11.7   Hyperplasia. The changes are more severe than in Fig. 11.6 with greater variation in nuclear size and shape. The presence of benign bipolar nuclei confirm the diagnosis of a benign lesion.

Changes of pregnancy and lactation
The aspirates are usually cellular, the cells show loss of cohesion. These features and the inconspicuous or absent pattern of benign bipolar nuclei may lead to a suspicious report if it is not known that the patient is pregnant or lactating.

Inflammation
1. Acute mastitis
2. Chronic mastitis (Fig. 11.8)
3. Duct ectasia
4. Fat necrosis.

To the radiologist the most important of these inflammatory lesions are duct ectasia and fat necrosis. In both, there may be a clinical suspicion of malignancy and microcalcification on mammography. The true diagnosis can readily be made by adequate aspiration.

Duct ectasia (Fig. 11.9) usually occurs in postmenopausal women. There is inflammation around the dilated ducts which contain amorphous material and frequently calcification. The aspirate appears 'cheesy' and contains amorphous material and cell debris with occasional cell outlines. Chronic inflammatory cells are present and a few giant macrophages. If only amorphous material is seen the aspirate should be repeated at the edge of the lesion to exclude necrotic carcinoma.

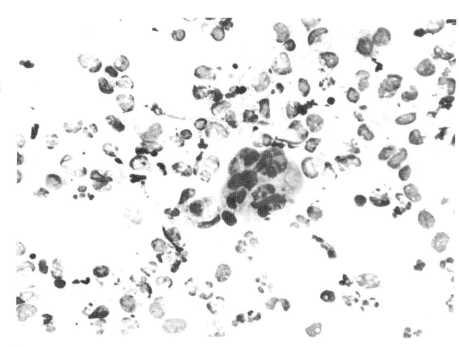

Fig. 11.8 Chronic mastitis. Benign epithelial cells, multinucleate giant cells and numerous polymorphs.

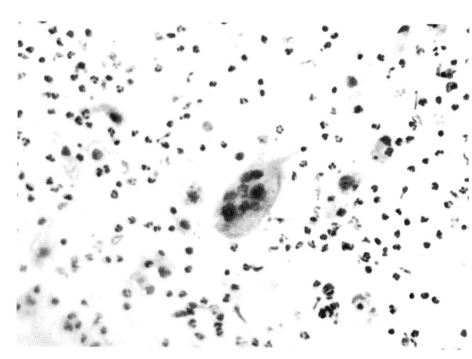

Fig. 11.9 Duct ectasia. Amorphous material and debris from the centre of a duct ectasis.

Fat necrosis (Fig. 11.10) This may occur following trauma to the breast, some 6 weeks prior to the patient presenting with a lump or microcalcification on the mammography. The aspirate is usually typical with a background of fat, and cell debris; chronic inflammatory cells; multinucleate giant cells. Foamy macrophages may be present but few or no epithelial cells.

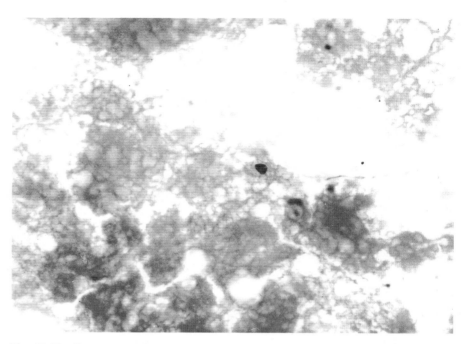

Fig. 11.10   Fat necrosis. Multinucleate giant cells, polymorphs, a background of degenerate fatty material.

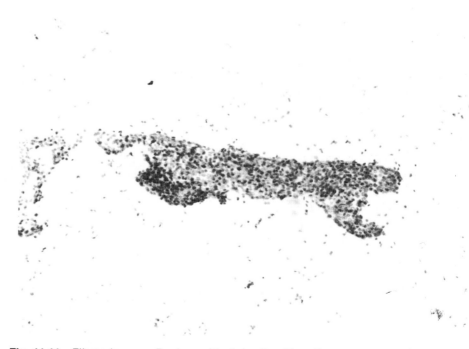

Fig. 11.11   Fibroadenoma. Benign epithelial cells with uniform arrangement.

Benign tumours

1. Fibroadenoma
2. Phylloides tumour
3. Duct papilloma
4. Lipoma
5. Granular cell tumours.

Fibroadenoma is the commonest benign tumour, usually occurring beween puberty and the menopause. It is usually easy to diagnose clinically and mammographically. The cytological diagnosis depends on a cellular aspirate and monolayer sheets of cells (Fig. 11.11). These may be branching and described as having a 'stag horn' appearance (Figs 11.12, 11.13). There may also be numerous single and pairs of benign bipolar nuclei. If there is insufficient material to make the diagnosis the aspirate should be repeated, although some clinicians will be content with a few benign cells in a lesion which is clinically a fibroadenoma. Problems in diagnosis may occur in cases where there is atypical hyperplasia or atypical apocrine metaplasia. In these cases an excision biopsy should be requested.

Phylloides tumour. These are usually benign tumours in an older age group but very similar to fibroadenoma. Rarely the stromal elements may become malignant. The histological sections from a fibroadenoma in post- and perimenopausal women should be carefully searched for any evidence of sarcomatous change before the tumour is reported as benign.

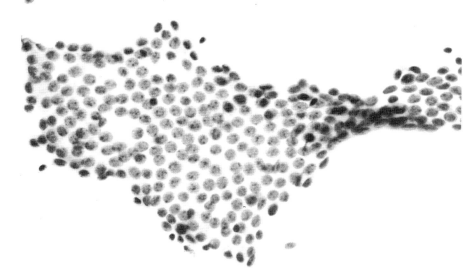

Fig. 11.12 Fibroadenoma. Sheets of benign cells with a 'stag horn' arrangement.

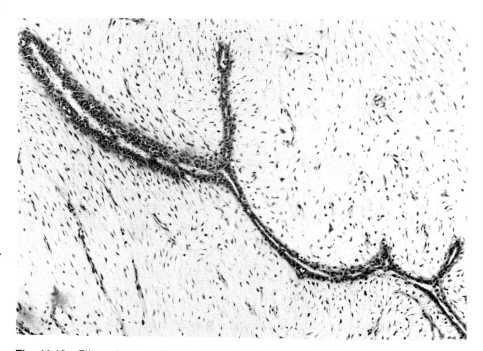

Fig. 11.13 Fibroadenoma. Histological section. Increase in ductal epithelium and fibrous tissue.

Duct papilloma. The solitary central duct papilloma arising within the large ducts of the subareolar area is a benign neoplasm. These may present with blood-stained nipple discharge at an early stage; in this there are small papillary groups of benign cells (Fig. 11.14). Unlike the multiple peripheral papilloma they do not have an increased risk of subsequent carcinoma. Multiple peripheral papillomata are precancerous and on aspiration they may show quite marked atypia.

The identification of this lesion is only possible by excision biopsy and careful examination of the tissue which may contain atypical features consistent with carcinoma-in-situ or an invasive lesion.

Granular cell tumour (granular cell myoblastoma). This tumour is rare, but should be mentioned as clinically and radiologically it can mimic cancer. The diagnosis can be made by FNA which is usually cellular with bland nuclei; the cytoplasm shows granularity quite clearly seen on the Diff Quik stain and is bright red with Schiff (PAS) stain, making the suspected diagnosis easy to confirm.

Malignant lesions

It is usual for the cytopathologist to make the diagnosis between benign and malignant lesions and to leave accurate typing to histopathological examination. However, with experience it may be possible to suggest the type of carcinoma and to identify lymphomas or metastatic carcinoma.

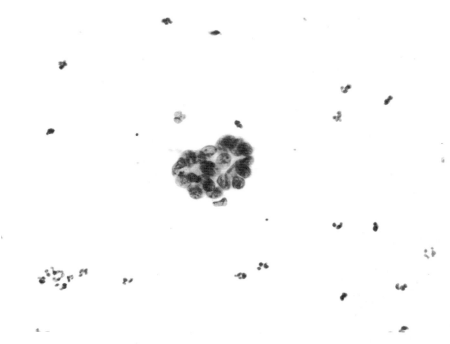

Fig. 11.14 Papilloma. Papillary group of epithelial cells in a blood-stained nipple discharge.

The histological classification is of some importance, because of the prognostic significance of the various types of carcinoma, and is therefore included here.

WHO classification 1981
Primary tumours of the breast:
1. Non-invasive
    a. Intraductal carcinoma
    b. Lobular carcinoma in situ
2. Invasive
    a. Invasive ductal carcinoma
    b. Invasive lobular carcinoma
    c. Mucinous
    d. Medullary
        e. Papillary
        f. Tubular
        g. Adenocystic
        h. Carcinoma with apocrine features
        i. Others
3. Paget's disease of the nipple

Non-intrinsic tumours
    a. Metastatic carcinoma
    b. Malignant melanoma
    c. Hodgkin's disease
    d. Myeloma and plasmacytoma
    e. Leukaemias
    f. Postradiation angiosarcoma.

It is essential to realize that other factors are of equal or greater importance in prognoses (Anderson et al 1986, Auer et al 1980). These are the tumour size, the hormone receptor status for both oestrogen and progestogen (Hogg et al 1988, Redard et al 1989, Ames et al 1990, Katz et al 1990, Scoog et al 1990), DNA profile (Renvikos et al 1988, Azavedo et al 1990) and NEU (or HER-2) oncogene expression (Van de Vigner et al 1988, Tandon et al 1989, Bacus et al 1990, Borg et al 1990, Read et al 1990).

Cytological features of malignancy
The main cytological features of malignancy are a high cellular yield, a single population of dissociated cells, an increase in nuclear cytoplasmic ratio and intact cytoplasm (Fig. 11.15). The nuclei show hyperchromasia and an irregular chromatin pattern and sometimes large macronucleoli (Fig. 11.16). An important feature is the absence of benign bipolar nuclei. If the majority of these features are present, the diagnosis of malignancy is easy, but when there are few it may not be possible to make a definite diagnosis (Pilotti et al 1982). A biopsy and histological confirmation are essential before proceeding to definitive treatment (Figs 11.17, 11.18).

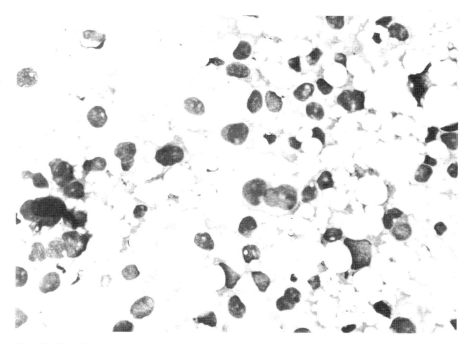

Fig. 11.15 Ductal carcinoma. Dissociation, the presence of cytoplasm. Variation in nuclear shape and size, irregular chromatin and hyperchromasia.

Fig. 11.16 Ductal carcinoma showing the features in Fig. 11.15 and showing macro nucleoli.

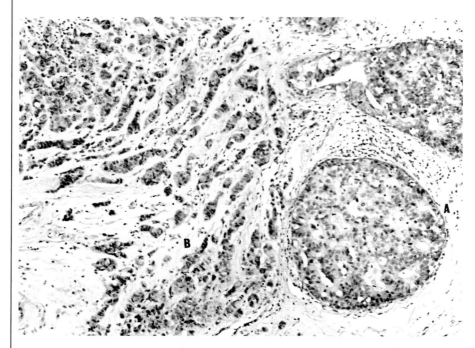

Fig. 11.17   Histological section. A, ductal in-situ (intraductal) carcinoma; B, invasive (infiltrating ductal) carcinoma.

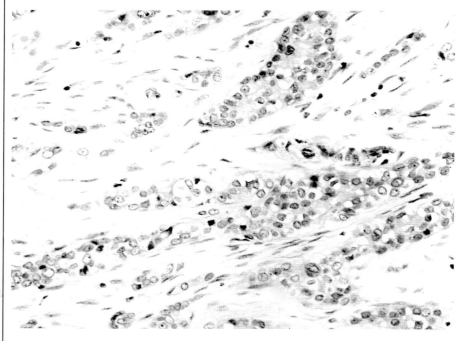

Fig. 11.18   Invasive ductal carcinoma.

The only types of carcinoma that will be discussed here are those in which there is difficulty in diagnosis from the FNA and those which have special features. It is important that the radiologist or clinician should understand the diagnostic problems.

Intraductal carcinomas (in-situ ductal) are of two main types: *cribriform*, which have small regular nuclei and which it may be difficult to make an unequivocal diagnosis from the FNA, and sometimes even from the histology without special stains (Fig. 11.19); the large-celled *comedo*, in which it is possible to make a diagnosis of malignancy, but it is only possible to suggest whether or not the lesion is in situ. Histology is essential to exclude invasion (Sneige et al 1989, Wang et al 1989).

Invasive ductal carcinoma is the commonest type of breast cancer and makes up approximately 70% of all breast malignancies (Anderson et al 1986). The FNAs from ductal carcinoma vary from the well-differentiated, with uniform regular cells, difficult to diagnose on the smears, to the large pleomorphic, poorly-differentiated which cause no diagnostic problem.

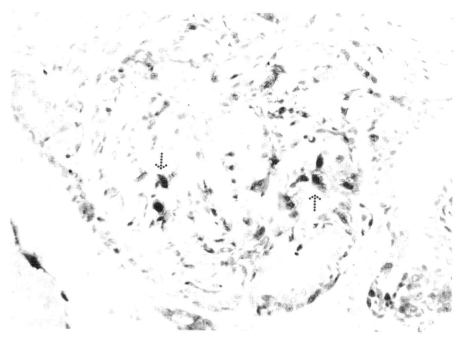

Fig. 11.19 Histological section showing S100 immunostain positive for myoepithelial cells (arrows), confirming a two-cell type and that this lesion is a hyperplasia, not carcinoma-in-situ.

Lobular carcinoma (Figs 11.20, 11.21) are approximately 10% of breast cancer. These may be difficult to diagnose from FNA cytology and are frequently missed. The smears are often poorly cellular. The cells are small. The nuclei may be all the same size but differ from benign bipolar nuclei, being round or square and showing a tendency to 'mould' together.

Mucinous carcinoma. It is possible to suggest the diagnosis from the sheets of monomorphic cells and the presence of mucin in the background.

Medullary carcinoma may feel soft, both clinically and to the aspirator. The smears are usually highly cellular with pleomorphic nuclei and many lymphocytes present. However, in the last two types the diagnosis may be suggested by cytology but should be confirmed by histological examination.

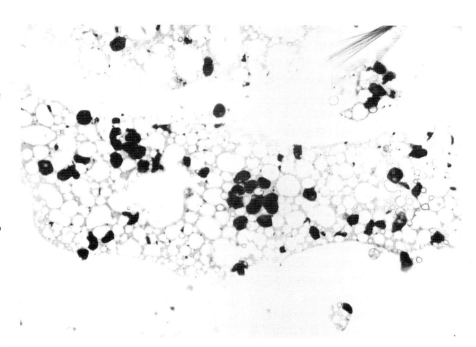

Fig. 11.20   Lobular carcinoma. Aspirates may be scanty. The small 'square' nuclei show dissociation.

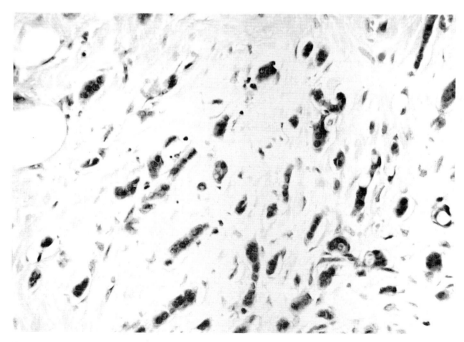

Fig. 11.21   Lobular carcinoma. Histological section shows rows of cells arranged in single file.

Tubular carcinoma (Figs 11.22, 11.23) more commonly found in screening patients than those with symptomatic lumps. The diagnosis by FNA may be difficult because the morphology is bland. The smears may be quite cellular and there may be tubule formation. There is usually little dissociation of the cells. Changes in the chromatin pattern are inconspicuous but there is usually a slight increase in nuclear cytoplasmic ratio. A definite diagnosis of malignancy from cytology can only be made in approximately 50% of these carcinomas (Bonderson & Lindholm 1990).

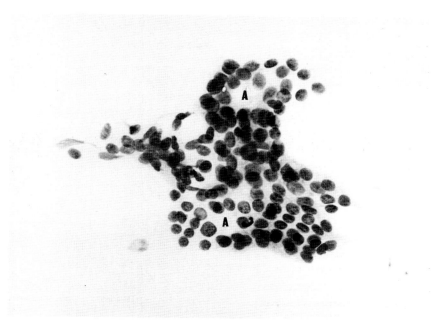

Fig. 11.22 Tubular carcinoma. A tubular formation. However, the cells do not have the features of malignancy. An unequivocal diagnosis is only possible in about half the cases.

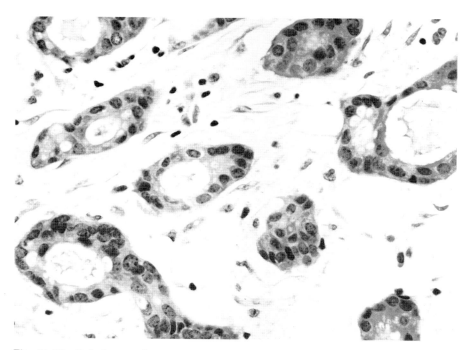

Fig. 11.23 Tubular carcinoma. Histological section.

Rare carcinomas include:

Adenocystic carcinoma. This has a better prognosis than most breast carcinomas. The smears are characteristic and show the same features as adenocystic carcinoma of the salivary gland.

Carcinoma with apocrine features. Pure apocrine carcinoma is rare. It may be difficult to make the diagnosis from the smear (Johnson & Kiwi 1989). Apocrine metaplasia can show many of the features of malignancy, with marked pleomorphism, while some well-differentiated carcinomas may resemble apocrine metaplasia and look quite benign. The diagnosis should therefore be guarded, and it is our policy never to make an unequivocal diagnosis of apocrine carcinoma but to report it as suggestive only.

Paget's disease of the nipple. First described in the mid-nineteenth century, the diagnosis is easy even in small lesions. A scrape will show large malignant cells (Paget's cells) (Figs 11.24, 11.25). In early cases the ductal carcinoma may still be in situ, but in more than 70%, the cells have spread along the ducts from an invasive lesion. It is therefore important to make the diagnosis as early as possible in the hope that the underlying carcinoma is still in situ.

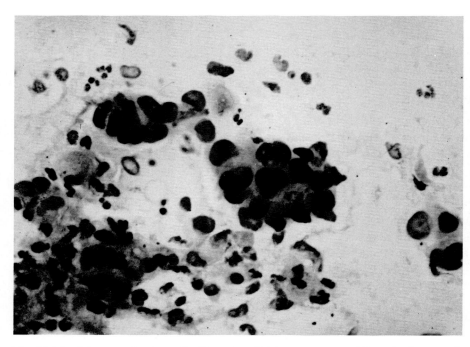

Fig. 11.24 Adenocarcinoma cells (Paget's cells) from a scrape of Paget's disease of the nipple.

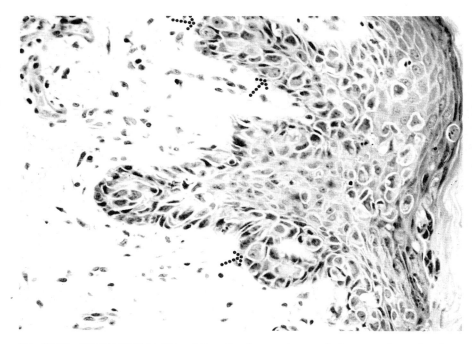

Fig. 11.25 Histological section of Paget's disease (arrows) shows malignant cells infiltrating the skin.

CONCLUSION

It may be of value to end this chapter by looking at the United Kingdom NHS BSP Guidelines for Pathologists produced by the Royal College of Pathologists Working Group (1989). This states that the aims of FNA cytology are:

1. To improve the identification of changes producing mammographic abnormalities. The changes in which a diagnosis can be made from the cytology have been discussed.

2. To maximize the number of women in whom accurate diagnosis can be made by FNA cytology without open biopsy.

3. That definitive surgery for carcinoma may be planned preoperatively on findings from mammography, clinical examination and cytology, thus avoiding the need for frozen sections.

They also state that the ratio of benign to malignant biopsies should be reduced to 2:1. In many centres this has been reduced to 1:1, and the aim should be to reduce it even more. Although as this ratio falls there is a greater risk of cancers being missed.

The statement that false-positives should be less than 5% is far too high and the aim should be never to report a false-positive. However, from time to time the smear from a fibroadenoma with atypical hyperplasia or atypical apocrine metaplasia may lead the inexperienced cytopathologist astray, and this should be remembered by the clinician and radiologist.

An acceptable false-negative rate is given as 10%. This is again too high. Providing there is sufficient material and the aspirate is from the lesion (it is sometimes difficult to be certain of this in deep-seated lesions, lesions of less than 1 cm, and densely fibrotic lesions) it should be possible to reduce this figure considerably. However, it must be realized that it is not difficult to report as negative the uniform regular cells with little nuclear atypia seen in a few of the well-differentiated ductal or tubular and lobular carcinomas, particularly if there is little material.

REFERENCES

Alberhasky M T 1989 Mammographic and gross pathologic analyses of breast needle localisation specimens. American Journal of Clinical Pathology, Oct, 92(4): 452–457

Anderson T J, Lamb J, Alexander F et al 1986 Comparative pathology of prevalent and incident cancers detected by breast screening. Lancet 1: 519–522

Auer G, Tribukait 1980 Comparative single cell and flow DNA analysis in aspiration biopsies of breast carcinomas. Acta Pathologica Microbiologica Scandinavia A 88: 355–358

Auer G, Caspersson T, Wallgren A 1980 DNA content and survival in mammary carcinoma. Analytical Quantitative Cytology 2: 161–165

Azavedo E, Svane G, Auer G 1989 Stereotactic fine needle biopsy in 2594 mammographically detected non-palpable lesions. Lancet, May 13, 1 (8646): 1033–1036

Azavedo E, Fallenus A, Svane G, Auer G 1990 Nuclear DNA content histological grade A clinical course in patients with non-palpable mammographically detected breast adenocarcinoma. American Journal of Clinical Oncology, Feb, 13(1): 23–27

Bacus S S, Ruby S G, Weinberg D S, Chin D, Ortiz R, Bacus J W 1990 Her-2/ Neu oncogene expression and proliferation in breast cancers. American Journal of Pathology, Jul, 137(1): 103–111

Baeter C G, Weidema W F, Lillebrand D, De-Jong R 1989 Granular cell tumour of the breast. Netherlands Journal of Surgery 41C5: 111–113

Barrows G H, Anderson T J, Lamb J L, Dixon J M 1986 FNA of breast. Cancer 158: 1493–1498

Bauermeister D E 1980 The role and limitations of frozen section and needle aspiration biopsy in breast cancer diagnosis. Cancer 46: 947–949

Bibbo M, Scheiber M, Cayulis R, Feebler C M, Weid G L, Dowlatshabi K 1988 Stereotaxic FNA cytology of clinically occult malignant and pre-malignant breast lesions. Acta Cytologica, March/ April, 32(2): 193–201

Bonderson L, Lindholm K 1990 Aspiration cytology of tubular breast carcinoma. Acta Cytologica, Jan–Feb,
341: 15–20

Borg A, Tandon A K, Sigurdsson H, Clark G M, Feund M, Fugua S A, Fillander D, McGuire W L 1990 Her-2/ Neu amplification predicts poor survival in node positive breast cancer. Cancer Research, Jul 15, JO(14): 4322–4337

Coleman D, Desai S, Dudley H, Hollowell S, Hulbert M 1975 Needle aspiration of palpable lesions: a new application of the membrane filter technique and its results. Clinical Oncology 1: 27–32

Cowen P N, Benson E A 1979 Cytologic study of breast cysts. British Journal of Surgery 66: 209–211

Curtin C T, Pertschuk L P, Mitchell V 1982 Histochemical determination of oestrogen and progesterone binding in fine needle aspirates of breast cancer. Correlation with conventional biochemical assays. Acta Cytologica 26: 841–846

Dent D M, Firkpatrick A F, McGoogan E, Chefty U, Anderson T J 1989 Stereotaxic localisation of aspiration cytology of impalpable breast lesions. Clinical Radiology, July, 40(4): 380–382

Dixon J M, Lamb J L, Anderson T J 1983 FNA of the breast: importance of operator. Lancet ii: 564

Dixon J M, Lee E C G, Crucioli V 1986 Frozen section of true cut biopsies versus cytology. British Journal of surgery 73: 4

Dowlatshabi K, Gent H J, Schmidt R, Jokich P M, Bibbo M, Sprenger E 1989 Non-palpable breast tumours diagnosis with stereotaxic localisation and FNA. Radiology, Feb, 170(2): 427–433

Duguid H L D, Wood R A B, Irving A D, Preece P E, Cuschieri A 1979 Needle aspiration of the breast with immediate reporting of material. British Medical Journal 2: 185–187

Falco M L, Vinaccia P, Camaturo G, Petuso L 1989 FNA cytology of the breast—a statistical evaluation of accuracy based on 1080 cases. Applied Pathology 7(6): 333–337

Frable W J 1984 Needle aspiration of the breast. Cancer 53: 671–676

Franzen S, Zajicek J 1968 Aspiration biopsy in diagnosis of palpable lesions of the breast: Critical review of 3479 consecutive biopsies. Acta Radiologica
7: 241–262

Gelabet H A, Hsin J G, Mullen J T, Jaffe A H, D'Amato N A 1990 Prospective evaluation of the role of FNA biopsy in the diagnoses and management of patients with palpable solid breast lesions. American Surgeon, April, 56(4): 263–267

Gent H J, Spranger E, Dowlatshabi K 1986 Stereotactic needle localisation and cytological diagnosis of occult breast lesions. Annals of Surgery 204: 580–584

Harper A B 1988 FNA biopsy of the breast using ultrasound techniques— superficial localisation and direct visualisation. Ultrasound Medical Biology 14 (suppl I): 5–11

Helvie M A, Baker D E, Adler D D, Anderson L, Naylor B, Buckwalter K A 1990 Radiologically guided FNA of non-palpable breast lesions. Radiology, March, 174(3 pt 1): 657–661

Hogbin B M, Melcher D H, Smith R, Lawrence W 1977 The value of breast aspiration to the general surgeon. Fifteenth Annual Meeting of British Society of Clinical Cytology. Symposium on Breast Cytology. Acta Cytologica 21: 711

Hogg J P, Harris K M, Skolnek L 1988 The role of ultrasound guided needle aspiration of breast masses. Ultrasound Medical Biology 14 (suppl 1): 13–21

Ingram D W, Sterrett G F, Sheiner H J, Shilkin K B 1983 Fine needle aspiration cytology in the management of breast masses. Medical Journal of Australia 2: 170–173

Johnson T L, Kiwi S R 1989 The significance of atypical apocrine cells in FNAs of the breast 5(3): 248–254

Katz R L, Patel S, Sneige N, Fritscke H A Jr, Hortobagyi G N, Ames F C, Brooke T, Ordones N G 1990 Comparison of immunocytochemical and biochemical assays for estrogen receptor in FNAs and histological sections from breast carcinoma. Breast Cancer Treatment, May, 15(3): 191–203

Kline T S 1979 Masquerades of malignancy. A review of 4,241 aspirates from the breast. Acta Cytologica 25: 263–266

Kreuzer G, Zajicek J 1972 Cytologic diagnosis of tumours from aspiration biopsy smears. III. Studies of 200 carcinomas with false negative or doubtful cytologic reports. Acta Cytologica 16: 249–252

Kwok D, Chan M, Gwi E, Law D 1988 Aspiration cytology in the management of breast lesions. Australian and New Zealand Journal of Surgery, April, 58(4): 295–299

Lamb J, Anderson T J 1989 Influences of cancer history on the success of FNA of the breast. Journal of Clinical Pathology 42(7): 733–735

Linsk J, Kreuzer G, Zajicek J 1972 Cytologic diagnosis of mammary tumours from aspiration biopsy smears. II. Studies on 210 fibroadenomas and 210 cases of benign dysplasia. Acta Cytologica 16: 130–138

McSwain G R, Valican J F, O'Brien P H 1978 Cytologic evaluation of breast cysts. Surgery Gynaecology and Obstetrics 146: 921–925

Martin H F, Ellis E B 1930 Biopsy by needle puncture and aspiration. Annals of Surgery 92: 169–185

Naylor B 1988 FNA cytology of the breast. An overview. American Journal of Surgical Pathology Suppl 1: 54–61

Nicholson S, Sainsbury J R, Wadehra V, Needham G K, Faundon J R 1988 Use of FNA cytology with immediate reporting in the diagnosis of breast disease. British Journal of Surgery, Sep 75(9): 847–850

Paget J 1853 Surgical lectures on pathology delivered at the Royal College of Surgeons, England

Palombini L, Fulcinitis F, Vetrani A et al 1988 FNA biopsies of breast masses. A critical analysis of 1956 cases in 8 years. Cancer, June 1, 61(11): 2273–2277

Pilotti S, Rilke F, Delpiano C, Di Pietro S, Guzzon A 1982 Problems in fine needle aspiration biopsy cytology of clinically or mammographically uncertain breast tumours. Tumori 68: 407–412

Preece P E, Hunter S M, Duguid H L, Wood R A 1989 Cytodiagnoses and other methods of biopsy in modern management of breast cancer. Seminars in Surgical Oncology 5(2): 69–81

Rangwala A F, Perez-Blanco M, Reitty J 1989 Cytological diagnosis of breast cancers. New England Journal of Medicine, Nov 86(11): 859–865

Read L D, Leith D Jr, Slamon D J, Katzenellenbogen B S 1990 Hormonal modulation of HER-2/Neu

prolooncogene messenger ribonucleic acid and P185 problem expression in human breast cancer. Cancer Research, Jul 1, 50(13): 3947–3951

Redard M, Vassilakos P, Werntraub J 1989 A simple method of oestrogen receptor antigen preservation in cytological specimens containing breast carcinoma cells. Diagnostic Cytopathology 5(2): 188–193

Renvikos Y, Magdelenal H, Zajdela A 1988 DNA flow cytometry applied to fine needle sampling of human breast cancer. Cancer, April 15, 61(8): 1629–1634

Royal College of Pathologists Working Group 1990 Guidelines for pathologists. NHS BSP Screening Publications, February 1990, ISBN 1871997 65 8

Shabot M M, Goldberg I M, Schick P, Nieberg R, Pilch Y H 1982 Aspiration cytology is superior to Tru-Cut needle biopsy in establishing the diagnosis of clinically suspicious breast masses. Annals of Surgery 196: 122–126

Silfversward C, Gustafsson J A, Gustafsson S A, Nordenskjöld B, Wallgren A, Wrange O 1980 Estrogen receptor analysis on fine needle aspirates and on histologic biopsies from human breast cancer. European Journal of Cancer 16: 1351–1357

Sneige N, White V A, Latr R H, Troncoso P, Libshitz H I, Hortobagyi G N 1989 Ductal carcinoma in situ of the breast. Diagnostic Cytopathology 5(4): 371–377

Strawbridge H T G, Bassett A A, Foldes I 1981 Role of cytology in management of lesions of the breast. Surgery, Gynecology and Obstetrics 152: 1–7

Svane G 1983 Stereotaxic needle biopsy of non-palpable breast lesions. A clinical and radiological follow up. Acta Radiologica Diagnostica 24: 385–390

Svane G, Silfversward C 1983 Stereotactic needle biopsy of non-palpable breast lesions. Cytologic and histologic findings. Acta Radiologica Diagnostica 24: 283–288

Tandon A F, Clark G M, Chaumness G C, Ullrich A, McGuire W L 1989 Her-2/Neu oncogene protein and prognosis in breast cancer. Journal of Clinical Oncology Aug 7(8): 120–128

Trott P A, McKinna J A, Gazet J C 1981 Breast aspiration cytology. Lancet 1: 40

Van de Vigner M J, Petersen J L, Mooi

W J et al 1988 Neu protein one expression in breast cancer. Association with comedo type ductal carcinoma in situ and limited prognostic value in stage II breast cancer. New England Journal of Medicine, Nov 10, 319(19): 1239–1245

Wallgren A, Arnes O, Bergström J et al 1978 Pre-operative radiotherapy in operable breast cancer. Cancer 42: 1120–1125

Walloch J 1989 Technique and interpretation of breast aspiration cytology. Clinic Obstetrics and Gynecology, Dec 32(4): 486–499

Wang H H, Ducatman B S, Eick D 1989 Comparative features of ductal carcinoma in-situ and infiltrating carcinoma of the breast on FNA biopsy. American Journal of Clinical Pathology, Dec 92(6): 736–740

Wilkinson E J, Schnettke C M, Ferrier C M, Franzins D A, Bland K L 1989 FNA of breast masses. An analysis of 276 aspirates. Acta Cytologica 33(5): 613–619

Zajicek J 1974 Aspiration biopsy cytology. Part I. Cytology of supradiaphragmatic organs. Monographs in Clinical Cytology. S Karger, Basel, vol 4

Zajicek J, Franzen S, Jakobsson P 1967 Aspiration biopsy of mammary tumours in diagnosis and research. A critical review of 2200 cases. Acta Cytologica 11: 169–175

Zuk J A, Maudsley G, Zakhour H D 1989 Rapid reporting in FNA of breast lumps in outpatients. Journal of Clinical Pathology, Sept, 42(9): 906–911

CHAPTER 12

Implications of population screening for breast cancer

Audrey K. Tucker

THE NEED FOR SCREENING

It is unequivocally accepted that breast cancer is the commonest form of cancer in the female population throughout the world. In the UK approximately 25 000 women will develop breast cancer per year, and only 65% of these will survive for 5 years. The incidence is even higher in the USA and is rising, particularly in younger women, although the figure for 5 year survival in the US is higher than in the UK. Countries which have a much lower incidence, such as Japan, have also been recording increasing incidence over recent years.

There is a great diversity of treatment for the condition, which varies from simple mastectomy with axillary clearance, to segmental mastectomy. Radiotherapy is sometimes used as primary treatment or in conjunction with limited resection. Chemotherapy and hormones are also used in conjunction with other treatments, and occasionally as a primary treatment in the elderly. One of the great advantages of the screening programme in the UK is that teams have been set up to discuss choice of treatment for the individual patient, tailored to the type and extent of the disease. Recent research (Badwe et al 1991) has shown that the timing of surgery in relation to the menstrual cycle in premenopausal women may influence the outcome, but little else has made significant change to survival since Halsted introduced the radical mastectomy 100 years ago. The challenge remains—how to improve prognosis.

THE EVIDENCE FOR SCREENING

In 1956 Gerschon-Cohen et al suggested that mass X-rays could be used in the detection of early breast cancer and that such occult cancers had a better prognosis than clinically obvious disease. Again in 1961 the same team published the results of a 5 year survey of detection of breast cancer by periodic X-rays (Gerschon-Cohen et al 1961). the Health Insurance Plan (HIP) Study for New York (Shapiro et al 1971) ran from 1963 until 1966 and was the first selective population study which demonstrated a mortality reduction. 31 000 women aged 40–64 years of age were offered breast screening by clinical examination and mammography at yearly inervals for 4 years. A control population of the same size was also taken from the female members of the insurance plan. The compliance with the screened group from the first screen was 67%, but dropped later so that only 40% of women attended all four screens.

Although more cancers were found in the screened group in the prevalent first screen, the numbers of cancers detected in the screened and non-screened groups were virtually equal at 5 years, indicating early detection of cancer, which would have become clinically obvious after an interval. The tumours found in the screened group were smaller in size and had less nodal involvement than in the control population.

Analysis of mortality at 5 years showed cumulative survival rates in the screened women were 38.1% better than in the controls, with subsequent 10 year and 18 year survival rates still giving a 30% and 23% difference, respectively. Survival rates in the 40–50-year-old age groups were not obviously improved in the earlier years, but by 9 years from the start of the trial the mortality in the screened group was less than in the control group, and improvement has been maintained up to the 18 year analysis (Shapiro et al 1988).

Following the HIP trial, many other screening programmes were instituted, some as service programmes rather than trials, but it was not until the Two Countries Study in Sweden in 1977 that further significant evidence of the benefit of screening and reduction of mortality was obtained. This study from Koppaberg and Ostergötland confirmed the findings of the HIP study, with similar results, which have maintained a 30% improvement in mortality up to 8 years (Tabar et al 1985). Compliance in the Swedish study was markedly better than in the HIP study with approximately 80% of invited women attending for screening. Other Swedish studies including those from Stockholm (Frisell et al 1989), Malmö (Andersson et al 1988) and Göteburg all obtained similar results in women over 50 years of age. Reports of the Gotenburg study also quote high compliance (88% in prevalent and 76% in incident rounds), and a low (0.02%) interval cancer rate (Bjurstam 1991).

Further case–control studies from Utrecht (Colette et al 1984) and Nijmegen (Verbeek et al 1985) in Holland and Florence (Palli et al 1986, 1989) have confirmed the mortality reduction in the screened population, particularly in the over-50-year age group.

The Breast Cancer Detection Demonstration Project (BCDDP) (Baker 1982) was initiated by the American Cancer Society and the National Cancer Institute in America to review screening programmes in 29 centres in North America. Screening was performed with clinical examination and mammography, and the results were reported on 283 222 women, the majority of whom attended all five screens offered. One major difference from the HIP study was the improvement in mammographic detection. In the HIP study 45% of cancers were found by clinical examination alone, whereas in the BCDDP study only 7% were found by clinical examination alone. There was a higher incidence of very small cancers and in-situ cancers, as well as a much higher incidence of axillary-node-negative disease, all of which have an improved prognosis and survival rate. The population screened in this study, with the bias towards surgery in all equivocal cases, also contributed to the difference from the HIP results.

The Gävleborg Screening Project, begun in Sweden in 1973, introduced a simplified concept of screening by a single oblique mammogram (Lundgren & Jakobsson 1976) with no clinical examination, and used mobile mammography units with central processing and central assessment. This approach has been followed by many of the subsequent screening programmes. Mobile units are of considerable advantage in covering widespread country populations, and provide accessability for women in remote places.

In the UK the Trial of Early Detection of Breast Cancer was undertaken by a working party chaired by Sir Richard Doll (UK Trial of Early Detection of Breast Cancer Group 1981). This trial was planned to compare screening by mammography and clinical examination with breast self-examination only (after suitable teaching and subsequent direct access to assessment). Both arms of the trial were compared and contrasted with four control districts.

Subsequent to this a working party was then established, chaired by Professor Sir Patrick Forrest, to study the information available on screening for breast cancer by mammography and to consider implementation of such a service, including planning, manpower and finance (Forrest 1986). The Forrest Committee recommended breast screening in the 50–64 year age group. Subsequent to this, breast screening has been made available to every woman aged 50 years or over in specialist units throughout the country.

THE SERVICE

To provide a satisfactory service, many aspects need to be considered.

1. The compliance must be high. Women who do not attend for breast screening cannot benefit. Adequate publicity, personal invitations and encouragement from family doctors all help to increase the numbers attending. A friendly centre with suitable decor and a relaxed atmosphere can also help. The screening centre should be easily accessible for the population. Both static and mobile centres can be used. Computerization of invitations and results with a suitable system for retrieval of results for final analysis is essential. Corrected lists from the family practitioners are important together with appropriate invitations for ethnic minorities.

2. Apparatus—the computerized invitation system as previously described will be needed. The apparatus for mammography must be specifically designed with adequate but comfortable compression. All edges must be suitably rounded with no sharp corners and there must be foot control of compression, with quick release available, although it must be possible to override this control for localization and stereotaxis. Machines with facilities for coning, magnification and possible stereotaxis will be needed for assessment units, though this will not be vital in a basic screening unit. Radiographers working on mobile units must be given sufficient space around the machine for adequate positioning. Ease and lightness of control and movement would be necessary for radiographers who may complete 100 examinations in a day. Dedicated processing will also be needed, preferably with automatic loading, in order to minimize dust and handling artefacts.

3. Training of radiographers to a high standard will be needed, both for care in dealing with the women screened and for the taking of films. Diagnosis can only be possible if lesions are demonstrated on the film. Knowledge of pattern recognition is invaluable for radiographers who are able to see their own films, in order to reduce recall visits for further films. This diagnostic element also adds interest and motivation for the radiographer, but radiographers should not be expected to give a definitive diagnosis and most mobile units rely on central processing rather than using on-board facilities. Recall of women for radiographic and technical faults should be less than 3%.

4. Training of radiologists is also mandatory for screening mammography. Although X-ray appearances are the same in both the screening and symptomatic situations, the low incidence of pathology in normal screening needs very careful assessment and vigilance. Sensitivity must be high, but specificity is equally important, and unnecessary recall or biopsy must not be incurred. Recall rates should be less than 10%.

Suitable viewing conditions are necessary for accurate diagnosis. Double reading of films will increase sensitivity.

Careful audit of performance is needed. Quality control is essential. Auditing and self-assessment will:

a. Improve the specificity in respect to the numbers and the smaller size of cancers detected
b. Lower the rate of recall
c. Improve the malignant to benign biopsy ratio.

Cancers detected in the UK in the prevalent round should be greater than 5/1000, while in the incident rounds the rate should be more than 3/1000. These figures were considered the very minimal acceptable (Muir Gray 1990), but more recent analyses show better results.

The interval and 'missed' cancers must also be calculated and this requires an accurate cancer registry.

Most centres use a classification of

a. Missed cancers, i.e. detected on a retrospective review of the films
b. Occult cancers, i.e. known cancer but not visible on films
c. Interval cancer, i.e. presenting after the original normal screen, but before the next screen.

Current malignant/benign ratios vary from 9 malignant/1 benign in Sweden, where the use of stereotaxis is widespread, to 1 malignant/5 benign biopsies in the UK centres without fine-needle aspiration. After some experience, most radiologists will achieve a 1 malignant/1 benign rate without stereotactic cytology. Follow-up with accurate figures for these ratios will also give the radiologist the false-positive rate. This will of course differ from the symptomatic patient situation where biopsy is sometimes necessary to remove benign masses for the patient's peace of mind. Aspiration with cytology should be available in all assessment centres.

Similar quality control criteria have been laid down for pathology, and a similar new manual for standards in cytology is in preparation.

The assessment unit must work as an integrated team and should consist of radiologist, radiographers, surgeon, pathologist, cytologist and a counsellor, usually a specially trained nurse. Ultrasound facilities must be available at the time of assessment, both for the differentiation of solid and cystic masses, and for guided fine-needle aspiration. The surgeon will need to assess the extent of the disease with the radiologist after his clinical evaluation, and after performing cytology on the palpable masses (though this must not be performed before any extra films are taken, because oedema or haematoma can obscure or simulate pathology). Communication with the patient is, of course, of paramount importance, and urgent communication with the family doctor is also necessary in order to provide relevant information for patient management.

The counsellor plays an important part, as asymptomatic women will react to a greater or lesser degree when informed of pathology and they need time to adjust. The counsellor should be available to answer questions at the time of consultation and also between then and any future procedures; many women do not take in all the information given in the first instance and certainly do not think of all the questions they want answered at the time. Facilities for urgent admission of patients with lesions found on screening must be available, though timing of admission for surgery, as previously mentioned, is said to be important (Badwe et al 1991). Psychiatric studies have shown that patients requiring mastectomy are less likely to have psychological problems if a short time, i.e. 7–10 days, is given to adjust before proceeding to the definitive operation.

THE COST

The cost of the service is difficult to assess. The life-years gained from various health care procedures puts breast screening high in the league table of cost, though by no means the highest, with estimates from the UK National Health Service at £3000 per life-year gained against a hip replacement at £700 and a coronary artery bypass graft at £12 000, all based on 1984 figures (Forrest 1990). There must be a significant reduction of mortality in order to achieve real benefit. Costs in the United States vary from $10 000–$100 000 per life saved. In Holland 12% of deaths are prevented at a cost of 73 guilders per screen, otherwise stated as 10 000 guilders per life-year gained or 100 000 guilders per prevented death (Van der Mass 1988).

Women who have smaller operations are likely to be ready to return to work after a much shorter interval, and given extra lifespan they will contribute to the economy for a much longer period, provided that significant reduction in mortality can be maintained.

RISKS AND BENEFITS FOR WOMEN 50 YEARS OF AGE AND OVER

The risks and benefits from any procedure must be calculated and few, if any, medical procedures are without an element of risk, though the benefits can be overwhelming. The risks include possible carcinogenesis from ionizing radiation. The evidence for the risk of radiation-induced breast cancer at the doses used in mammography is theoretical; the risk is exceedingly small and has been extensively reviewed in the Forrest Report (HMSO 1987). It suggests that among 2 million women above the age of 50 years receiving a mean dose of radiation of 1.5 mGy to the breast, one extra breast cancer might develop each year after a latent interval of 10 years. This is less than 1/1000 of the incidence of naturally occurring breast cancer in women over 50 years of age. The improved quality of mammography incorporating grids has increased the radiation dose and therefore the theoretical risk might be doubled to two extra cancers per 2 million women, after a latent period of 10 years, but as was stated in the Forrest Report, the magnitude of possible risk from low-dose mammography appears negligible. Other risks include the possibility of psychological worries, although recent investigation has shown that the only people who suffer permanent psychological impairment are those found to have breast cancer. There is a

lead-time bias, which means that cancers should be found earlier in a screening programme than if they were left to develop until there were clinical manifestations, which would give the women a longer time to worry. There is also a length-time bias to be considered, which is that the tumours that will do well when found on screening would be those which grow slowly and therefore would have done well whether diagnosed on screening or left until clinical presentation.

The false-positive diagnosis will also cause considerable psychological upset until proven negative, and false-negative results, which are inevitable in any programme although they should be kept to a minimum, will cause doubt as to the effectiveness of the programme.

RISKS AND BENEFITS FOR WOMEN OVER 40 YEARS OF AGE

The evidence for the benefit of population breast screening for the 40–50-year-old age group is controversial at present. One-fifth of the women developing breast cancer in the United Kingdom will be under 50 years of age at the time of diagnosis. Detection in the younger dense breast is more difficult, although it appears that the age of natural involution of the glandular tissue is increasing and the time of menopause is also becoming later. The widespread use of hormone replacement therapy also influences continuing breast density, so this is not a problem confined to women under 50. Present techniques can undoubtedly detect the majority of cancers occurring in the young breast, but the decreased sensitivity and specificity in dense breasts must be

recognized. Complimentary ultrasound examination can be helpful in doubtful cases and careful clinical examination is important.

If regular screening is instituted from 40 years of age the theoretical induction of breast cancer by radiation would be greater, both from increased sensitivity of the young glandular tissue and the larger doses of accumulated radiation.

An extensive review of risk versus benefit in relation to mammography (Feig 1990) concluded that 'possible' years of life expectancy lost from annual mammography beginning at 40 years of age may be calculated, and are negligible compared with the estimates for life expectancy gained from such screening.

CURRENT ANALYSES AND PROBLEMS

It has been suggested that mortality is higher in the screened than the control group in the under 50-year-old population (Gullberg et al 1991). The Malmö trial, however, was not designed to show differences in age, and the numbers in this age group are small. Results from the Canadian national trials (Miller 1991) show an increased mortality in the screened population, but a relatively large proportion of the tumours detected were over 1.5 cm in size, as opposed to the much larger percentages of small tumours and in-situ tumours in the Swedish trials. Feasibility studies for a larger trial on the 40–50-year-old age group are being undertaken in the UK. This should be followed by the trial, which will involve sufficient women to give an answer to this difficult problem.

The types of treatment must also be considered in relationship to mortality. Analysis on the time of operation, the type of operation, adjuvant chemotherapy and radiotherapy, will be necessary before relative advantages or disadvantages can be calculated.

Individual screening

Although population screening in the 40–50-year-old group must be considered in relation to cost and resources, personal screening either for anxiety or significant risk factors should be considered in a different light, and it must also be remembered that reducing mortality in various age groups is not the only consideration that should be taken into account. Possible improvements in morbidity are also worthwhile, particularly when considered on an individual basis.

Breast awareness in the population undoubtedly leads to the detection of smaller tumours which may in turn well mean less mutilating surgery and better prognosis. A case can be established for screening higher risk groups at earlier ages.

Controversies

While breast screening will always have protagonists and antagonists, analysis of the nine major studies demonstrates undeniable benefit to the women in the screened groups of age 50 years or over (Cuckle 1991). Population screening or feasibility studies for population screening are now being undertaken throughout Europe, particularly in the UK, the Irish Republic, France, Germany, The Netherlands, Belgium, Italy, Spain and Portugal.

The questions which still need investigation, as well as the age of onset of screening, are the optimal interval between screens and the necessity for more than one view in the prevalent screen. Large trials are at present being undertaken in the UK, in an attempt to solve these problems, but regrettably finance will always play a dominant part in the final decision.

The benefit of screening to older women is the hope of longer life, less mutilation to those diagnosed, and reassurance and peace of mind to the rest. The so-called psychological stresses, especially of the positive and false-negative patient, should be balanced by the morbidiy and stress to the non-diagnosed cancers, whose final years can be disastrous for the family as well as the patient.

REFERENCES

Andersson I, Aspergen K, Janzon L et al 1988 Mammographic screening and mortality from breast cancer: the Malmo mammographic screening trial. British Medical Journal 297: 934–938

Badwe R A, Gregory W M, Chaudary M A et al 1991 Timing of surgery during menstrual cycle and survival of premenopausal women with operable breast cancer. Lancet 337: 1261–1264

Baker L H 1982 Breast Cancer Detection Demonstration Project—five year preliminary report. Cancer 32: 194–225

Bjurstam N 1991 The Göteburg results. Communication given at the 2nd International Cambridge Conference on Breast Cancer Screening, April 1991

Collette H J A, Day N E, Rombach J J, DeWaard F 1984 Evaluation of screening for breast cancer in a non-randomized study (The DOM Project) by means of a case control study. Lancet 1: 1224–1226

Cuckle H 1991 Breast cancer screening by mammography: an overview. Clinical Radiology 43: 77–80

Feig S A 1990 Estimation of radiation risk from screening mammography. Recent trends and comparisons with expected benefits. Radiology 174(3): 638–647

Forrest P 1990 Breast cancer: the decision to screen. Fourth HM Queen Elizabeth The Queen Mother Fellowship. The Nuffield Provincial Hospitals Trust, London

Frisell J, Eklund G, Hellstrom L, Glas U, Somell A 1989 The Stockholm Breast Cancer Screening Trial—5 year results and state at discovery. Breast Cancer Research and Treatment 13: 79–87

Gerschon-Cohen J, Ingolby H, Moore L 1956 Can mass X-ray surveys be used in the detection of early cancer of the breast? Journal of the American Medical Association 161:1069–1072

Gerschon-Cohen J, Hermal M B, Berger S M 1961 Detection of breast cancer by periodic examinations—5 year survey. Journal of the American Medical Association 176: 1114–1116

Gullberg B, Andersson I, Janzon L, Ranstam J 1991 Screening mammography. Lancet 337: 224

HMSO 1987 Breast cancer screening. Report to the Health Ministers of England, Wales, Scotland and Northern Ireland by a working group chaired by Professor Sir Patrick Forrest

Lundgren B, Jakobsson S 1976 Single view mammography a single and efficient approach to breast cancer screening. Cancer 38: 1124–1129

Miller A 1991 The Canadian results. Communication given at the 2nd International Cambridge Conference on breast Cancer Screening, April 1991

Muir Gray J A 1990 A draft set of criteria for evaluation and quality assurance. NHS Breast Screening Programme. Oxford Breast Screening Publications

Palli D, Roselli del Turco M, Buiatti E et al 1986 A case control study of the efficacy of a non-randomized breast cancer screening programme in Florence (Italy). International Journal of Cancer 38: 501–504

Palli D, Rosselli del Turco M, Buiatti E, Ciatto S, Crochetti E, Paci E 1989 Time interval since last test in a breast cancer screening programme—a case controlled study in Italy. Journal of Epidemiological Community Health 43: 241–248

Shapiro S, Strax P, Venet L 1971 Periodic breast cancer screening in reducing mortality from breast cancer. Journal of the American Medical Association 215: 1777–1785

Shapiro S, Venet W, Strax P, Venet L 1988 Periodic screening for breast cancer. The Health Insurance Plan Project and its sequelae 1963–1986. The John Hopkins University Press, Baltimore and London, 1988

Tabar L, Gad A, Holmberg L H et al 1985 Reduction in mortality after mass screening with mammography—randomized trial from the breast cancer screening working group of the Swedish National Board of Health and Welfare. Lancet 1: 829–832

UK Trial of Early Detection of Breast Cancer Group 1981 Trial of Early Detection of Breast Cancer: description of method. British Journal of Cancer 44: 618–627

Van Der Mass D J 1988 The costs and effects of mass screening for breast cancer. Medical Technology Assessment, The Netherlands

Verbeek A L H, Hendricks J H C L, Holland R 1985 Mammographic screening and breast cancer mortality: age specific effects in the Nijmegan project 1975–1982. Lancet 1: 865–866

CHAPTER 13

Epidemiology

J. Chamberlain

INTRODUCTION

Epidemiology is the study of the distribution of disease in a population, and is relevant to screening in three ways. The first is that it provides information on trends in disease frequency, thus enabling public health policy-makers to decide whether the disease is a sufficiently large and continuing problem to justify screening as a means of control. Second, epidemiology is used to generate and test hypotheses about risk factors and thus to identify subgroups of the population at high risk on whom screening may be concentrated. Third, because screening is a population-based method of disease control, evaluation of its effectiveness requires epidemiological methods. These three aspects of epidemiology will each be reviewed in the context of breast cancer screening.

THE SIZE OF THE PROBLEM

Worldwide, breast cancer is the commonest female malignancy (Parkin et al 1984) and this is true also within the UK, with nearly 25 000 women developing the disease each year. In most countries breast cancer is increasing in frequency, the increase being most marked in previously low-incidence developing countries, and least in countries like the US which have been affluent over several decades (Kalache, 1990). The *incidence* of breast cancer is best measured by population-based cancer registries which record all new diagnoses of cancer in a given population in a given time period. As far as screening is concerned, however, the appropriate measure of the size of the problem is not incidence but *mortality*. This is because screening for breast cancer cannot reduce incidence—indeed in

the early years of a screening programme incidence will apparently increase—but is aimed at reducing mortality.

Mortality rates from breast cancer in the UK are the highest in the world, although some other countries such as the US have higher incidence rates; Fig. 13.1 (Cancer Research Campaign 1988) shows the rank order of mortality in 13 different countries, expressed as age-standardized mortality rates which adjust for the different age structure in different countries. Moreover, like incidence, mortality rates have been slowly increasing over the past half-century, the increase being most marked in women over the age of 55.

The reasons why UK mortality rates are greater than those in other countries with comparable or higher incidence have not yet been elucidated and a number of possible explanations can be advanced. Prime among these is the probability that UK women present with breast cancer at a more advanced stage, less amenable to treatment, than do patients in most other developed countries. Even though the extent of this problem is not accurately known, the high mortality rates alone indicate that breast cancer is a major public health problem and, in the absence of effective primary prevention and only relatively minor advances in treatment efficacy, screening warrants serious consideration as a means of reducing

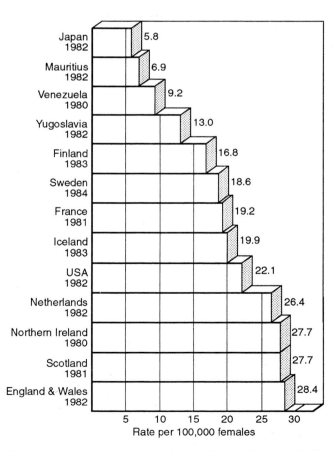

Fig. 13.1 International comparisons. Standardized mortality rates for breast cancer for a number of countries. [Redrawn from Cancer Research Campaign (1988).]

the 15 000 deaths from breast cancer each year in the UK.

HIGH-RISK GROUPS

The aetiology of breast cancer has been very extensively researched but as yet no precise cause has been identified. A variety of risk factors has been established, the majority of them clearly pointing to a hormonal role in causation of breast cancer. The risk factors may be classified into the nine categories shown in Table 13.1.

Table 13.1 Risk factors for breast cancer

Demographic
Menstrual history
Reproductive history
Exogenous hormones
Diet
Genetic
Ionizing radiation
Past medical history
Other

Demographic factors

The most obvious of these is *sex*; breast cancer occurs in men as well as women but the incidence in women is about 100 times that in men. *Age* is another very important demographic factor, with older women being at much greater risk than younger. Unlike most other carcinomas, however, age-specific incidence does not rise steadily with increasing age, but levels off to a greater or lesser exent at about age 50. There are interesting differences between high- and low-risk countries in the shape of the age-specific incidence curve. In all countries, there is a steep increase in sucessive age groups from about 25 to 50; thereafter low-risk countries plateau with little increase in risk at older ages, but in high-risk countries incidence continues to increase in each successive age group although at a less steep rate than in young women.

As already mentioned *country of residence* is a most important determinant of risk, and migrant studies, principally among low-risk Japanese migrating to the high-risk US, have shown that second generation migrants acquire the incidence pattern of their host country. *Socio-economic status* is a risk indicator, breast cancer being one of the few diseases that is more common in upper classes than lower, although the difference in risk is not large. Less important demographic factors include *race*, white women being more at risk than black; *marital status*, single women being at greater risk than those ever married; and *place of residence*, urban women being at greater risk than rural. Many of these demographic factors can be largely explained by the various other aetiological factors described below.

Menstrual history

An *early menarche* puts a woman at slightly greater risk of breast cancer, as does a *late menopause*. It is known that in athletic girls menarche is often delayed (e.g. to age 16 or 17) and this has led some to advocate vigorous exercise during adolescence as a protection against breast cancer in later life. However the 'cause and effect' relationship between exercise and menarche has not been established, and it may be that an underlying imbalance of androgenic and oestrogenic hormones causes both late menarche and development of muscle power leading to prowess in sport; hence sport, per se, is not necessarily protective. Women who have had a *premenopausal oophorectomy* are at substantially reduced risk of subsequent breast cancer, and, interestingly, women who smoke are also at decreased risk, the presumed mechanism being that the

menopause occurs earlier in heavy smokers.

Reproductive history

It has long been known that *nulliparous women* are at greater risk than those who have had children, and within the latter group there also seems to be a slight association with *number of children*, those who have had five or more being at decreased risk. The most important reproductive risk factor, however, is a woman's *age at first full-term pregnancy*. It has been shown that a pregnancy at an early age is protective against breast cancer in later life, and that for every year of increase in age at first pregnancy, the relative risk of developing breast cancer increases by 3.5% (Trichopoulos et al 1983). This protective effect of early pregnancy is restricted to the risk of developing breast cancer at age 40 or over (93% of all cases). For the few women destined to develop breast cancer at younger ages, women who have been pregnant are at greater risk than the nulliparous, and it has been postulated that hormonal changes in pregnancy promote the growth of a cancer that has already been initiated. *Lactation* was in the past thought to be the mechanism whereby pregnancy protected against breast cancer. Multivariate analytical techniques have now shown that it is a much less important contribution to decreasing risk than early pregnancy, but some recent studies from the developing world indicate that prolonged lactation may have a small protective effect independent of other variables (Rosero-Bixby et al 1987).

Exogenous hormones

The above findings suggest that oestrogenic hormones may play a major part in the aetiology of breast cancer, and this has led to concern about the possible carcinogenic effect of *oral contraceptives* (OCs) and *hormone replacement therapy* (HRT). Numerous case–control studies have been done comparing use of OCs in breast cancer cases and age-matched controls. When OCs were first introduced, in the 1960s, they were largely used by women who had already had children and needed a reliable contraceptive to control their family size; among these women, taking OCs in their late 20s and 30s after one or more pregnancies, it is now clearly established that there is *no* association between use of OCs and breast cancer; moreover OCs seem to have a protective effect against benign breast disease. But recently a number of studies have looked specifically at the risk of breast cancer in women who have used OCs from a young age and before their first pregnancy. The conclusion is that OC use at young ages does increase the risk of breast cancer, particularly if used continuously for several years (UK National Case–Control Study Group 1989). Because OCs have only been widespread for 20–25 years these studies have necessarily limited their cases to women who have developed breast cancer under the age of 40. It is not yet known whether the excess risk will persist at older ages. Moreover the situation is complicated by the changes in dose and preparation of different OCs that have occurred over time.

Similar methodological difficulties beset the study of HRT. Not only have the drug preparations changed over time (principally from unopposed to opposed oestrogens), but daily doses may vary widely, current users may be at different risk from ex-users, and adjustments may have to be made for whether or not the woman previously used OCs. Most of the studies of HRT have shown a modest increase in risk among users, concentrated among women with long (e.g. 10 years) duration of use.

Diet

Average levels of consumption of various dietary constituents have been explored as an explanation for the international differences in incidence. There is a close correlation between different countries' consumption of *fat*, and to a lesser exent meat, and their breast cancer incidence. Case–control studies of individuals have, however, been inconclusive in implicating dietary fat, possibly because of the difficulty of collecting valid retrospective dietary information on a substance as ubiquitous in various foodstuffs as fat. However, it has been shown that obese women are at greater risk than lean women, particularly after the menopause. Androstenedione in adipose tissue is the main source of oestrogen in postmenopausal women and it is postulated that the higher mass of adipose tissue in obese women accounts for their greater risk. It is possible that diet in early life also plays a role in that a high-calorie diet is associated with an early menarche. One statistical analysis has concluded that 70% of the difference in risk between Japan and the US can be accounted for by two risk factors, age at menarche and postmenopausal weight (Pike et al 1983).

Another dietary constituent which is an established risk factor for breast cancer, but whose mode of action is unclear, is *alcohol*. The association between alcohol and breast cancer applies particularly to premenopausal thin women (IARC 1988).

Genetic factors

A history of *breast cancer in a first-degree female relative,* on either the maternal or paternal side of the family, is well-known to be a risk factor for breast cancer. As with other inherited cancer syndromes, familial breast cancer tends to occur at younger ages and therefore a history of premenopausal breast cancer in one or more relatives is particularly relevant, risk being increased by a factor of four or more, over that of women without such a family history.

Ionizing radiation

Follow-up of survivors of the nuclear bombings in Japan has demonstrated an excess risk of breast cancer in those exposed. A number of other studies of women who received large doses of ionizing radiation for medical reasons have also shown increased risk. The relevance of these findings to current mammography is discussed elsewhere in Chap. 2.

Past medical history

A history of a *benign breast biopsy* indicates slightly increased risk of breast cancer. It is now established that risk is dictated by the histology found at biopsy, being limited to cases showing epithelial proliferation, particularly those with cellular atypia (Dupont & Page 1985). A past history of *endometrial or ovarian cancer* also indicates increased risk, and there is a suggestion that *large bowel and gall bladder cancers* are also indicators of risk of subsequent breast cancer. Previously breast cancer was thought to be more likely in women receiving long-term medication with *reserpine* and/or *vallium*, but these drugs have now been discounted as risk factors, as has a postulated association with *thyroid disease*.

Other risk factors

A number of other factors have been investigated, generally with inconclusive or negative findings. A possible relationship exists between suppression of emotions during psychological stress and breast cancer. Other postulated risk factors include abortion, infertility, male sex of first child, use of hair dyes, and viral infections.

SELECTIVE SCREENING OF RISK GROUPS

The purpose of selective screening applied only to high-risk women is to reduce the human and financial costs of a programme which would otherwise be applied to the whole population. This can only be done at the price of reduced sensitivity, because cancers occurring in the low-risk group will be missed. The proportion of cancers which fall into the high-risk group depends on the prevalence of the risk factor, and the magnitude of risk in those women with the factor relative to those without it. Apart from age and sex, the relative risk of most of the factors described above is between 1.5 and 3, and the prevalence of the factors is low, indicating that a sizeable majority of breast cancers would be missed if only women with the risk factor were screened. Combining risk factors into a risk score by multiple discriminant analysis works better than the most preponderant single factor on its own. The cut-off point on the scoring system for defining high-risk can be varied in order to identify a group sufficiently small to make a substantial cost saving, (bearing in mind that there is a cost in identifying which women fall into the group), but which will include most of the cancers. Development of these risk scores for

breast cancer indicate that, at best, one would have to screen 79% of the population in order to detect 67% of the cancers, and this sensitivity level is generally regarded as unacceptably low (Soini & Hakama 1978).

EFFECTIVENESS OF SCREENING

The only way to measure the contribution of screening to saving lives is to compare the mortality rate from breast cancer in a screened population with that in an unscreened population. Intermediate indicators such as a high yield of cancers, a shift to an earlier stage distribution and improved survival of screen-detected cases are necessary concomitants of a successful screening programme but, because of various biases are insufficient evidence of its effectiveness (Chamberlain 1984). Several prospective epidemiological trials have now been conducted in which a population of women has been randomly allocated to be offered screening or to be in an unscreened control group, and deaths from breast cancer in both groups have been recorded over 7–18 years. Forrest (1990), in a summary of the evidence, points out the consistency of their finding that, among women aged 50 or over when first invited for screening, there are fewer deaths from breast cancer in the invited group than in the control group. The size of the mortality reduction varies between different studies from about 15% to more than 30%, and some reported differences were not statistically significant.

One of the principal determinants of efficacy is that a high proportion of invited women should be screened, and in studies where compliance has been relatively low, the reduction in

population mortality underestimates the proportional effect on the women who were screened. An alternative method of evaluation is a retrospective case–control approach that compares the screening history of women who have died of breast cancer and age-matched living controls, and derives the relative protection afforded by screening. Several such studies have now been performed and show that screened women are 50–60% less likely to die of breast cancer than unscreened women from the same population. However, the latter group include those who reject the invitation, who are usually found to be at greater risk of dying from breast cancer than women in a completely unscreened control group (Moss et al 1991). Thus the selection of bias affecting this study design gives an overestimate of the effect of screening.

A consistent finding of both types of study is the lack of effect among women aged under 50 when first screened, and the relatively poor sensitivity of all screening methods in this age-group. Because death from breast cancer is a rare event in young women a large number of such women would require to be enrolled in order to give a trial sufficient statistical power to demonstrate a difference, and none of the trials so far published has had a large enough sample of women under 50. The case for screening younger women is therefore still unproven, but—because of poorer sensitivity—is probably less strong than that for women aged 50 and over.

In summary, epidemiological evidence on the effectiveness of screening indicates that it can achieve a modest reduction in mortality among women over 50, this reduction starting to appear 5–7 years after the introduction of the programme. Until further, larger studies of screening younger women are completed there is no case for providing a population screening programme for women under 50.

REFERENCES

Cancer Research Campaign 1988 Factsheet 6.3. Breast cancer

Chamberlain J 1984 Planning of screening programmes for evaluation. In: Prorok P, Miller A B (eds) Screening for cancer. UICC Technical Report 78: 5–17

Dupont W D, Page D L 1985 Risk factors for breast cancer in women with proliferative breast disease. New England Journal of Medicine 312: 146–151

Forrest A P M 1990 Breast cancer: the decision to screen. Nuffield Provincial Hospitals Trust

IARC 1988 Monographs on the evaluation of carcinogenic risks to humans: alcohol drinking. International Agency for Research on Cancer, Lyon. IARC Scientific Publication 44: 387

Kalache A 1990 Risk factors for breast cancer, with special reference to developing countries. Health Policy and Planning 5: 1–22

Moss S M 1991 Case–control studies of screening. International Journal of Epidemiology 20 (in press)

Parkin D M, Stjernswaard J, Muir C S 1984 Estimates of the worldwide frequency of twelve major cancers. Bulletin of the World Health Organization 62: 163–182

Pike M C, Krailo M D, Henderson B E, Casagrande J T, Hoel D G 1983 'Hormonal' risk factors, 'breast tissue age' and the age-incidence of breast cancer. Nature 303: 767

Rosero-Bixby L, Oberle M W, Lee N C 1987 Reproductive history and breast cancer in a population of high fertility Costa Rica 1984–5. International Journal of Cancer 40: 747–754

Soini I, Hakama M 1978 Failure of selective screening for breast cancer by combining risk factors. International Journal of Cancer 22: 275–281

Trichopoulos D, Hsieh C C, MacMahon B et al 1983 Age at any birth and breast cancer risk. International Journal of Cancer 31: 701–704

UK National Case–Control Study Group 1989 Oral contraceptive use and breast cancer risk in young women. Lancet 1: 973–982

CHAPTER 14

Breast imaging in other modalities

Elizabeth Wylie, Yin Y. Ng

INTRODUCTION

Mammography is currently the most sensitive and specific imaging modality for the detection of breast cancer, since it alone demonstrates microcalcification which may be the only sign of malignancy. Other modalities such as ultrasound or magnetic resonance imaging (MRI) may be used to further elucidate a mass lesion seen on mammography.

Pneumocystography and ductography may also be used for further assessment of a lesion detected on mammography. Thermography and transillumination have been in vogue but their value in screening for breast cancer is limited unless spatial resolution can be improved so that smaller lesions may be detected. Computed tomography (CT) is not a practical alternative to mammography because of the high radiation dose (Homer 1985) and inferior spatial resolution (Feig 1986): microcalcification is not easily detected, and carcinomas less than 1 cm may be overlooked. Malignant lesions enhance more markedly than benign lesions after intravenous contrast medium administration, but this increases the cost and risk of the examination (Martin 1983).

Other techniques such as digital subtraction angiography (DSA), digital enhancement of the image, and magnetic resonance spectroscopy (MRS) are still experimental at the time of writing.

PNEUMOCYSTOGRAPHY

The technique involves the injection of air into a breast cyst immediately following aspiration of the cyst contents, in order to exclude an intracystic tumour. This may be suspected if on mammography the cyst is extremely dense, or there is cyst wall distortion or flattening. Alternatively ultrasound may show an intracystic tumour. The index of suspicion is raised if the cyst aspirate is blood-stained, particularly in the absence of previous aspiration (Logan & Janus 1988).

DUCTOGRAPHY

Opacification of the duct system with radiographic contrast medium is useful for accurate preoperative localization of a discharging duct, and to identify any intraductal tumour.

Spontaneous serous and blood-stained nipple discharge should be investigated, because an underlying cancer may be present in up to 12% of cases (Treatt 1987). However, Reid et al (1989) suggest that ductography be limited to those patients with serous or blood-stained discharge from a single duct orifice, in order to reduce patient discomfort and unnecessary irradiation. In their series of 60 ductograms, no patient with a green discharge required surgical intervention, the cause of the discharge being duct ectasia or fibrocystic disease. Cytology of the discharge may be helpful in some cases.

Using a sterile technique, the discharging duct orifice, which is usually enlarged, is cannulated with a lymphographic needle and 0.5–3 ml of intravenous contrast medium is injected (Egan 1988). The patient will normally experience a feeling of fullness at the end of the injection, more severe pain usually indicating extravasation of contrast medium. Mammography is then performed with the needle taped in place at the nipple. The normal subareolar ducts are 2–3 mm in diameter, and show regular branching and arborization more distally in the breast substance. The walls of the ducts should be smooth without evidence of narrowing, displacement or beading.

Solitary filling defects are most often intraduct papillomas, which appear smoothly outlined or finely lobulated. The presence of ductal epithelial hyperplasia or papillomatosis may be suggested by multiple filling defects. Carcinomas may cause stricturing or distortion of a duct with focal obstruction and intramural filling defects.

THERMOGRAPHY

The rationale for the use of thermography in breast imaging is based on the observation that the skin overlying a malignant breast lesion may be 1–3°C warmer than other areas of the breast (Martin 1983). The technique has been in use for over 30 years. However, the tumour has to be fairly large for detection by this method alone (Homer 1985), and in one series (Martin 1983) only 42% of patients with breast cancers detected by mammography had an abnormal thermogram.

Contact thermography

A plastic sheet containing heat-sensitive liquid cholesterol esters is placed on the skin of the breast. The black cholesteric crystals change colour in response to the varying emitted infra-red energies (Milbrath 1987). The colour image may be photographed as a permanent record.

Telethermography

An electronic infra-red detector measures infra-red radiation emitted from the breast. The examination takes place in a cooled room at 20°C. Photographs of the cathode ray tube signal are obtained as a permanent record.

BREAST TRANSILLUMINATION

This is also known as transmission spectroscopy or diaphanography. The rationale for the use of transillumination is that in theory breast cancers absorb light in the red and infra-red portion of the electromagnetic spectrum because of tumour hypervascularity.

The light source is placed against the breast and light is pulsed through the breast while a modified video camera recording of the transmitted signal is obtained (Dowle et al 1987). Abnormal areas with increased blood flow appear as dark shadows on the image due to differential light absorption.

The detectability of a lesion depends on its size and position within the breast. Lesions can only be detected to a depth slightly more than twice their size (Dexler et al 1985). Very dense or very large breasts are difficult to transilluminate adequately (Gisvoid 1986). The technique is further limited by a high false-positive rate: many benign lesions produce positive light scans.

Compared with mammography, transillumination is an insensitive technique. In one series (Dexler et al 1985), mammography detected 96% of the breast cancers present, whereas transillumination detected only 58%. In another series, Monsees et al (1988) found that 70% of non-palpable cancers detected by mammography were not visible with light scanning.

Only large lesions are demonstrated, and carcinoma-in-situ cannot be seen.

MAGNETIC RESONANCE IMAGING (MRI)

The development of dedicated surface coils for the breast has permitted improved spatial resolution of MR images (Wolfman et al 1985). These surface coils improve the signal-to-noise ratio and have the added advantage of reducing motion artefact from cardiac and respiratory movement. In one series (Heywang et al 1986) MRI proved comparable to mammography and superior to sonography in the fatty to medium dysplastic breast, but inferior to the combined examination by mammography and sonography in the dense breast. To date, the best images show a resolution of approximately 2 mm (Powell & Stelling 1988), but this is inadequate for the demonstration of proliferative patterns of fibrocystic disease and carcinoma-in-situ.

On MRI, the normal breast fat provides signal contrast with the fibroglandular tissue and pathologic processes. Breast carcinoma may appear as a spiculated mass with associated architectural distortion, skin thickening and nipple retraction, but these signs are relatively insensitive indicators of malignancy (Turner et al 1988a). Microcalcification is not seen on MRI.

T1-weighted images (short TR/short TE spin echo) provide predominantly morphological information. T2-weighted images (long TR/long TE spin echo) may show an increase in signal intensity for malignant lesions relative to the normal fibroglandular tissue, but this high signal is not specific for malignancy, and cysts and fibroadenomas may show similar hyperintensity. Fibrous tissue shows low signal on T2-weighted images, and MRI may have a role in the assessment of patients with suspected recurrent breast carcinoma (Lewis-Jones et al 1991).

MRI may be used to further evaluate a mass if sonography has failed to identify the mass as a cyst, particularly if the mass lies adjacent to the chest wall, deep within a very large breast, or is obscured by a breast prosthesis (Turner et al 1988b). Malignant lesions may be undetectable in dense breasts (Heywang et al 1986).

Recent advances with the use of gadolinium diethylenetriamine pentaacetic acid (Gd-DTPA) have shown potential for distinguishing a stellate carcinoma from scar tissue—the latter does not seem to enhance with intravenous Gd-DTPA (Turner et al 1988b, Lewis-Jones et al 1991). Gd-DTPA is a paramagnetic contrast agent which causes T1-shortening, thus increasing the signal intensity on T1-weighted images of regions of increased vascularity or abnormal capillary permeability. However, enhancement wih gadolinium may be seen in fibroadenomas and proliferative dysplasia as well as carcinomas (Heywang et al 1989). Preliminary studies using gradient echo sequences and dynamic imaging suggest that malignant lesions show a different pattern of enhancement from benign lesions. Kaiser & Zeitler (1989) used fast low-angle shot (FLASH) and fast imaging with steady precession (FISP) sequences in combination with intravenous Gd-DTPA to show carcinomas as small as 3 mm in diameter in dense breast tissue. Dynamic studies in 25 patients showed a different pattern of enhancement for malignant compared with benign lesions. These preliminary findings need to be confirmed. Experiments with human breast carcinoma implanted in mice showed that the strongly-enhancing areas corresponded with richly vascularized connective tissue and apparently viable tumour tissue, whereas the weakly enhancing areas corresponded to non-vascularized necrotic tissue (Revel et al 1986).

Much work has been done on the measurement of T1 and T2 relaxation times in excised breast tissue samples or mastectomy specimens, in an attempt to distinguish benign from malignant disease. The results do not conclusively demonstrate a clear separation based on these values alone (Powell & Stelling 1988). There is overlap between fibroadenomas, carcinoma and fibrocystic disease. Martin & el Yousef (1986) showed no significant alteration in breast T2 relaxation times during the menstrual cycle of normal young volunteers.

Magnetic resonance spectroscopy

Some groups have been studying the role of in-vivo phosphorus spectroscopy in the tissue characterization of breast tumours. Preliminary results suggest that ^{31}P spectroscopy may be useful in monitoring tumour response to therapy (Sijens et al 1988, Glaholm et al 1989) but tumours less than 2 cm in diameter cannot be studied with present technology, thus currently limiting the technique to a research tool.

COMPUTED TOMOGRAPHY (CT)

As with mammography, a malignant lesion appears as an area of increasd density with radiating spicules extending into the mammary fat (Muller et al 1983). Secondary signs include skin thickening, enlarged axillary and internal mammary lymph nodes, and involvement of the adjacent chest wall. CT is useful for the evaluation of the retromammary space and axilla in postmastectomy patients with local recurrence (Chang et al 1982). CT may also be of value in the assessment of patients with associated intrathoracic problems (Fig. 14.1).

DIGITAL SUBTRACTION ANGIOGRAPHY (DSA)

DSA of the breast may be performed by central venous or intra-arterial injection of low concentrations of radiographic contrast medium. A malignant lesion may show abnormal vascularity (Watt et al 1986). However, the technique is not sufficiently sensitive or specific to be used routinely in the evaluation of breast masses, and lesions smaller than 2 cm cannot be easily demonstrated (Dean & Sickles 1987).

DIGITAL ENHANCEMENT OF CONVENTIONAL MAMMOGRAMS

Digital imaging is currently experimental, showing great promise in terms of improved exposure latitude and computer manipulation of image contrast and enhancement. Digitized images currently provide less spatial resolution than conventional mammograms.

A laser scanning system can digitize a mammographic film into a chosen number of pixels which are then displayed on a cathode ray tube monitor (Kopans 1987). When the image has been copied into this digital form, the window width and centre of the displayed image can be varied, permitting a greater range of display of the radiographic contrast within the image. Standard 512-line cathode ray tubes provide inadequate spatial resolution for the display of microcalcifications on digitized images. Cathode ray tubes with a 2000×2000 matrix, required for a 100 μm resolution, are more expensive (Merritt 1988).

Direct digital mammography is now possible using a europeum-doped barium fluorohalide plate in a special cassette that can be used in a conventional X-ray unit. The image is edge-enhanced similar to a xeromammogram, but has the added advantage of post-processing. Very fine microcalcification is difficult to see, and at present a mass and associated microcalcification cannot be demonstrated simultaneously. Processing of the image currently requires several minutes, which would be impracticable in a large screening programme. Algorithms have been developed for diagnosis, and it is probable that dose can be reduced considerably.

In conclusion, mammography is the best technique currently available for the detection of breast carcinoma, although other techniques may be helpful in tissue characterization.

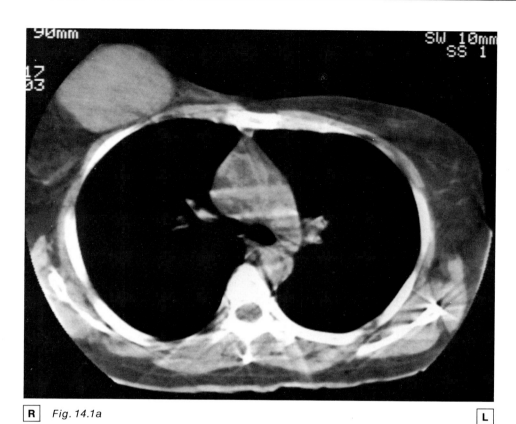

R *Fig. 14.1a* L

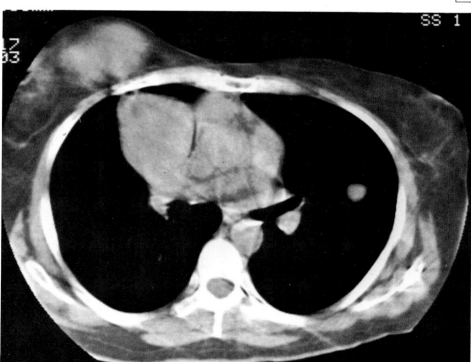

R   *Fig. 14.1b*   L

Fig. 14.1   Axial CT image showing abnormal soft tissue mass in the right breast (a) in a woman with recurrent malignant fibrous histiocytoma in the anterior mediastinum. (b) Note left-sided intrapulmonary metastasis. (Reproduced by courtesy of Dr M Rubens.)

REFERENCES

Chang C H, Nesbit D E, Fisher D R et al 1982 Computed tomographic mammography using a conventional body scanner. American Journal of Roentgenology 138: 553–558

Dean P B, Sickles E A 1987 Critical review — breast lesions examined by digital angiography. Investigative Radiology 22: 698–699

Dexler B, Leonard Davis J, Schofield G 1985 Diaphanography in the diagnosis of breast cancer. Radiology 157: 41–44

Dowle C S, Caseldine J, Tew J et al 1987 An evaluation of transmission spectroscopy (lightscanning) in the diagnosis of symptomatic breast lesions. Clinical Radiology 38: 375–37

Egan R L 1988 Breast imaging: diagnosis and morphology of breast diseases. W B Saunders, Philadelphia

Feig S A 1986 The breast. In: Grainger R, Allison D (eds) Diagnostic radiology. An Anglo-American textbook of imaging. Churchill Livingstone, Edinburgh, pp 1631–1668

Gisvoid J J, Brown L R, Swee R G et al 1986 Comparison of mammography and transillumination light scanning in the detection of breast lesions. American Journal of Roentgenology 147: 191–194

Glaholm J, Leach M O, Collins D J et al 1989 In-vivo 31-P magnetic resonance spectroscopy for monitoring treatment response in breast cancer (letter). Lancet i: 1326–1327

Heywang S H, Fenzl G, Hahn D et al 1986 MR imaging of the breast: comparison with mammography and ultrasound. Journal of Computer Assisted Tomography 10: 615–620

Heywang S H, Wolf A, Pruss E, Hilbertz T, Eiermann W, Permanetter W 1989 MR imaging of the breast with Gd-DTPA: use and limitations. Radiology 171: 95–103

Homer M J 1985 Breast imaging: pitfalls, controversies and some practical thoughts. Radiologic Clinics of North America 23: 459–471

Kaiser W A, Zeitler E 1989 MR imaging of the breast: fast imaging sequences with and without Gd-DTPA. Preliminary observations. Radiology 170: 681–686

Kopans D B 1987 Nonmammographic breast imaging techniques: current status and future developments. Radiologic Clinics of North America 25: 961–971

Lewis-Jones H G, Whitehouse G H, Leinster S J 1991 The role of magnetic resonance imaging in the assessment of local recurrent breast carcinoma. Clinical Radiology 43: 197–204

Logan W W, Janus J 1988 Fine needle aspiration biopsy, ductography and pneumocystography. American Roentgen Ray Society Categorical Course Syllabus in Breast Imaging, 97–104

Martin J E 1983 Breast imaging techniques, mammography, ultrasonography, computed tomography, thermography and transillumination. Radiologic Clinics of North America 21: 149–153

Martin B, el Yousef S J 1986 Transverse relaxation time values in MR imaging of normal breast during menstrual cycle. Journal of Computer Assisted Tomography 10: 924–927

Merritt C R 1988 Digital mammography. American Roentgen Ray Society Categorical Course Syllabus in Breast Imaging, 153–160

Milbrath J R 1987 Thermography. In: Bassett L W, Gold R H (eds) Breast cancer detection. Grune & Stratton, Florida

Monsees B, Destouet J M, Gersell D 1988 Light scanning of nonpalpable breast lesions: reevaluation. Radiology 167: 352

Muller J W, van Waes P F, Koehler P R 1983 Computed tomography of breast lesions: comparison with X-ray mammography. Journal of Computer Assisted Tomography 7: 650–654

Powell D E, Stelling C B 1988 Magnetic resonance imaging of the human female breast. Current status and pathologic correlations. Pathology Annual 23: 159–194

Reid A W, McKellar N J, Sutherland G R 1989 Breast ductography: its role in the diagnosis of breast disease. Abstract, British Journal of Radiology 62 (suppl): 11

Revel D, Brasch R C, Paajanen H et al 1986 Gd-DTPA contrast enhancement and tissue differentiation in MR imaging of experimental breast carcinoma. Radiology 158: 319–323

Sijens P E, Wijrdeman H K, Moerland M A, Bakker C J, Vermeulen J W, Luyten P R 1988 Human breast cancer in vivo: H-1 and P-31 MR spectroscopy at 1.5T. Radiology 169: 615–620

Treatt B 1987 Ductography. In: Bassett L W, Gold R H (eds) Breast cancer detection. Grune & Stratton, Florida, pp 119–129

Turner D A, Alcorn F S, Shorey W D et al 1988a Carcinoma of the breast: detection with MR imaging versus xeromammography. Radiology 168: 49–58

Turner D A, Alcorn F S, Adler Y T 1988b Nuclear magnetic resonance in the diagnosis of breast cancer. Radiologic Clinics of North America 26: 673–687

Watt A C, Ackerman L V, Windham J P et al 1986 Breast lesions: differential diagnosis using digital subtraction angiography. Radiology 159: 39–42

Wolfman N T, Moran R, Moran P R, Karstaedt N 1985 Simultaneous MR imaging of both breasts using a dedicated receiver coil. Radiology 155: 241–243

Appendix

With the increasing worldwide access to mammography, a knowledge of Right and Left in various languages is helpful, and the following list has been compiled for reference:

Country	Right	Left	Medial	Lateral	Superior	Inferior
Belgium (French)	Droit	Gauche	Intérieur	Extérieur	Supérieur	Inférieur
Belgium (Flemish)	Rechts	Links	Mediaal	Lateraal	Boven	Onder
Belgium (German)	Rechts	Links	Medial	Lateral	Über	Unter
Bolivia	Derecho	Izquierdo	Al centro	Lateral	Superior	Inferior
Botswana	Right	Left	Medial	Lateral	Superior	Inferior
Canada	Right	Left	Medial	Lateral	Superior	Inferior
Chile	Derecha	Izquierda	Media	Lateral	Superior	Inferior
China	右	左	中央	側面	上	下
Colombia	Right	Left	Medial	Lateral	Superior	Inferior
Costa Rica	Derecho	Izquierdo	Centro	Lateral	Superior	Inferior
Cuba	Derecho	Izquierdo	Medial	Lateral	Superior	Inferior
Cyprus	Right	Left	Medial	Lateral	Cranial	Caudal
Czechoslovakia	Pravý	Levý	Strední	Postranní	Vrchní	Spodní
Denmark	Højre	Venstre	Medial	Lateral	Superior	Inferior
Egypt	Right	Left	Medial	Lateral	Superior	Inferior
El Salvador	Derecha	Izquierda	Medial	Lateral	Superior	Inferior
Esperanto	Dekstra	Maldeketra	Meza	Hanka	Supra	Malsupra
France	Droite	Gauche	Mediane	Laterale	Superieure	Inferieure
Germany	Rechts	Links	Medial	Lateral	Über	Unter
Ghana	Right	Left	Medial	Lateral	Superior	Inferior
Greece	Dexios	Aristeros	Meso-eso	Plagios	Ano	Kato
Greece	ΔΕΞΙΟΣ	ΑΡΙΣΤΕΡΟΣ	ΜΕΣΟ-ΕΣΩ	ΠΛΑΓΙΟΣ	ΑΝΩ	ΚΑΤΩ
Guatemala	Derecha	Izquierda	Media	Lateral	Superior	Inferior
Guyana	Right	Left	Medial	Lateral	Superior	Inferior
Hungary	Jobb	Bal	Középsö	Oldalsó	Felsö	Alsó
Iceland	Haegri	Vinstri	Naer midju	Fjaer midju	Ofar	Neðar
India	दाहिना	बायाँ	मध्य	पार्श्व	ऊपरी	निचला
Indonesia	Kanan	Kiri	Tengah	Sisi	Diatas	Dibawah
Irish Republic	Right	Left	Medial	Lateral	Superior	Inferior

Country	Right	Left	Medial	Lateral	Superior	Inferior
Israel	Right	Left	Medial	Lateral	Superior	Inferior
Israel (Hebrew rare)	ימין	שמאל	מרכזי	צדדי	עליון	תחתון
Italy	Destra	Sinistra	Mediale	Laterale	Superiore	Inferiore
Japan	Migi	Hidari	Naisoku	Gaisoku	Jyobu	Kabu
Japan (formerly)	Right	Left	Medial side	Lateral side	Superior part	Inferior side
Japan (characters)	右 (MIGI)	左 (HIDARI)	内側 (NAISOKU)	外側 (GAISOKU)	上部 (JYOBU)	下部 (KABU)
Korea	오른 쪽	왼 쪽	중간	옆, 측면	상위	하위
Lebanon	يمــين	يســار	وســط	جـانبي	الجهة العليا	الجهة السفلى
Madagascar	Ankavia	Ankavanana	Anivony	Anilany	Ambony	Ambany
Mexico	Derecho	Izquierdo	Medio	Lateral	Superior	Inferior
Morocco	Yamine	Yassar	Wasat	Janb	Fawq	Taḫt
Nicaragua	Derecho	Izquierdo	Medial	Lateral	Superior	Inferior
Norway	Høyre	Venstre	Mot midten	Til siden	Den øvre	Den nedre
Norway (English)	Right	Left	Medial	Lateral	Superior	Inferior
Panama	Derecho	Izquierdo	Medio	Lateral	Superior	Inferior
Paraguay	Derecho	Izquierdo	Medial	Lateral	Cranial	Caudal
Peru	Derecha	Izquierda	Medio	Lateral	Superior	Inferior
Poland	Prawa	Lewa	Środkowa	Bocza	Wyższa	Niższa
Portugal	Direito	Esquerdo	Médio	Lateral	Superior	Inferior
Quatar	Right	Left	Medial	Lateral	Superio/Cranial	Inferior/Caudal
Saudia Arabia	Yamin	Shemal	Wassat	Janibi	Fouk	Asfall
Saudia Arabia	يمــين	يســار	وســط	جـانبي	الجهة العليا	الجهة السفلى
Sierra Leone	Right	Left	Medial	Lateral	Superior	Inferior
S. Africa (English)	Right	Left	Medial	Lateral	Superior	Inferior
S. Africa (Afrikaans)	Regs	Links	Lateraal	Mediaal	Superior	Inferior
Spain	Derecha	Izquierda	Medial	Lateral	Superior	Inferior
Sweden	Höger	Väntser	Medial	Lateral	Superio/Cranial	Inferior/Caudal
Switzerland (French)	Droit	Gauche	Medial	Lateral	Cranial	Caudal
Switzerland (German)	Rechts	Links	Medial	Lateral	Cranial	Caudal
Syria	Yamin	Yassar	Tebi	Janebi	Afdal	Adna
Syria	يمــين	يســار	وســط	جـانبي	الجهة العليا	الجهة السفلى

Country	Right	Left	Medial	Lateral	Superior	Inferior
Thailand	ด้านขวา	ด้านซ้าย	ตรงกลาง	ด้านข้าง	ด้านบน	ด้านล่าง
Tunisia	Droite	Gauche	Médiales	Latérale	Supérieure	Inférieure
Turkey	Sağ	Sol	Orta	Yan	Üst	Alt
Uganda	Right	Left	Medial	Lateral	Superior	Inferior
United Arab Emirates	يمين	يسار	وسط	جانبي	الجهة العليا	الجهة السفلى

Index